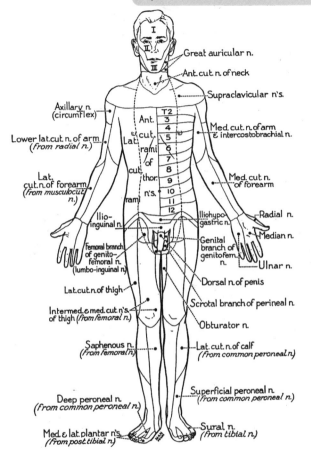

Second of four views. See comment opposite regarding the lower lateral cutaneous nerve of the arm. Reproduced with permission from Haymaker, W. and Woodhall, B. (1998). *Peripheral Nerve Injuries: Principles of Diagnosis*, 2nd edn. American Association of Neurological Surgeons.

OXFORD MEDICAL PUBLICATIONS

Oxford Handbook of
Neurology

BARCODE ON
PREVIOUS PAGE

Published and forthcoming Oxford Handbooks

Oxford Handbook for the Foundation Programme 3e
Oxford Handbook of Acute Medicine 3e
Oxford Handbook of Anaesthesia 3e
Oxford Handbook of Applied Dental Sciences
Oxford Handbook of Cardiology 2e
Oxford Handbook of Clinical and Laboratory Investigation 3e
Oxford Handbook of Clinical Dentistry 5e
Oxford Handbook of Clinical Diagnosis 2e
Oxford Handbook of Clinical Examination and Practical Skills
Oxford Handbook of Clinical Haematology 3e
Oxford Handbook of Clinical Immunology and Allergy 3e
Oxford Handbook of Clinical Medicine – Mini Edition 8e
Oxford Handbook of Clinical Medicine 9e
Oxford Handbook of Clinical Pathology
Oxford Handbook of Clinical Pharmacy 2e
Oxford Handbook of Clinical Rehabilitation 2e
Oxford Handbook of Clinical Specialties 9e
Oxford Handbook of Clinical Surgery 4e
Oxford Handbook of Complementary Medicine
Oxford Handbook of Critical Care 3e
Oxford Handbook of Dialysis 3e
Oxford Handbook of Emergency Medicine 4e
Oxford Handbook of Endocrinology and Diabetes 3e
Oxford Handbook of ENT and Head and Neck Surgery 2e
Oxford Handbook of Epidemiology for Clinicians
Oxford Handbook of Expedition and Wilderness Medicine
Oxford Handbook of Gastroenterology and Hepatology 2e
Oxford Handbook of General Practice 4e
Oxford Handbook of Genetics
Oxford Handbook of Genitourinary Medicine, HIV and AIDS 2e
Oxford Handbook of Geriatric Medicine 2e
Oxford Handbook of Infectious Diseases and Microbiology
Oxford Handbook of Key Clinical Evidence
Oxford Handbook of Medical Dermatology
Oxford Handbook of Medical Imaging
Oxford Handbook of Medical Sciences 2e
Oxford Handbook of Medical Statistics
Oxford Handbook of Neonatology
Oxford Handbook of Nephrology and Hypertension 2e
Oxford Handbook of Neurology 2e
Oxford Handbook of Nutrition and Dietetics 2e
Oxford Handbook of Obstetrics and Gynaecology 3e
Oxford Handbook of Occupational Health 2e
Oxford Handbook of Oncology 3e
Oxford Handbook of Ophthalmology 2e
Oxford Handbook of Oral and Maxillofacial Surgery
Oxford Handbook of Orthopaedics and Trauma
Oxford Handbook of Paediatrics 2e
Oxford Handbook of Pain Management
Oxford Handbook of Palliative Care 2e
Oxford Handbook of Practical Drug Therapy 2e
Oxford Handbook of Pre-Hospital Care
Oxford Handbook of Psychiatry 3e
Oxford Handbook of Public Health Practice 3e
Oxford Handbook of Reproductive Medicine and Family Planning 2e
Oxford Handbook of Respiratory Medicine 2e
Oxford Handbook of Rheumatology 3e
Oxford Handbook of Sport and Exercise Medicine 2e
Oxford Handbook of Tropical Medicine 4e
Oxford Handbook of Urology 3e

Oxford Handbook of
Neurology

Second edition

Hadi Manji

Consultant Neurologist and Honorary Senior Lecturer
National Hospital for Neurology and Neurosurgery
Queen Square, London; and Consultant Neurologist
Ipswich Hospital NHS Trust, UK

Seán Connolly

Consultant in Clinical Neurophysiology
St Vincent's University Hospital, Dublin, Ireland

Neil Kitchen

Consultant Neurosurgeon, National Hospital for
Neurology and Neurosurgery, Queen Square, London, UK

Christian Lambert

Clinical Lecturer in Neurology
St George's University of London, London, UK

Amrish Mehta

Consultant Neuroradiologist, Charing Cross Hospital
NHS Trust, London, UK

OXFORD
UNIVERSITY PRESS

OXFORD
UNIVERSITY PRESS

Great Clarendon Street, Oxford, OX2 6DP,
United Kingdom

Oxford University Press is a department of the University of Oxford.
It furthers the University's objective of excellence in research, scholarship,
and education by publishing worldwide. Oxford is a registered trade mark of
Oxford University Press in the UK and in certain other countries

First Edition published in 2007
Second Edition published in 2014

Impression: 1

Published in the United States of America by Oxford University Press
198 Madison Avenue, New York, NY 10016, United States of America

British Library Cataloguing in Publication Data
Data available

Library of Congress Control Number: 2013942201

ISBN 978–0–19–960117–2

Printed in China by
C&C Offset Printing Co. Ltd

Foreword to second edition

Although the methods of clinical neurology are well tried and tested, the busy medical practitioner faces challenges in analysing symptoms and signs in the context of an ever-expanding spectrum of diseases affecting the nervous system and in managing those illnesses. Is it reassuring—we may ask—for the patient to be greeted by a doctor thumbing through one or other of the thirty-six Oxford Handbooks, some now in their seventh editions, when assessing that person's particular complaints?

The Oxford Handbook of Neurology appeared in 2007, drawing on a team of experts in clinical neurology, neurosurgery, neurophysiology, and neuroradiology under the expert editorship of Hadi Manji. Two have moved on, with Christian Lambert now joining the other contributors—Seán Connolly, Neil Kitchen, and Amrish Mehta—for the second edition. The authors have responded to constructive criticism by updating sections where knowledge has advanced, especially in neuroimmunology and disease mechanisms involving ion channels. They have added chapters on managing emergencies in neurological and neurosurgical practice, and on the neurology of general medicine. There are new appendices and references that supplement the pithy contents of this Handbook.

As before, this is not a book to be read for rich and discursive prose narratives of the eloquent clinical expositor, nor, equally, one in which to be ensnared by the weeds of descriptive reflexology or shackled by the competitive impedimenta of eponymous hagiography. Rather, it is a book for both the specialist and generalist to consult when faced with the typical, but nonetheless complex, presentations of neurological disease; in which to be reminded how best to investigate and manage the many conditions that affect the central and peripheral nervous systems and muscle; and which wisely sets out what to expect from laboratory investigations, and how these inform the clinical formulations that are the substance of clinical neurology. Bullet points, lists, and algorithms for diagnosis and management may not make for bedtime reading but they do provide an economic and invaluable synthesis for others of what needs to be known in order to manage diseases of the nervous system effectively, and they serve as checklists that the right bases have been covered.

Having done this successfully for themselves on many occasions in the clinic and on the wards, the authors now pass on their experience and understanding of neurological and neurosurgical disease to a wider readership. The wisdom that pervades the well-constructed text and tables, together with occasional personal asides and interpolations, reassure the reader that behind each list stands a well-informed commentator conveying the nuances of experience and judgement on how to function safely and efficiently as a specialist in neurological medicine.

In the preface to this second edition, Hadi Manji replaces a typically whimsical quote from Richard Asher on common sense in medicine with a more philosophical portrait from the writings of Mahatma Gandhi on the responsibilities and attitude of doctors to their patients. Mr Gandhi was not always well himself: 'Mahatma Gandhi is now threatened with an impending danger of apoplexy due to high blood-pressure condition as a result of continuous overwork. He must have absolute rest in a cool climate for some time to come. He is also advised to cancel all his present programmes till his condition decidedly improves'. We can be confident that, in seeking neurological advice, Mahatma Gandhi would have placed confidence in a doctor well versed in the contents of the *Oxford Handbook of Neurology* and one who had no compunction in openly displaying a well-thumbed copy by the bedside or on the consulting desk.

Alastair Compston
University of Cambridge
July 2013

Foreword to first edition

Pass any young doctor in the corridor of a busy general hospital and the chances are that person will be carrying an Oxford Handbook relevant to their current clinical attachment. Surprise any consultant reviewing notes from a recent clinic in the office and the same book may also be (more discreetly) close at hand. Previously, those dealing with the intricacies of clinical neurology were disadvantaged. Now, Hadi Manji, Seán Connolly, Neil Dorward, Neil Kitchen, Amrish Mehta, and Adrian Wills have put right this defect. The team offers expertise in clinical neurology, neurosurgery, neurophysiology, and neuroradiology. And, as consultants working in busy clinical neuroscience centres, each brings to his contribution the discipline of a classical approach to the neurological encounter together with pragmatism, much common sense, and a good deal of clinical experience.

This is not a book to read expecting the rich and discursive prose narratives of the eloquent clinical expositor; nor, equally, one in which to be ensnared by the weeds of descriptive reflexology or shackled by the competitive impedimenta of eponymous hagiography—although a useful appendix lists some names that have echoed through the corridors of neurological establishments down the ages. Rather, it is a book for both the specialist and generalist to consult when faced with the typical, but nonetheless complex, presentations of neurological and neurosurgical disorders; one from which to be reminded of how best to investigate and manage the many conditions—common and otherwise—that affect the central and peripheral nervous systems and muscle; and one that wisely sets out what to expect from laboratory investigations, and how these inform clinical formulations that remain the substance of clinical neurology. Bullet points, lists, and algorithms for diagnosis and management may not make for bedtime reading but they do provide an economic and invaluable synthesis for others of what needs to be known in order to manage diseases of the nervous system effectively. Having done this successfully for themselves on many occasions in the clinic and on the wards, the team of experts now passes on its experience and understanding of neurological and neurosurgical disease to a wider readership.

Do not look for copies of the *Oxford Handbook of Neurology* sitting undisturbed on dusty office shelves. This book will only be found alongside the many dog-eared and well-thumbed copies of its 35 companion volumes in the pockets and on the desktops of busy students of neurological disease.

Professor Alastair Compston
University of Cambridge
October 2006

Foreword to first edition

Preface to second edition

Since the first edition seven years ago, in order to introduce new young blood, Christian Lambert, who is a research registrar at the National Hospital was drafted into the team. Also, in 2010 the US version of the book was published with Professor Sid Gilman as editor. Apart from changes in layout, since no significant changes were made to the content, we must have got it right for our US colleagues.

Even in the short period since the publication of the first edition in 2007, there have been further developments in diagnosis and treatment of neurological disorders. Newer syndromes have been increasingly recognized and delineated, including the MuSK antibody myasthenic syndrome, NMDA receptor antibody encephalitis, and neuromyelitis optica (NMO). Newer treatments have emerged for stroke, epilepsy, Parkinson's disease, and multiple sclerosis, and these sections have been updated.

The feedback from the first edition suggested a need for new sections on neurological and neurosurgical emergencies as well as neurology and general medicine. We have duly obliged and filled in these 'lacunes'. A further addition has been to add references to each chapter.

Amidst all our strife and tribulation of working as neurologists we would do well to take heed:

> 'A customer is the most important visitor on our premises. He is not dependent on us. We are dependent on him. He is not an interruption to our work. He is the purpose of it. He is not an outsider to our business. He is part of it. We are not doing him a favour by serving him. He is doing us a favour by giving us an opportunity to do so.'

Mahatma Gandhi

Hadi Manji
May 2014

Preface to first edition

General physicians have always found neurology difficult and perhaps intimidating. This is a reflection of inadequate training and perhaps perpetuated by the neurologists of a bygone era. Neurology still remains the most clinical of the medical subspecialities—investigative tools such as MRI and DNA analysis will never replace the basic neurological history-taking and examination which, when performed skilfully, is wonderful to watch. This is not some voodoo technique revealed to the chosen few but can be learnt from good role models and practice.

Even today, neurological training remains a clinical apprenticeship with hints and 'clinical handles' that are passed down from teacher to pupil and are not in the standard textbooks. In this book we have tried to pepper these in when appropriate. In keeping with the style of the Oxford Handbook series the format is necessarily didactic and hopefully clear for the reader when faced with a patient with neurological symptoms and signs.

Neurology and neurologists have had a reputation for 'being elephantine in their diagnostic skills but murine in their therapeutic strategies'. This has changed with numerous treatment options now being available. Although neither dramatic in their benefit nor curative, options now exist for patients with multiple sclerosis, Alzheimer's disease, motor neuron disease, Parkinson's disease, and ischaemic stroke.

Our hope is that this book will go some way to smooth the neurological pathways for juniors in training and perhaps even some senior colleagues!

> '…few patients oblige with the symptoms it is their duty to have and not many refrain from complaining of those they ought not to have. When I tried to teach the art of medical diagnosis to students, I often used to ask them this riddle: "what runs about farm yards, flaps its wings, lays eggs and barks like a dog?"…the answer is a hen! Usually one of the more earnest and innocent of the students would say: "But sir! I don't understand the bit about barking like a dog". Ah yes, I must explain. That was just put in to make it difficult.'

> [Richard Asher quoted in British Medical Association (1984). *A sense of Asher; a new miscellany*. BMA, London.]

Hadi Manji
September 2006

Acknowledgements

Michael Hawkes, Viki Mortimer and colleagues at OUP in continuing to support us in the preparation of this second edition.

With thanks to Neil Dorward and Adrian Wills for their contributions on the first edition.

Dedication

To my Father, Akbarali Rahim Manji (1922–2010)
'Nothing lasts forever.'

Contents

Symbols and abbreviations *xv*

1 Neurological history and examination 1
2 Neuroanatomy 31
3 Neurological emergencies 53
4 Common clinical presentations 135
5 Neurological disorders 177
6 Neurology in medicine 395
7 Neurosurgery 459
8 Clinical neurophysiology 523
9 Neuroradiology 569

Appendix 1: Neurological disability scales *595*
Appendix 2: Clinical pearls *599*
Appendix 3: Neurological eponyms *603*
Appendix 4: Useful websites *611*
Index *613*

Symbols and abbreviations

📖	cross-reference
⌀	internet reference
≥	greater than or equal to
≤	less than or equal to
↓	decreased
↑	increased
±	plus/minus
♂	male
♀	female
A&E	accident and emergency (department)
ABG	arterial blood gas
ACA	anterior cerebral artery
AC	air conduction
ACE	angiotensin-converting enzyme
ACh	acetylcholine
AChI	acetylcholinesterase inhibitor
AChR	acetylcholine receptor
ACom	anterior communicating (artery)
ACST	Asymptomatic Carotid Surgery Trial
ACTH	adrenocorticotrophic hormone
AD	Alzheimer's disease or autosomal dominant
ADC	apparent diffusion coefficient (map)
ADCA	autosomal dominant cerebellar ataxia
ADEM	acute disseminated encephalomyelitis
ADH	antidiuretic hormone
ADL	activities of daily living
ADM	abductor digiti minimi (muscle)
ADP	adductor pollicis (muscle)
AED	anti-epileptic drug
AF	atrial fibrillation
AFO	ankle foot orthosis
AHB	abductor hallucis brevis
AIC	anterior iliac crest
AICA	anterior inferior cerebellar artery
AIDP	acute inflammatory demyelinating polyneuropathy

AIDS	acquired immune deficiency syndrome
AION	anterior ischaemic optic neuropathy
ALL	anterior longitudinal ligament
ALS	amyotrophic lateral sclerosis
AMAN	acute motor axonal neuropathy
AMSAN	acute motor and sensory axonal neuropathy
ANA	antinuclear antibody
ANCA	anti-neutrophil cytoplasmic antibody
AP	anteroposterior
APAS	antiphospholipid antibody syndrome
APB	abductor pollicis brevis (muscle)
ApoE	apolipoprotein E
APP	amyloid precursor protein
APTT	activated partial thromboplastin time
AR	autosomal recessive
ART	anti-retroviral (therapy)
ASA	anterior spinal artery
ASDH	acute subdural haematoma
ATLS	Advanced Trauma Life Support (protocol)
AV	arteriovenous
AVF	arteriovenous fistula
AVM	arteriovenous malformation
BAER	brainstem auditory evoked response
BBB	blood–brain barrier
BC	bone conduction
bd	twice a day
BE	bacterial endocarditis
BETS	benign epileptiform transients of sleep
BHCG	beta human chorionic gonadotrophin
BIH	benign intracranial hypertension
BMD	Becker muscular dystrophy
BMI	body mass index
BP	blood pressure
BPPV	benign paroxysmal positional vertigo
BSAEP	brainstem auditory evoked potential
BSE	bovine spongiform encephalopathy
BSEP	brainstem evoked potential
bvFTD	behavioural variant frontotemporal dementia

CADASIL	cerebral autosomal dominant arteriopathy with subcortical infarcts and leucoencephalopathy
CAN	chronic axonal neuropathy
c-ANCA	cytoplasmic anti-neutrophil cytoplasmic antibody
cART	combination antiretroviral therapy
CASPR2	contactin-associated protein 2
CB	conduction block
CBD	corticobasal degeneration
CCA	common carotid artery
CCF	carotid cavernous fistula
CE	contrast-enhanced (MRI)
CEA	carcinoembryonic antigen
CEO	chronic external ophthalmoplegia
CH	cluster headache
CIDP	chronic inflammatory demyelinating polyneuropathy
CJD	Creutzfeldt–Jakob disease
CK	creatine kinase
CMAP	compound muscle action potential
CMCT	central motor conduction time
CMT	Charcot–Marie–Tooth disease
CMV	cytomegalovirus
CNE	concentric needle electrode
CNS	central nervous system
COC	combined oral contraceptive
COMT	catechol-O-methyltransferase
COX	cyclo-oxygenase
CPA	cerebellopontine angle
CPAP	continuous positive airway pressure
CPEO	chronic progressive external ophthalmoplegia
CPK	creatine phosphokinase
CPN	common peroneal nerve
CPP	cerebral perfusion pressure
CR	controlled-release
CRP	C-reactive protein
CSF	cerebrospinal fluid
CT	computed tomography
CTA	computed tomography angiography
CTS	carpal tunnel syndrome

CV	conduction velocity
CVLM	caudal ventrolateral medulla
CVS	cardiovascular system
Cx	cervical (spine)
CXR	chest X-ray
DA	dopamine or dopamine agonist
DAI	diffuse axonal injury
DaT	dopamine transporter
dAVF	dural arteriovenous fistula
DBS	deep brain stimulation
DCLB	dementia with cortical Lewy bodies
ddC	zalcitabine
ddI	didanosine
DHE	dihydroergotamine
DI	diabetes insipidus
DIC	disseminated intravascular coagulation
DILS	diffuse inflammatory lymphocytosis syndrome
DIO	dorsal interosseous (muscle)
DIP	distal interphalangeal
DIPJ	distal interphalangeal joint
DLB	dementia with Lewy bodies
DM	diabetes mellitus or dermatomyositis
DMD	Duchenne muscular dystrophy
DML	distal motor latency
DMT	disease-modifying treatment
DNET	dysembryoplastic neuroepithelial tumour
DRD	dopa-responsive dystonia
DRG	dorsal respiratory group
DRPLA	dentatorubral pallidoluysian atrophy
DSA	digital subtraction angiography
d4T	stavudine
DVA	developmental venous anomaly
DVLA	Driver and Vehicle Licensing Agency
DVT	deep vein thrombosis
DWI	diffusion-weighted image (MRI)
DXT	deep X-ray therapy
EA	episodic ataxia (EA1, EA2)
EAM	external auditory meatus

EBV	Epstein–Barr virus
ECG	electrocardiogram
ECT	electroconvulsive therapy
EDB	extensor digitorum brevis (muscle)
EDH	extradural haematoma
EDP	extensor digitorum profundus
EEG	electroencephalogram
EHL	extensor hallucis longus (muscle)
EMG	electromyography
ENA	extractable nuclear antigen
ENT	ear, nose, and throat
EOM	eye movement channel (in EEG)
EP	evoked potential
EPC	epilepsia partialis continua
EPP	endplate potential
ERG	electroretinography
ESR	erythrocyte sedimentation rate
ET	essential tremor
EVD	extraventricular drain
FAP	familial amyloid polyneuropathy
FBC	full blood count
FCU	flexor carpi ulnaris (muscle)
FDG	fluorine-18 labelled deoxyglucose
FDIO	first dorsal interosseous (muscle)
FDP	flexor digitorum profundus (muscle)
FDS	flexor digitorum superficialis (muscle)
FEV_1	forced expiratory volume in 1 second
FH	family history
FLAIR	fluid attenuated inversion recovery (MRI)
FLARE	fast low-angle recalled echoes (MRI)
FM	foramen magnum
fMRI	functional magnetic resonance imaging
FPB	flexor pollicis brevis
FP-CIT	fluoropropyl-2β-carbomethoxy-3β-(4-iodophenyl)tropane
FPL	flexor pollicis longus
FS	functional system
FSH	facioscapulohumeral (dystrophy) or follicle-stimulating hormone
FTD	frontotemporal dementia

FVC	forced vital capacity
GAD	glutamic acid decarboxylase
GBS	Guillain–Barré syndrome
GCS	Glasgow Coma Scale
Gd	gadolinium
GE	gradient echo
GEN	gaze-evoked nystagmus
GH	growth hormone
GI	gastrointestinal
GP	general practitioner
GPi	globus pallidus internus
GRN	progranulin
GSS	Gerstmann–Sträussler–Scheinker (syndrome)
GT	glutamyl transferase
GTN	glyceryl trinitrate
GTP	guanosine triphosphate
GTT	glucose tolerance test
HAD	HIV-associated dementia
Hb	haemoglobin
HD	Huntington's disease
HDL	high-density lipoprotein
HDU	high-dependency unit
HHV6	human herpesvirus 6
HI	head injury
HIV	human immunodeficiency virus
HLA	human leucocyte antigen (system)
HNPP	hereditary neuropathy with liability to pressure palsies
HMSN	hereditary motor and sensory neuropathy
HOCM	hypertrophic obstructive cardiomyopathy
HRT	hormone replacement therapy
HSAN	hereditary sensory and autonomic neuropathy
HSE	herpes simplex encephalitis
HSN	hereditary sensory neuropathy
HSV	herpes simplex virus
5-HT	5-hydroxytryptamine
HTLV-1	human T-cell lymphocytotrophic virus type 1
hyperKPP	hyperkalaemic periodic paralysis
hypoKPP	hypokalaemic periodic paralysis

IAC	internal auditory canal
IBD	inflammatory bowel disease
IBM	inclusion body myositis
ICA	internal carotid artery
ICH	intracerebral haemorrhage
ICP	intracranial pressure
ICU	intensive care unit
Ig	immunoglobulin (IgA, IgM, etc.)
IHD	ischaemic heart disease
IHS	International Headache Society
IIH	idiopathic intracranial hypertension
IM	intramuscular
INO	internuclear ophthalmoplegia
INR	international normalized ratio
IO	inferior oblique (muscle)
IP	interphalangeal (joint)
IPD	idiopathic Parkinson's disease
IPNV	isolated peripheral nerve vasculitis
IQ	intelligence quotient
IR	inferior rectus (muscle)
ISC	intermittent self-catheterization
ISH	idiopathic stabbing headache
ITU	intensive therapy unit
IV	intravenous
IVDU	intravenous drug user
JME	juvenile myoclonic epilepsy
KRIT1	Krev interaction trapped protein 1
KSS	Kearns–Sayre syndrome
LA	local anaesthetic
LDL	low-density lipoprotein
LEMS	Lambert–Eaton myasthenic syndrome
LFT	liver function test
LGI1	leucine-rich, glioma-inactivated protein 1
LGMD	limb–girdle muscular dystrophy (LGMD1A, LGMD1B, etc.)
LH	luteinizing hormone
LHON	Leber's hereditary optic neuropathy
LMN	lower motor neuron
LOC	loss of consciousness

LP	lumbar puncture
LOS	lower oesophageal sphincter
LR	lateral rectus (muscle)
LVF	left ventricular failure
MAG	myelin-associated glycoprotein
MAPT	microtubule-associated protein tau
MAOI	monoamine oxidase inhibitors
MCA	middle cerebral artery
MCV	mean corpuscular volume or motor conduction velocity
MD	myotonic dystrophy
MELAS	mitochondrial encephalopathy with lactic acidosis and stroke-like episodes
MEN	multiple endocrine neoplasia
MERRF	mitochondrial epilepsy with ragged red fibres
MG	myasthenia gravis
MGUS	monoclonal gammopathy of unknown significance
MI	myocardial infarction or myoinositol
min	minute(s)
MIP	maximum intensity projection (MRI)
MMA	methylmalonic acid
MMN	multifocal motor neuropathy
MMNCB	multifocal motor neuropathy with conduction block
MMSE	Mini-Mental State Examination
MND	motor neuron disease
MNGIE	mitochondrial myopathy–neuropathy–GI dysmotility–encephalopathy
MoCA	Montreal Cognitive Assessment
MP	metacarpophalangeal (joint)
MPR	multiplanar reformation (CT)
MPTP	1-methyl-4-phenyl-1,2,3,6-tetrahydropyridine
MR	medial rectus (muscle) or magnetic resonance
MRA	magnetic resonance angiography
MRC	Medical Research Council
MRI	magnetic resonance imaging
MRS	magnetic resonance spectroscopy
MRSA	meticillin-resistant *Staphylococcus aureus*
MRV	magnetic resonance venography
MS	multiple sclerosis

MSA	multiple system atrophy
MSA-C	multiple system atrophy, olivo-ponto-cerebellar variant
MSA-P	multiple system atrophy, parkinsonian variant
MSLT	multiple sleep latency test
MSU	midstream urine
MUAP	motor unit action potential
MUP	motor unit potential
MuSK	muscle-specific kinase
NAA	N-acetyl aspartate
NAP	nerve action potential
NARP	neuropathy–ataxia–retinitis pigmentosa
NBCA	N-butyl-cyanoacrylate (glue)
NCS	nerve conduction studies
NCT	non-contrast computed tomography or nerve conduction tests
NEAD	non-epileptic attack disorder
neuro obs	neurological observations
NF	neurofibromatosis (NF1, NF2)
NG	nasogastric (tube)
NH_3	ammonia
NINDS	National Institute of Neurological Disorders and Stroke (USA)
NIV	non-invasive ventilation
NMDA	N-methyl-D-aspartate
NMJ	neuromuscular junction
NMO	neuromyelitis optica
NPH	normal pressure hydrocephalus
NSAID	non-steroidal anti-inflammatory drug
NTD	neural tube defect
NTS	nucleus tractus solitarius (nucleus of the solitary tract)
O_2 sat	oxygen saturation
OA	optic atrophy
OCB	oligoclonal band
OCT	optical coherence tomography
od	once a day
ON	optic neuritis
OP	opening pressure
OPB	opponens pollicis brevis
OPCA	olivopontocerebellar atrophy
OPMD	oculopharyngeal muscular dystrophy

OSAHS	obstructive sleep apnoea/hypopnoea syndrome
OT	occupational therapist
$PaCO_2$	arterial carbon dioxide tension
p-ANCA	perinuclear anti-neutrophil cytoplasmic antibody
PANK	pantothenate kinase
PAS	periodic acid–Schiff
PaO_2	arterial oxygen tension
PC	phase contrast
PCA	Purkinje cell antibody
PCNSL	primary CNS lymphoma
PCO_2	carbon dioxide tension
PCOS	polycystic ovarian syndrome
PCom	posterior communicating (artery)
PCR	polymerase chain reaction
PD	Parkinson's disease or proton density
PDD	Parkinson's disease dementia
PE	pulmonary embolism or plasma exchange
PEG	percutaneous endoscopic gastrostomy
PET	positron emission tomography
PFO	patent foramen ovale
PICA	posterior inferior cerebellar artery
PIPJ	proximal interphalangeal joint
PK	protein kinase
PLD	peripheral labyrinthine disorder
PLEDs	periodic lateralizing epileptiform discharges
PLL	posterior longitudinal ligament
PM	polymyositis
PMA	progressive muscular atrophy
PMH	past medical history
PML	progressive multifocal leucoencephalopathy
PNET	primitive neuroectodermal tumours
PNFA	progressive non-fluent aphasia
PNS	peripheral nervous system
PO	orally, by mouth
PO_2	oxygen tension
POEMS	polyneuropathy–organomegaly–endocrinopathy–monoclonal gammopathy–skin changes
POP	progestogen-only pill

PPMS	primary progressive multiple sclerosis
PPN	pedunculopontine nucleus
PPRF	paramedian pontine reticular formation
PR	per rectum (via the rectum)
PRN	pro re nata (whenever necessary)
PROGRESS	Perindopril Protection Against Recurrent Stroke Study
PROMM	proximal myotonic myopathy
PrP	prion protein
PSA	prostate-specific antigen
PSP	progressive supranuclear palsy
PV	per vagina (via the vagina)
PWI	perfusion-weighted imaging (MRI)
qds	four times a day
RAPD	relative afferent pupillary defect
RAR	rapid adapting receptor
RAS	reticular activating system
RBC	red blood cell
RBD	REM sleep behaviour disorder
RCT	randomized controlled trial
REM	rapid eye movement (sleep)
RhF	Rheumatoid factor
RIG	radiologically inserted gastrostomy
RNS	repetitive nerve stimulation
RR	relative risk or respiratory rate
RRMS	relapsing–remitting multiple sclerosis
RTA	road traffic accident
rt-PA	recombinant tissue plasminogen activator
RVLM	rostral ventrolateral medulla
Rx	treatment
SA	sinoatrial (node)
SAD	seasonal affective disorder
SAH	subarachnoid haemorrhage
SALT	speech and language therapist
SANDO	sensory ataxic neuropathy, dysarthria, and ophthalmoparesis
SAP	sensory action potential
SAR	slow reacting receptor
SaO_2	arterial oxygen saturation
SC	subcutaneous

SCA	spinocerebellar ataxia
SCLC	small cell lung cancer
SCM	sternocleidomastoid (muscle)
SCV	sensory conduction velocity
SD	semantic dementia
SDH	subdural haematoma
SE	spin echo
SERMS	selective (o)estrogen receptor modulator
SFEMG	single fibre electromyography
SIADH	syndrome of inappropriate antidiuretic hormone
$SjvO_2$	jugular venous oxygen saturation
SLE	systemic lupus erythematosus
SM	sensorimotor
SMA	spinal muscular atrophy
SN	substantia nigra
SNAP	sensory nerve action potential
SO	superior oblique (muscle)
SOD1	superoxide dismutase 1
SOMI	sterno-occipito-mandibular immobilizer (brace)
SPECT	single-photon emission computed tomography
SPMS	secondary progressive multiple sclerosis
SR	superior rectus (muscle) or slow-release
SRS	stereotactic radiosurgery
SSEP	somatosensory evoked potential
SSPE	subacute sclerosing panencephalitis
SSRI	selective serotonin-reuptake inhibitor
STICH	Surgical Trial in Intracerebral Haemorrhage
STN	subthalamic nucleus
SUDEP	sudden unexpected death in epilepsy
SUNCT	short-lasting unilateral neuralgiform headache with conjunctival injection and tearing
SWI	susceptibility weighted imaging
SWJ	square wave jerk
SXR	skull X-ray
T_4	thyroxine
TB	tuberculosis
T/C	tonic–clonic (seizure)

TCA	tricyclic antidepressant
tds	three times a day
TFT	Thyroid Function tests
TG	trigeminal
TGN	trigeminal neuralgia
TIA	transient ischaemic attack
TLE	temporal lobe epilepsy
TM	tympanic membrane or transverse myelitis
TMJ	temporomandibular joint
TOE	transoesophageal echocardiogram
TOF	time of flight (in MRI)
TOS	thoracic outlet syndrome
TPHA	*Treponema pallidum* haemagglutination assay (syphilis)
TPMT	thiopurine methyltransferase
TSH	thyroid-stimulating hormone
TVO	transient visual obscuration
T_1W	T_1-weighted (MRI)
T_2W	T_2-weighted (MRI)
U&E	urea and electrolytes
UMN	upper motor neuron
UPDRS	Unified Parkinson's Disease Rating Scale
UPSIT	University of Pennsylvania Smell Identification Test
URTI	upper respiratory tract infection
USS	ultrasound scan
UTI	urinary tract infection
UV	ultraviolet
VA	visual acuity or ventriculo-atrial
VC	vital capacity
vCJD	variant CJD
VDRL	Venereal Disease Research Laboratory (test for syphilis)
VEP	visual evoked potential
VEGF	vascular endothelial growth factor
VER	visual evoked response
VGKC	voltage-gated potassium channel
VHL	von Hippel–Lindau disease
VIM	ventral intermediate (thalamic nucleus)
VLCFA	very-long-chain fatty acid
VLDL	very-low-density lipoprotein

VM	vacuolar myelopathy
VMA	vanillylmandelic acid
VP	ventricular peritoneal
VRG	ventral respiratory group
VZV	varicella zoster virus
WBC	white blood cell
WCC	white cell count
WFNS	World Federation of Neurological Surgeons
XL	extended release (drug)

Neurological history and examination

Principles of neurological history-taking 2
The general examination 3
Cranial nerve 1 (olfactory nerve) 4
Cranial nerve 2 (optic nerve and visual pathway) 6
Cranial nerves 3 (oculomotor), 4 (trochlear),
    and 6 (abducens) 10
Cranial nerves 5 and 7–12 14
Examination of the upper and lower limbs 16
Bedside cognitive testing, including language 24
The Mini-Mental State Examination (MMSE) 29

Principles of neurological history-taking

> 'The primary role of the examination becomes the testing of the hypotheses derived from the history'
>
> (William Landau)

The usual approach to a clinical problem is to ask the following:
- Where is the lesion, e.g. brain, spinal cord, anterior horn cell, peripheral nerve, neuromuscular junction, muscle?
- What is the aetiology, e.g. vascular, degenerative, toxic, infective, genetic, inflammatory, neoplastic, functional?
- What is the differential diagnosis?
- Is treatment possible?
- What is the prognosis?

A detailed history will usually yield more information than the neurological examination and ancillary tests.
- Family members and eyewitness accounts are essential, e.g. in patients with dementia and blackouts. Obtain a history by telephone if necessary.
- A review of the case notes, if available, is very useful.
- Analysis of symptoms will follow a similar plan:
  - date/week/month/year of onset;
  - character and severity;
  - location and radiation;
  - time course;
  - associated symptoms;
  - aggravating and alleviating factors;
  - previous treatments;
  - remissions and relapses.

Past medical history
Do not always accept the patient's diagnostic terms—enquire into specific symptoms, e.g. 'migraine', 'seizure', 'stroke'.

Family history
Draw a family tree. Document specific illnesses and cause of death if known. In certain communities enquire about consanguinity.

Social history
This should include:
- occupation;
- alcohol;
- smoking;
- recreational drug use;
- risk factors for HIV;
- detailed travel history;
- dietary habits, e.g. vegetarian or vegan.

The general examination

This starts on first meeting the patient—it is useful practice to collect patients from the waiting room.

- Assess gait—broad-based, unsteady, reduced arm swing on one side?
- Look for tremor—may only be evident when walking.
- Look for loss of facial expression.
- Assess speech—dysarthria.

General examination is essential: ideally all patients should be stripped to their underclothes.

- Cardiovascular system. Pulse, heart sounds, blood pressure (lying down and standing after 3 minutes if any suggestion of autonomic involvement).
- Respiratory system. Diaphragmatic movement. May need to measure forced vital capacity (FVC) not FEV_1, e.g. in GBS, MG.
- Gastrointestinal (GI) system. Palpate for hepatosplenomegaly or abdominal masses.
- Genitalia. In men testicular examination should be considered. PR examination if malignancy suspected, or assessment of anal tone and sensation if cord or cauda equina compression in differential diagnosis.
- Breasts. Essential if neoplastic or paraneoplastic conditions are considered.
- Examine the spine—hairy patch may indicate underlying spinal disorder or a dermal sinus. Auscultation over spine may reveal the bruit of a dural AVM.
- Skin—melanoma. Vitiligo indicating underlying autoimmune disorder, e.g. MG.
- Head. Remember to palpate the temporal arteries in elderly headache patients; auscultation may reveal a bruit. Palpate the trapezii for evidence of tenderness in muscle tension and cervicogenic headache.

Cranial nerve 1 (olfactory nerve)

- Patients may not recognize a problem unless it is essential for work or hobbies, e.g. chef. Therefore question specifically.
- History may indicate local nasal or sinus disease, preceding URTI, or head injury.
- The nose is supplied by the olfactory and trigeminal nerves. Irritants like NH_3 stimulate the trigeminal nerve and may be misleading.
- Use the University of Pennsylvania Smell Identification Test (UPSIT) if available (℘ <http://www.smelltest.com>).
- Otherwise use bedside products, e.g. orange peel, coffee, chocolate. Ask if there is a smell (perception, peripheral process) and then identify it (cognitive, central process).
- Anosmia commonly occurs after viral infections and head injury.
- In idiopathic Parkinson's disease (80%) and Alzheimer's disease, loss of sense of smell may be an additional early feature.
- Other causes of anosmia:
  - Refsum's disease;
  - olfactory groove meningioma;
  - superficial siderosis;
  - Kallman's syndrome (anosmia + hypogonadism, X-linked recessive);
  - paraneoplastic disorders;
  - Sjögren's syndrome.

Cranial nerve 2 (optic nerve and visual pathway)

Visual acuity (VA)

- Distance VA of each eye is tested using the Snellen chart. This compares what a normal person can see at 6 m. Below the age of 40 years most should see better than 6/6. In older patients VA < 6/9 needs explanation.
- Correction for refractive errors with glasses or using a pinhole.
- Near VA assessed with Jaeger reading charts.
- In papilloedema VA preserved unless chronic. In optic neuritis or infiltration VA impaired.
- Colour vision tested with Ishihara colour plates.

Visual field

- Visual field is assessed by confrontation with each eye in turn using a red pin (5 mm red target). Finger waving is too crude.
- Goldmann perimeter is a bowl-shaped device and uses small light targets (kinetic).
- Humphrey is an automated technique (static).
- Visual inattention indicates parietal lobe dysfunction.
- Uncooperative or aphasic patients—observe reaction to menace.

Visual field defects

- Monocular field defect—ocular, retinal, or optic nerve disorders.
- Constricted fields—glaucoma, chronic papilloedema.
- Tunnel vision—retinitis pigmentosa.
- Tubular vision—non-organic.
- Central scotoma—optic nerve or macular disease.
- Altitudinal defects are due to retinal vascular lesions as no vessels cross the horizontal raphe.

Defects affecting both eyes may indicate a lesion of or behind the optic chiasm (vertical meridian). The common patterns of field loss are shown in Table 1.1. Figure 1.1 shows a diagram of visual field defects.

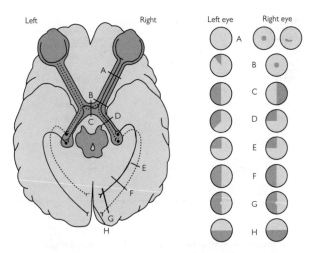

Fig. 1.1 Patterns of visual field loss due to lesions at different locations along the visual pathway: A, optic nerve lesions result in a central scotoma or arcuate defect; B, optic nerve lesions just before the chiasm produce a junctional scotoma due to ipsilateral optic nerve involvement with the inferior contralateral crossing fibres (dashed lines) producing a central or circuate defect in the ipsilateral eye and a superior temporal defect in the contralateral eye; C, chiasmal lesions produce bitemporal hemianopia; D, optic tract lesions result in incongruous hemianopic defects; E, F lesions of the optic radiation result in either homonymous quadrantanopia or hemianopia depending on the extent and location of the lesion (upper quadrant, temporal lobe; lower quadrant, parietal lobe); G, lesions of the striate cortex produce a homonymous hemianopia, sometimes with macular sparing, particularly with vascular disturbances; H, lesions of the superior or inferior bank of the striate cortex result in inferior or superior altitudinal defects, respectively. Reproduced from *Oxford Textbook of Medicine*, edited by David A. Warrell, Timothy M. Cox, John D. Firth (2010), with permission from Oxford University Press.

Table 1.1 Common patterns of visual field loss

Field defect	Site of lesion(s)	Aetiology
Homonymous hemianopia	Optic tract, optic radiation, occipital lobe	Stroke, tumour
Superior quadrantanopia	Temporal lobe	Stroke, tumour
Inferior quadrantanopia	Parietal lobe	Stroke, tumour
Bitemporal hemianopia	Optic chiasm	Pituitary adenoma, craniopharyngioma
Binasal hemianopia	Perichiasmal	Bilateral internal carotid artery aneurysms
Junctional scotoma	Junction of optic nerve and chiasm	Tumour
Bilateral scotomas	Occipital pole	Head injury

Clinical points
- Complete homonymous hemianopia indicates only that the lesion is behind the optic chiasm. The more posterior the lesion, the more congruous the defect.
- Macular sparing occurs because the middle cerebral artery supplies the occipital pole and the posterior cerebral artery supplies the rest of the lobe.
- Junctional lesions between the optic nerve and chiasm affect ipsilateral optic nerve fibres and fibres from the inferior nasal retina of the opposite optic nerve as they loop after decussation (Wilbrand's knee).

Pupillary reactions
- Test reaction to light: direct and consensual with a bright pen torch; ophthalmoscope light is not strong enough.
- Accommodation reflex is observed by watching the pupil as gaze is shifted from a distant object to a near object.
- Marcus Gunn pupil (afferent pupillary defect) results from optic nerve dysfunction or, if extensive, retinal disease. Detected by the 'swinging torch test'—a bright light is quickly moved back and forth between the eyes. The affected eye dilates rather than constricts when the light is swung to it because less light is perceived by the damaged pathway.

Fundoscopy with the direct ophthalmoscope
- Confirm the red reflex and assess the clarity of the media.
- Assess disc colour for pallor.

Fundoscopic findings
- Pigmented temporal crescent seen in myopes.
- 80% of normal discs will have venous pulsation. May be elicited by gentle eyeball pressure.
- Papilloedema:
  - hyperaemia of disc margin;
  - blurring of margins;

- raised optic disc;
- engorged veins;
- haemorrhages;
- cotton wool spots and exudates;
- retinal folds.
- Retinal abnormalities:
  - hard and soft exudates;
  - microaneurysms and new vessel formation;
  - pigmentary changes (bone spicules in retinitis pigmentosa).
- Macular changes (star, cherry-red spot).
- Drusen or hyaline bodies are shiny bodies on the surface near or buried in the disc, elevating it and resembling papilloedema.
- Medullated nerve fibre layer (pearly white) is myelin from the optic nerve that continues into the nerve fibre layer. May be confused with papilloedema.

See Table 1.2 for pupillary abnormalities.

Table 1.2 Pupillary abnormalities

Abnormality	Pupils	Other features	Tests
3rd nerve palsy	Dilated; no response to light or accommodation	Weakness: MR, IO, IR, SR. Ptosis (complete/ partial)	—
Horner's syndrome (miosis, ptosis, enophthalmos, anhidrosis)	Constricted pupil; reacts to light and accommodation	Partial ptosis, also upside-down ptosis (lower lid elevation), anhidrosis, enophthalmos	10% cocaine dilates normal pupil but not sympathetic denervated pupil. 1% hydroxyamphetamine dilates pupil in first- or second-order neuron damage
Argyll Robertson pupil	Small, horizontally elongated pupil. Response to accommodation but not to light	Syphilis, diabetes	—
Tonic pupil (Adie). Usually unilateral	Dilated pupil constricts slowly to accommodation. Unreactive to light but will constrict on prolonged and intense illumination. Vermiform movements visible on slit lamp	+ Generalized areflexia = Holmes–Adie syndrome	0.125% pilocarpine constricts pupil

Cranial nerves 3 (oculomotor), 4 (trochlear), and 6 (abducens)

Figure 1.2 shows the muscles innervated by cranial nerves 3, 4, and 6.

Extra-ocular eye movements

- Monocular diplopia due to refractive error, cataract, media opacity, macular disease, visual cortex disorder (bilateral), or functional.
- Horizontal diplopia is due to weakness of medial or lateral rectus.
- Oblique separation with one image slightly tilted is due to superior or inferior oblique weakness.
- Images are maximally separated when direction of gaze is towards the site of maximal action of the paretic muscle.
- The outer image comes from the paretic eye.
- In 4th nerve lesions, head tilts away from lesion; in 6th towards lesion.

Eye movements: pursuit and saccadic

- Fixation—observe the fixed eye for 30 seconds: horizontal square wave jerks (SWJs) seen in cerebellar disease, PSP, and MSA.
- Saccades (rapid conjugate eye movements) tested by asking the patient to fixate between two targets (fist right hand, and fingers left hand).
  - Observe for speed of initiation (latency).
  - Saccadic velocity.
  - Accuracy. (Undershoot = hypometria found in cerebellar disorders, PD and HD. Overshoot = hypermetria caused by cerebellar dysfunction.)
  - Helps detect subtle internuclear ophthalmoplegia (INO)—lesion of medial longitudinal fasciculus. In a partial lesion, slowing of adduction ipsilateral to the lesion and nystagmus in contralateral abducting eye. In complete lesion adduction is absent. Causes: demyelination or vascular.

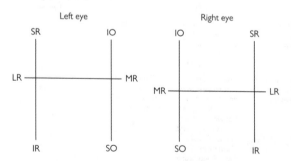

Fig. 1.2 Diagram showing muscles innervated by cranial nerves 3, 4, and 6. Cranial nerve 3: medial rectus (MR); inferior oblique (IO); superior rectus (SR); inferior rectus (IR). Cranial nerve 4: superior oblique (SO). Cranial nerve 6: lateral rectus (LR).

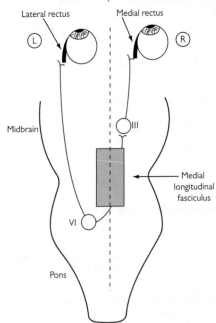

Horizontal eye movements

Lateral rectus   Medial rectus

Midbrain

Medial longitudinal fasciculus

Pons

Fig. 1.3 Horizontal eye movements.

See Fig. 1.3.
- Smooth pursuit. Test horizontal and vertical movements by tracking a target keeping the head still. Broken pursuit non-specific sign due to cerebellar disease, drugs (e.g. anticonvulsants, sedatives). If only in one direction indicates posterior cortical lesion ipsilateral to the direction of broken pursuit.

Nystagmus
- Involuntary oscillation is initiated by a slow drift of the eye. If followed by a corrective fast phase = jerk nystagmus; if both phases have equal velocity = pendular nystagmus. Direction of nystagmus is described by fast phase.
- Jerk nystagmus due to vestibular damage—peripheral (labyrinth, vestibular nerve) or central (brainstem). See Table 1.3.

Table 1.3 Features of peripheral and central vestibular nystagmus

Peripheral	Central
Unidirectional fast phase beating away from affected labyrinth	Uni- or multidirectional
Associated with severe vertigo, vomiting, nausea	Mild symptoms. Other neurological signs, e.g. disconjugate eye movements, pyramidal signs
Amplitude increases with gaze towards the direction of the fast phase	May be gaze-evoked
Various components—horizontal, torsional, vertical	
Suppressed by fixation (Fresnel goggles remove fixation)	No change with fixation

Other types of jerk nystagmus (central vestibular)
- Downbeat nystagmus:
  - present in the primary position;
  - accentuated on lateral gaze;
  - due to disturbance of vestibulocerebellum caused by Arnold–Chiari malformation, cerebellar degeneration, drug toxicity (e.g. lithium).
- Upbeat nystagmus:
  - present in primary position;
  - due to lesion in the tegmental grey matter of brainstem;
  - causes—MS, vascular, cerebellar degeneration.
- Gaze-evoked nystagmus (GEN):
  - only present on eccentric gaze not primary position;
  - may be horizontal, upbeating on upgaze and/or downbeating on downgaze;
  - bilateral horizontal GEN due to cerebellar and brainstem disorders, drugs, alcohol, diffuse metabolic disorders.

Cranial nerves 5 and 7–12

Cranial nerve 5 (trigeminal)

Sensory via three divisions (ophthalmic V^1, maxillary V^2, mandibular V^3).
- Ophthalmic (V^1). Extends posteriorly to the vertex.
- Sensation but not taste to anterior two-thirds of the tongue also supplied by TG nerve.
- Motor fibres to muscles of mastication (temporalis, masseter, and pterygoids via mandibular division).
- Jaw deviates to side of weak pterygoid muscle.
- Corneal reflex has a consensual component. Useful in the presence of an ipsilateral facial palsy.
- Jaw jerk—if brisk indicates pathology above midbrain level.
- Roger's sign = numb chin syndrome due to metastatic deposit around inferior alveolar branch. Breast cancer, lymphoma.

Cranial nerve 7 (facial)

- Supplies the muscles of facial expression and taste to anterior two-thirds of the tongue (via chorda tympani branch).
- Lower motor neuron (LMN) facial palsies result in complete ipsilateral facial weakness.
- The upper face is bilaterally innervated—frontalis and to a lesser extent orbicularis oculi are spared in upper motor neuron (UMN) palsies.

Cranial nerve 8 (acoustic nerve)

- Two divisions:
  - cochlear (hearing);
  - vestibular (balance).
- Hearing is crudely tested by whispering numbers in one ear whilst blocking the other.
- Rinne's test—256 Hz tuning fork first held in front of the external auditory meatus and then placed firmly on the mastoid.
  - Normal (positive test), air conduction louder > bone conduction.
  - Conductive deafness, BC > AC, Rinne's negative.
  - Sensorineural deafness, Rinne's test positive.
- Weber's lateralization test—tuning fork placed in middle of forehead.
  - Unilateral conductive deafness—louder to the ipsilateral side.
  - Sensorineural deafness—louder to contralateral side.
- Vestibular function tested using:
  - Hallpike's test (📖 see Fig. 5.20 in Chapter 5, 'Benign paroxysmal positional vertigo (BPPV)', pp. 344–7).
  - Unterberger's test—with eyes closed and arms extended, patient marches on the spot for 1 minute. Rotation towards vestibular hypofunctioning side. (Does not differentiate central from peripheral.)

Cranial nerve 9 (glossopharyngeal nerve)

- Taste fibres from posterior third of the tongue.
- General sensation tympanic membrane, mucous membranes from posterior pharynx, tonsils, and soft palate.
- Afferent part of the gag reflex.

Cranial nerve 10 (vagus nerve)

- Motor fibres innervate the striated muscles of palate, pharynx, larynx.
- Soft palate observed as patient says 'aahh':
  - deviation away from side of lesion.
- Lesions of recurrent laryngeal branch cause ipsilateral vocal cord paralysis with dysphonia and a weak cough.
- Parasympathetic autonomic fibres travel in the vagus nerve to the respiratory, GI, and cardiovascular systems.

Cranial nerve 11 (accessory nerve)

- Innervation to sternocleidomastoid (SCM) and trapezius.
- SCM (supplied by ipsilateral hemisphere) assessed by asking patient to twist the head against resistance and palpate contralateral SCM.
- Trapezius assessed by shoulder shrug and palpating muscle.

Cranial nerve 12 (hypoglossal nerve)

- Observe for fasciculations—may be difficult. Observe with tongue inside the mouth.
- Tongue strength assessed by asking patient to push inside the mouth against cheek.
- Tongue movement dexterity assessed by asking patient to move tongue side to side. Slowness without wasting suggests spasticity.
- In LMN lesions tongue deviates to the side of the lesion.

Examination of the upper and lower limbs

Ideally, the patient should be stripped to their underclothes.

General points
- Document hand dominance.
- Look for wasting—first dorsal interosseous muscle easiest (ulnar).
- Examine scapular muscles (winging of the scapula due to lesions of long thoracic nerve).
- Palpate extensor digitorum brevis (EDB) on the foot.
- Observe for fasciculation—may need to spend a few minutes in good light.
- Screening test—ask patient to hold arms outstretched, palms up, with eyes closed.
  - Pronator drift indicates mild pyramidal weakness.
  - Pseudoathetosis (involuntary movements of fingers) indicates loss of position sense.
  - Postural tremor may be caused by essential and dystonic tremor, demyelinating neuropathy, drugs (sodium valproate, steroids), $\uparrow T_4$, coffee, and alcohol.

Tone
↑ Spastic (pyramidal) assessed by the following:
- Upper limbs:
  - rapid flexion/extension movement at the elbow (clasp knife);
  - supinator catch (rapid supination movement at wrist);
  - Hoffman's sign (rapid flexion at DIPJ of middle finger results in brisk flexion movements at other fingers) positive in upper motor lesions.
- Lower limbs:
  - a brisk flick at the knee when legs extended results in a catch if tone increased;
  - test for clonus at ankles.

↑ Extrapyramidal increase in tone:
- assessed by slow flexion/extension movements at the wrist;
- may be enhanced by synkinesia (ask patient to move contralateral limb).

Muscle strength
All that is required is maximal strength for 1 second—useful in patients with 'give-way weakness'. Table 1.4 lists the muscles to be tested and Table 1.5 gives a grading system for evaluating the results.

Table 1.4 Important myotomes

Muscle*	Roots	Nerve	Action
Trapezius	C3, 4	Spinal accessory	Shrug shoulder
Rhomboids	C4, 5	Dorsal scapular	Brace shoulders back
Supraspinatus	C5, 6	Suprascapular	Abduct shoulder 15°
Deltoid	C5, 6	Axillary	Abduct shoulder 15–90°
Infraspinatus	C5, 6	Suprascapular	External rotation of arm
Biceps	C5, 6	Musculocutaneous	Flex forearm
Triceps	C6, 7	Radial	Extend forearm
Extensor carpi	C5, 6	Radial	Extend wrist
Finger extensors	C7, 8	Posterior interosseous	Extend fingers
FDP I and II	C8, T1	Median	Flex DIPJ
FDP III and IV	C8, T1	Ulnar	Flex DIPJ
FDS	C8, T1	Median	Flex PIPJ
APB	C8, T1	Median	Abduct thumb
OPB	C8, T1	Median	Thumb to 5th finger
ADM	C8, T1	Ulnar	Abduct 5th finger
First DIO	C8, T1	Ulnar	Abduct index finger
Iliopsoas	L1, 2	Femoral	Flex hip
Hip adductors	L2, 3	Obturator	Adduct hip
Hip extensors	L5, S1	Inferior gluteal	Extend hip
Quadriceps	L2, 3	Femoral	Extend knee
Hamstrings	L5, S1	Sciatic	Flex knee
Tibialis anterior	L5, S1	Deep peroneal	Dorsiflex foot
Gastrocnemius	S1, 2	Tibial	Plantarflex foot
Tibialis posterior	L4, 5	Tibial	Invert foot
EHL	L5, S1	Deep peroneal	Dorsiflex hallux
Peroneus longus	L5, S1	Superficial peroneal	Evert foot

*Muscles in bold type are essential in a basic neurological examination.

Table 1.5 MRC grading system for muscle strength

MRC grade	Observed muscle power
0	No movement
1	Flicker of movement
2	Movement with gravity eliminated
3	Movement against gravity
4, 4+, or 4−	Weak
5	Normal power

Coordination

Upper limbs
- 'Finger–nose' testing: ask the patient to touch their nose and then your finger which is held at least an arm's length away. Look for intention tremor with increased amplitude nearing the target ('hunting' tremor) or a kinetic tremor which is present through the action.
- Dysdiadokinesia (rapid pronation/supination movements of one hand on the palm of contralateral hand).
- Tapping to elicit rhythm.

Lower limbs
- Heel/shin testing.
- With eyes open and closed to assess for sensory ataxia (worse with eyes closed).
- Tap right heel on left knee and vice versa—rhythm.

Sensory testing
- Do not spend an excessive length of time on this.
- Map out abnormality for pain (pinprick), light touch (cotton wool), vibration (128 Hz tuning fork), joint position (at DIPJ) in fingers and toes and working proximally (upper limb) from DIP → MCP → wrist → elbow → shoulder. (Lower limb) MTP ankle → knee → hips.
- Cortical sensory assessment tested with eyes closed (parietal lobe lesions).
  - Extinction: ask patient which hand or foot is being touched—left, right, or both. Patient will fail to register stimulus in contralateral limb when both sides are touched.
  - Astereognosis: inability to identify objects (e.g. coins).
  - Agraphaesthesia: inability to identify numbers drawn on patient's palm.

Figure 1.4 shows the dermatomes of the upper and lower limbs.

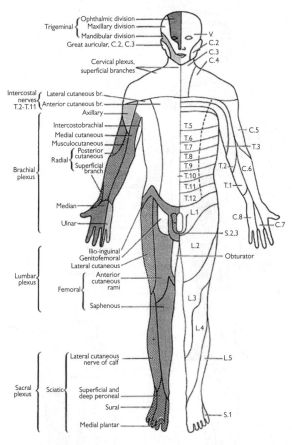

Fig. 1.4 (a) Dermatomes of the anterior of the body. Note the axial lines. Reproduced from Longmore, Murray, et al., *Oxford Handbook of Clinical Medicine*, 8th edn, pp. 458–9 (2010), with permission from Oxford University Press.

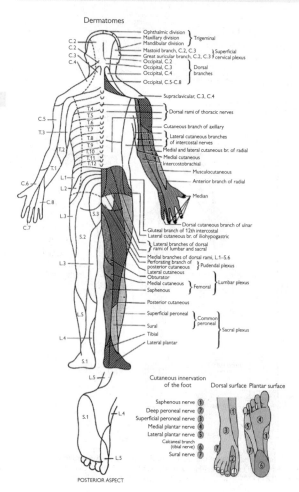

Fig. 1.4 (b) Dermatomes of the posterior of the body. Note the axial lines. Reproduced from Longmore, Murray, et al., *Oxford Handbook of Clinical Medicine*, 8th edn, pp. 458–9 (2010), with permission from Oxford University Press.

Deep and superficial tendon reflexes

Deep tendon reflexes

- The deep tendon reflexes are graded as follows: 0 (absent), ± (present with reinforcement), + (depressed), ++ (normal), +++ (increased).
- Reinforcement can be obtained by jaw clenching or Jendrassik's manoeuvre (patient links hands and pulls).
- Deep tendon reflexes may also be inverted—the tested reflex is absent but there is spread to a lower level. This indicates a lower motor neuron lesion at the level of the reflex but an upper motor neuron lesion below (most common at C5/C6).

See Table 1.6.

Main superficial reflexes

- Abdominal (upper T8/9; lower T10/11)—absent in some UMN lesions.
- Cremasteric (L1/2)—elicited by stroking inner thigh with reflex ipsilateral testicular elevation.
- Anal (S4/5)—scratch anal margin with reflex contraction visible.

Table 1.6 Deep tendon reflexes

Reflex	Nerve	Root
Biceps	Musculocutaneous	C5/6
Supinator	Radial	C5/6
Triceps	Radial	C7
Finger flexors	Median/ulnar	C8
Knee	Femoral	L3/4
Ankle	Tibial	S1/2

Gait examination

• Romberg's sign. Patient standing with eyes open. On closure of eyes, swaying or fall suggesting disturbance of proprioception. Also bilateral vestibular failure. Useful in non-organic disorders.

The various gait disturbances encountered in clinical practice are shown in Table 1.7.

Table 1.7 Gait disturbances encountered in clinical practice

Gait disturbance	Description	Common causes
Gait apraxia	Small shuffling steps (*marche à petits pas*); difficulty in starting to walk; cycling on bed significantly better	Small vessel disease, hydrocephalus
Parkinsonian	Shuffling; loss of arm swing	Parkinsonism
Spastic paraparesis	Stiff—'walking through mud'	Cord lesion, parasaggital lesion
Myopathic	Waddling	Myopathic, dystrophic disorders
Foot drop	Foot slapping	Neuropathy, radiculopathy, rarely UMN
Cerebellar ataxia	Wide-based; 'drunken'	Any cerebellar pathology
Sensory ataxia	Wide-based; foot slapping; deteriorates with eye closure	Neuropathy, subacute combined degeneration of cord, posterior column disorders (e.g. MS)

Bedside cognitive testing, including language

There is no point in attempting a cognitive assessment in a patient who is drowsy or uncooperative.

1 Alertness

Record the level of wakefulness and reactivity.

2 Orientation

- Time (time of day; day of the week, month, and year). Disorientation in time common in delirium, moderate dementia, and amnestic syndromes.
- Place (building, town, county, country).
- Person (name, age, date of birth). Dysphasic patients may appear confused due to an inability to understand or express themselves.

3 Attention and concentration

- Count backwards from 20.
- Months of the year backwards.
- Digit span. Ask patient to repeat string of increasing digits—two trials at each level. Record highest level at which either trial correct, e.g.

3	4	8				
4	7	9				
2	3	6	7			
1	4	5	9			
2	7	9	5	6		
1	8	7	2	3		
2	6	5	7	8	1	
3	2	4	9	5	3	
5	1	7	3	9	4	2
7	8	6	4	2	5	9

Normal 6

4 Memory

Anterograde memory

- Name and address, e.g. John Green, 157 Church Lane, Cambridge.
- Assess immediate recall and after 5 minutes.

Retrograde memory

- Dates for Second World War.
- Recent world events—sports, royal family news, prime minister.
- Autobiographical memory—parents, childhood events.

5 Frontal executive function (frontal lobe)

Initiation—verbal fluency test

- Ask patient to generate as many words as possible in 1 minute beginning with the letter F, A, or S, excluding names of people or places. Normal: 15 depending on age and intellect.
- Name as many animals or fruit as possible in 1 minute. > 20, normal; < 10, abnormal.

Abstract thought

Interpretation of proverbs (frontal lobe disorders result in concrete interpretations), e.g. 'a stitch in time saves nine'; 'too many cooks spoil the broth'.

Cognitive estimates

Frontal patients give bizarre and illogical answers to unusual questions such as the following:

- How many camels are there in Holland?
- What is the height of an average English woman?
- What is the population of London?

Alternating hand movements

- With arms out, fingers of one hand extended; the other with fist clenched. Reverse positions rhythmically. See Fig. 1.5.
- Luria three-step test. See Fig. 1.6. Difficulties with complex motor movements associated with left frontal lesions.

6 Dominant (usually left) hemisphere function

Language

Aphasia (Table 1.8) and dysphasia are impairments of language function. Dysarthria is the abnormal motor production of speech.

- Spontaneous speech assessed during conversation and description of a picture.
  - Articulation (abnormal in bulbar, cerebellar, and basal ganglia disorders).
  - Fluency—in non-fluent speech reduced rate of word production and short phrases.
  - Grammar—lack of pronouns, prepositions, and errors of tense. Correlates with non-fluent language.
  - Paraphasic errors—word substitution, e.g. black for blank (similar sounding = phonemic) or apple for pear (meaning-based = semantic).
  - Prosody—loss of intonation, pitch, and stress occur in right hemisphere lesions but also in non-fluent speech and articulatory disorders.
- Naming: record 10 items—a mixture of common and uncommon objects, e.g. pen, watch, sleeve, watch winder, buckle.
- Comprehension:
  - single words—point to objects in the room, e.g. door, ceiling;
  - complex instructions—'pick up the piece of paper, fold it in half and give it to me';

- conceptual—'What is the colour of a banana?' 'What is the name of the item in the kitchen that enables you to cut?'
- Repetition, e.g. 'The band played and the audience clapped', 'No ifs, ands, or buts'.
- Reading a passage (see example in Box 1.1) usually parallels spoken language problems. Occasionally alexia can occur without aphasia.
- Writing—ask patient to write any novel sentence. Dictate a sentence, e.g. 'The cat sat on the mat'.

Calculation
Simple arithmetic (addition, subtraction).

Praxis skills
Apraxia is the inability to carry out complex motor tasks despite intact motor, sensory, and coordination abilities, as well as comprehension.
- Ideomotor apraxia (left parietal or frontal lobe)—e.g. wave goodbye; 'Show me how you would use a toothbrush/comb'.
- Oral–buccal (oral) apraxia (left inferior frontal lobe)—e.g. blow a kiss, suck a straw.
- Ideational apraxia (corpus callosum, extensive left-hemisphere disease in e.g. Alzheimer's disease). Inability to carry out a complex sequence of movements (e.g. making a cup of tea) or to use real objects, such as a toothbrush, even though miming as in ideomotor apraxia is retained.

Table 1.8 Types of aphasia and their characteristics

Type of aphasia	Fluency	Repetition	Comprehension	Naming
Broca's aphasia (inferior frontal lobe)	Non-fluent	Affected	Not affected	Affected
Wernicke's aphasia (posterior superior temporal lobe)	Fluent	Affected	Affected	Affected

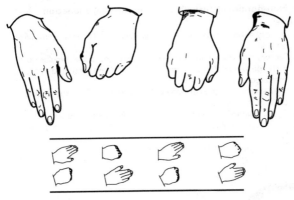

Fig. 1.5 Alternating hand movements test. The hand positions (above) and the sequence of movements to the patient (below) are shown.

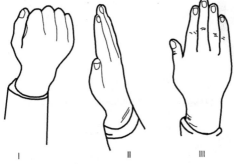

Fig. 1.6 Luria three-step test sequence of hand positions (fist–edge–palm).

Box 1.1 Example of a passage for reading

On an early autumn Monday morning, Dr David Gordon, driving his Mercedes convertible, reflected upon the weekend that he had spent relaxing at his seaside cottage in Aldeburgh on the Suffolk coast. As a busy general practitioner in Peckham, his morning surgery consisted of the usual mixture of patients with headaches, coughs and colds, and intractable social problems. Lunch, as always, was a cheese baguette accompanied by a yogurt drink. Driving home, exhausted but fulfilled, he looked forward to a quiet supper with his wife Rachel followed by watching Coronation Street on the TV.

7 Non-dominant (usually right) hemisphere function
Neglect
- Sensory neglect: patient ignores visual, tactile, and auditory stimuli from left side.
- Sensory extinction: patient responds to visual or tactile stimulus from each side separately, but when bilateral stimuli are presented ignores neglected side.
- Hemispatial neglect: in drawing a clock face, one side of the clock is omitted (see Fig. 1.7).
- Dressing apraxia: patient unable to dress, e.g. shirt inside out.
- Constructional ability: copy shapes, e.g. overlapping pentagons (see Fig. 1.8).
- Prosopagnosia: impaired facial recognition.

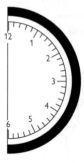

Fig. 1.7 When drawing a clock face a patient with hemispatial neglect will omit one side.

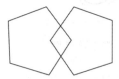

Fig. 1.8 Overlapping pentagons from the Mini-Mental State Examination.

The Mini-Mental State Examination (MMSE)

Commonly used bedside test[1]. Caveats include the following:
- Take into account age, education, culture.
- Insensitive to focal deficits especially frontal lobe.
- Cut-off score 24/30, but patients with superior background IQ may perform well despite significant cognitive impairment.

Other tests increasingly used include the Montreal Cognitive Assessment (MoCA) (⌘ <http://www.mocatest.org>).

Further reading

Brazis P, Masdeu J, Biller J (2011). *Localization in Clinical Neurology* (6th edn). Philadelphia, PA: Lippincott Williams & Wilkins.

Hodges J (2007). *Cognitive Assessment for Clinicians* (2nd edn). Oxford: Oxford University Press.

Reference

1 Folstein MF, Folstein S, McHugh PR (1975). 'Mini-mental state': a practical method for grading the cognitive state of patients for the clinician. *J. Psychiatric Res.*, **12**: 189–98.

The Mini-Mental State Examination (MMSE)

Chapter 2

Neuroanatomy

The cranial cavity 32
Dermatomes of the upper and lower limbs 34
Innervation of the upper limbs 36
Innervation of the lower limbs 42
Cross-sections of the brain and spinal cord 48

The cranial cavity

For the interior of the cranial cavity see Fig. 2.1. For the ventricular anatomy, see Fig. 2.2.

(a)

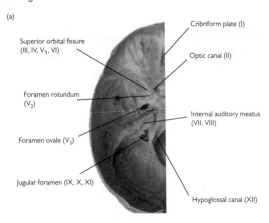

Superior orbital fissure (III, IV, V_1, VI)

Cribriform plate (I)

Optic canal (II)

Foramen rotundum (V_2)

Internal auditory meatus (VII, VIII)

Foramen ovale (V_3)

Jugular foramen (IX, X, XI)

Hypoglossal canal (XII)

(b)

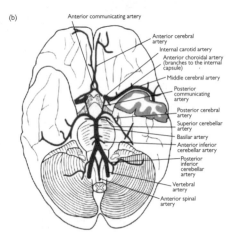

Anterior communicating artery

Anterior cerebral artery

Internal carotid artery

Anterior choroidal artery (branches to the internal capsule)

Middle cerebral artery

Posterior communicating artery

Posterior cerebral artery

Superior cerebellar artery

Basilar artery

Anterior inferior cerebellar artery

Posterior inferior cerebellar artery

Vertebral artery

Anterior spinal artery

Fig. 2.1 (a) The basal aspect of the brain. Only some of the cranial nerves are shown. (b) The main arteries of the brain. Anastomoses occur between the branches of the internal carotid artery and the vertebral artery, and between the two anterior cerebral arteries, forming an arterial circuit at the base of the brain. Reproduced from Per Brodal, *The Central Nervous System* (3rd edn) (2010), Figs 3.13 and 3.40, with permission from Oxford University Press.

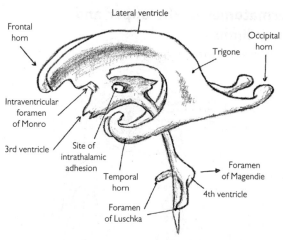

Fig. 2.2 Ventricular anatomy.

Dermatomes of the upper and lower limbs

For the dermatomes on the anterior and posterior of the body, see Fig. 2.3.

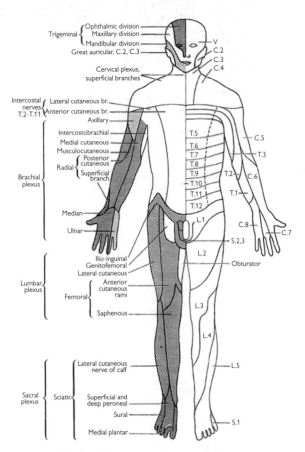

Fig. 2.3 (a) Dermatomes of the body: anterior aspect. Reproduced from Longmore, Murray, et al., *Oxford Handbook of Clinical Medicine* (8th edn), pp. 458–9 (2010), with permission from Oxford University Press.

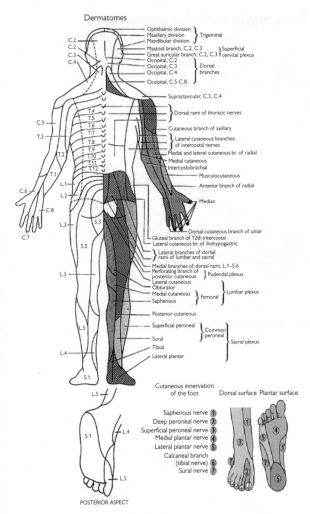

Fig. 2.3 (b) Dermatomes of the body: posterior aspect. Reproduced from Longmore, Murray, et al., *Oxford Handbook of Clinical Medicine* (8th edn), pp. 458–9 (2010), with permission from Oxford University Press.

Innervation of the upper limbs

For a schematic diagram of the brachial plexus, see Fig. 2.4. For the course of the musculocutaneous nerve to muscles, see Fig. 2.5. For the course of the median nerve to muscles, see Fig. 2.6. For the course of the ulnar nerve to muscles, see Fig. 2.7. For the course of the posterior cord, axillary, and radial nerves to muscles, see Fig. 2.8.

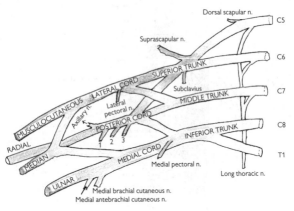

Fig. 2.4 Brachial plexus: schematic diagram of trunks, cords, and branches.

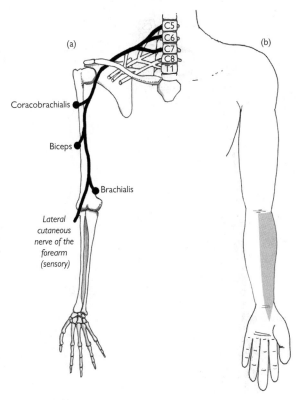

Fig. 2.5 Course of musculocutaneous nerve. (a) Supply to muscles. (b) Supply to skin.

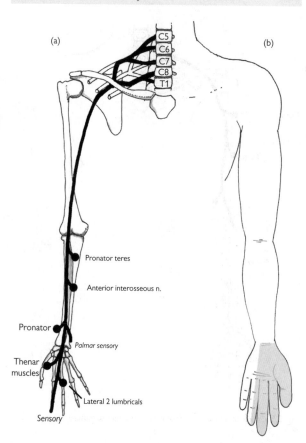

Fig. 2.6 Course of median nerve. (a) Supply to muscles. (b) Supply to skin. Note: anterior interosseous nerve supplies flexor pollicis longus; flexor digitorum profundus to first and second digits, and pronator quadratus. Thenar muscles = APB, FPB, and OPB.

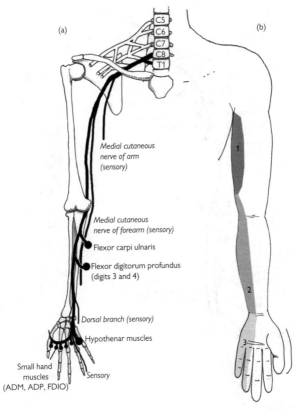

Fig. 2.7 Course of ulnar nerve. (a) Supply to muscles. (b) Supply to skin: 1=Medial cutaneous nerve of the arm, 2=Medial cutaneous nerve of the forearm, 3=Palmar and dorsal branches of the ulnar nerve.

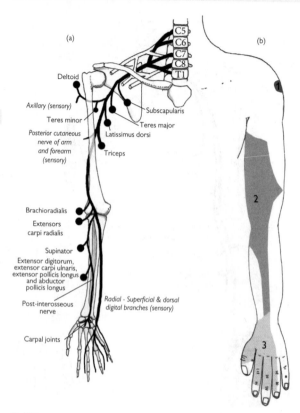

Fig. 2.8 (a) Posterior cord, axillary, and radial nerves: supply to muscles. Note: posterior interosseous branch supplies extensor digitorum communis, extensor pollicis longus, extensor carpi ulnars. (b) Supply to skin: 1=Axillary nerve (supplies lateral aspect of shoulder), 2=Radial n. (sensory) above origin of posterior interosseous nerve, 3=Radial—Superficial and dorsal branches below origin of the posterior interosseous nerve.

Innervation of the lower limbs

For the upper lumbosacral plexus, see Fig. 2.9. For a diagram of the lower lumbosacral plexus, see Fig. 2.10. For the course of the femoral and obdurator nerve supply, see Figs 2.11 and 2.12. For the course of the sciatic and tibial nerve supply, see Fig. 2.13. For the course of the common peroneal nerve supply, see Fig. 2.14.

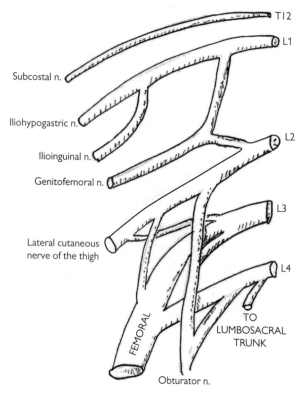

T12
L1
Subcostal n.
Iliohypogastric n.
Ilioinguinal n.
L2
Genitofemoral n.
L3
Lateral cutaneous nerve of the thigh
L4
FEMORAL
TO LUMBOSACRAL TRUNK
Obturator n.

Fig. 2.9 The upper lumbosacral plexus.

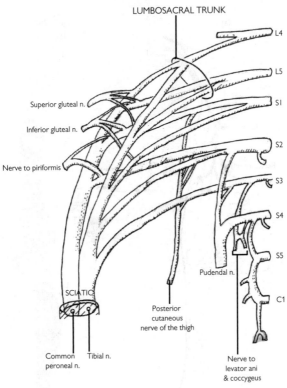

Fig. 2.10 Components and major branches of the lower lumbosacral plexus.

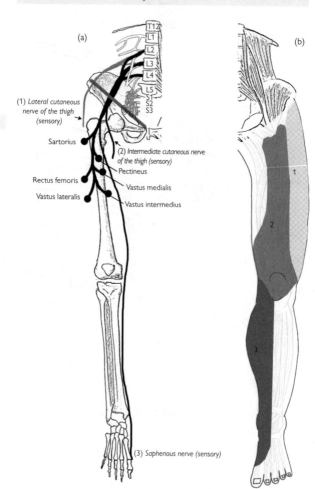

Fig. 2.11 (a) Femoral nerve: supply to muscles. (b) Femoral nerve: supply to skin; 1=Lateral cutaneous nerve of the thigh (L2-3), 2=Anterior (intermediate) cutaneous femoral nerve (L2-3), 3=Saphenous nerve (L3-4).

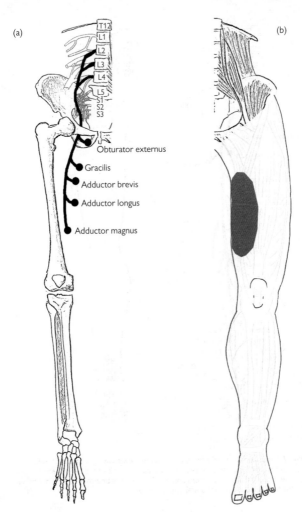

(a)

(b)

Obturator externus

Gracilis

Adductor brevis

Adductor longus

Adductor magnus

Fig. 2.12 Obturator nerve. (a) Supply to muscles. (b) Supply to skin (L2–4).

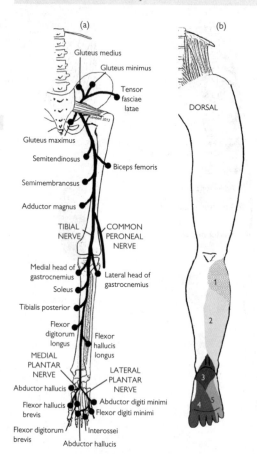

Fig. 2.13 Sciatic and tibial nerves. (a) Posterior view showing sciatic and tibial supply to muscles. (b) Supply to skin: 1=Lateral cutaneous nerve of the calf (from common peroneal n.), 2=Sural nerve (from tibial n.), 3=Calcaneal branches of the tibial nerve, 4=Medial plantar nerve, 5=Lateral plantar nerve.

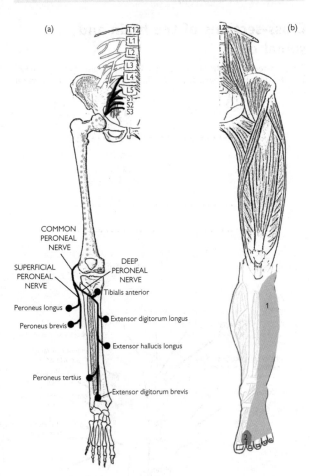

Fig. 2.14 Common peroneal nerve: (a) supply to muscles; (b) supply to skin.
1=Sensory branch of superficial peroneal nerve; 2=Deep peroneal nerve.

Cross-sections of the brain and spinal cord

For cross-sections of the brain, see Fig. 2.15. For vascular anatomy, see Fig. 2.16. For the rule of fours, see Fig. 2.17. For a cross-section of the spinal cord, see Fig. 2.18.

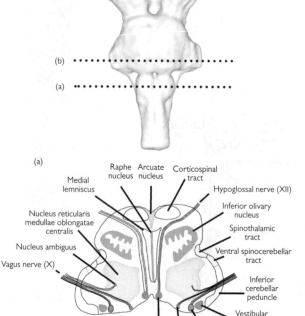

Fig. 2.15 Cross sectional anatomy of the brainstem. (a) Medulla at the level of the inferior olive showing CN 9–12.

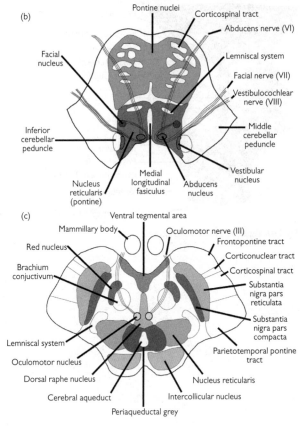

Fig. 2.15 (b) Mid-pons at the level of CN 6–7. (c) Midbrain at the level of CN 3.

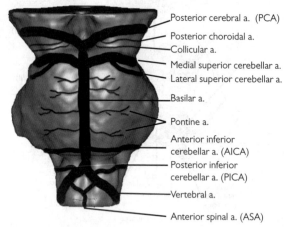

Posterior cerebral a. (PCA)

Posterior choroidal a.

Collicular a.

Medial superior cerebellar a.

Lateral superior cerebellar a.

Basilar a.

Pontine a.

Anterior inferior cerebellar a. (AICA)

Posterior inferior cerebellar a. (PICA)

Vertebral a.

Anterior spinal a. (ASA)

Fig. 2.16 Brainstem: vascular anatomy.

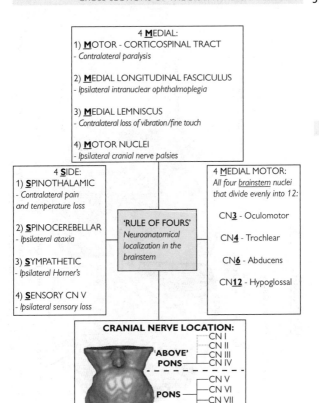

4 MEDIAL:
1) **M**OTOR - CORTICOSPINAL TRACT
- *Contralateral paralysis*

2) **M**EDIAL LONGITUDINAL FASCICULUS
- *Ipsilateral intranuclear ophthalmoplegia*

3) **M**EDIAL LEMNISCUS
- *Contralateral loss of vibration/fine touch*

4) **M**OTOR NUCLEI
- *Ipsilateral cranial nerve palsies*

4 SIDE:
1) **S**PINOTHALAMIC
- *Contralateral pain and temperature loss*

2) **S**PINOCEREBELLAR
- *Ipsilateral ataxia*

3) **S**YMPATHETIC
- *Ipsilateral Horner's*

4) **S**ENSORY CN V
- *Ipsilateral sensory loss*

'RULE OF FOURS'
Neuroanatomical localization in the brainstem

4 MEDIAL MOTOR:
All four brainstem nuclei that divide evenly into 12:

CN**3** - Oculomotor

CN**4** - Trochlear

CN**6** - Abducens

CN**12** - Hypoglossal

CRANIAL NERVE LOCATION:

'ABOVE' PONS —
CN I
CN II
CN III
CN IV

PONS —
CN V
CN VI
CN VII
CN VIII

MEDULLA —
CN IX
CN X
CN XI
CN XII

Fig. 2.17 Rule of 4. Reproduced from P. Gates (2005). The rule of 4 of the brainstem: a simplified method for understanding brainstem anatomy and brainstem vascular syndromes for the non-neurologist. *Intern. Med. J.*, **35**, 263–6.

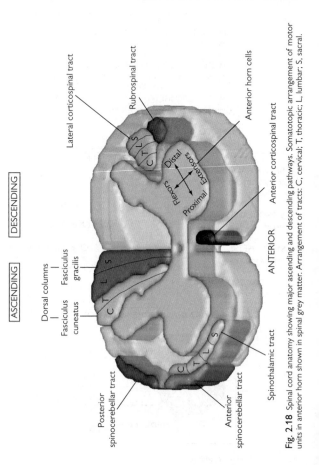

Fig. 2.18 Spinal cord anatomy showing major ascending and descending pathways. Somatotopic arrangement of motor units in anterior horn shown in spinal grey matter. Arrangement of tracts: C, cervical; T, thoracic; L, lumbar; S, sacral.

Further reading

Brazis P, Masdeu J, Biller J (2011). *Localization in Clinical Neurology* (6th edn). Philadelphia, PA: Lippincott Williams & Wilkins.

Gates P (2011). Work out where the problem is in the brainstem using 'the rule of 4'. *Pract. Neurol.*, **11**, 167–72.

Chapter 3

Neurological emergencies

Status epilepticus 54
Acute neuromuscular weakness 56
Guillain–Barré syndrome (GBS) 60
Acute headache (thunderclap headache) 64
Subarachnoid haemorrhage (SAH) 66
Imaging of SAH: examples 70
Acute focal neurological syndromes 78
Management of acute ischaemic stroke 80
Spontaneous intracranial haemorrhage (ICH) 84
Imaging of ICH: examples 86
Delirium 90
Head injury (HI) 94
Management of specific head injuries 98
Imaging of head injuries: examples 104
Spinal injuries 112
Imaging spinal injuries: examples 116
Meningitis 122
Spinal cord disorders 126
Raised intracranial pressure 128
Acute encephalitis (including limbic encephalitis) 130
Anti-NMDA receptor encephalitis 132

Status epilepticus

Definition
- Continuous seizures.
- Two or more seizures with incomplete recovery inbetween.
- Duration > 30 minutes.

Presentation
More common in those with mental handicaps or structural lesions, especially children. In established epilepsy, recent medication reduction/withdrawal, intercurrent illness, metabolic derangement, or progressive disease should be considered. Ensure any withdrawn/reduced AEDs are restarted. If no history of epilepsy consider the following:
- Febrile illness (children).
- Cerebral infections (e.g. encephalitis, meningitis).
- Space-occupying lesion (e.g. tumour, haematoma).
- Subarachnoid haemorrhage.
- Cerebrovascular disease—haemorrhagic/ischaemic infarcts.
- Metabolic derangement: ↓ glucose, ↓ Na, ↓↑Ca^{++}.
- Alcohol intoxication/withdrawal.
- Toxicity (e.g. cocaine, carbon monoxide, tricyclic antidepressants).
- Pseudo-status epilepticus—may have a previous history/normal EEG.
- Note: mortality 10–20%.

Complications and management
See Table 3.1 for cerebral, cardiorespiratory, and systemic complications of status epilepticus. See Fig. 3.1 for management.

Table 3.1 Complications of status epilepticus

Cerebral	Cardiorespiratory	Systemic
Cerebral oedema + ↑ ICP	Hyper/hypotension	Dehydration
Cerebral damage secondary to hypoxia, seizure, or metabolic derangement	Cardiac arrhythmias	Electrolyte derangement (especially ↓ glucose, ↓ Na, ↓ Mg, ↑ K)
Cerebral venous thrombosis	Cardiogenic shock	Metabolic acidosis
Cerebral haemorrhage and infarction	Cardiac arrest	Hyperthermia
	Hypoxia (often severe)	Rhabdomyolysis
	Aspiration pneumonia	Pancreatitis
	Pulmonary oedema	Acute renal failure (often acute tubular necrosis)
	Pulmonary embolism	Acute hepatic failure
	Respiratory failure	Disseminated intravascular coagulation
		Fractures

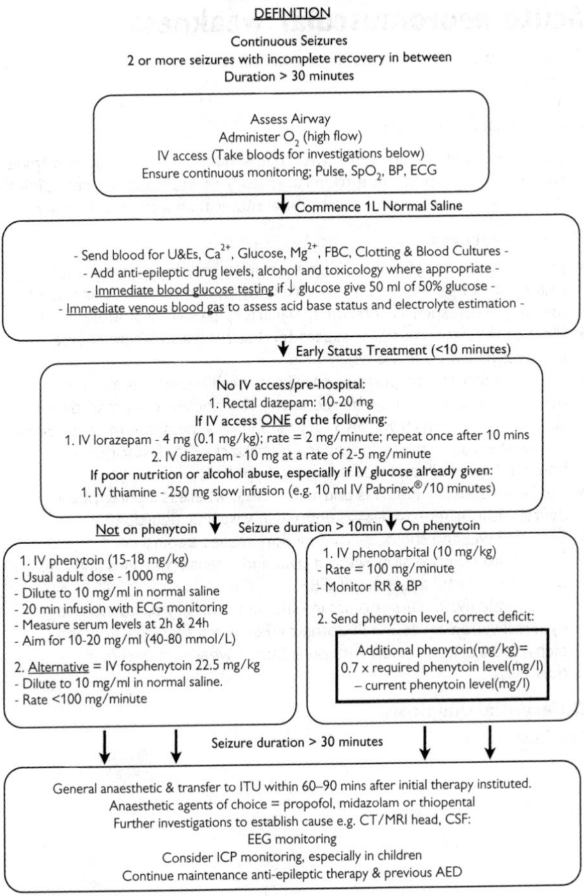

DEFINITION

Continuous Seizures
2 or more seizures with incomplete recovery in between
Duration > 30 minutes

Assess Airway
Administer O_2 (high flow)
IV access (Take bloods for investigations below)
Ensure continuous monitoring; Pulse, SpO_2, BP, ECG

↓ Commence 1L Normal Saline

- Send blood for U&Es, Ca^{2+}, Glucose, Mg^{2+}, FBC, Clotting & Blood Cultures -
- Add anti-epileptic drug levels, alcohol and toxicology where appropriate -
- Immediate blood glucose testing if ↓ glucose give 50 ml of 50% glucose -
- Immediate venous blood gas to assess acid base status and electrolyte estimation -

↓ Early Status Treatment (<10 minutes)

No IV access/pre-hospital:
1. Rectal diazepam: 10-20 mg
If IV access ONE of the following:
1. IV lorazepam - 4 mg (0.1 mg/kg); rate = 2 mg/minute; repeat once after 10 mins
2. IV diazepam - 10 mg at a rate of 2-5 mg/minute
If poor nutrition or alcohol abuse, especially if IV glucose already given:
1. IV thiamine - 250 mg slow infusion (e.g. 10 ml IV Pabrinex®/10 minutes)

Not on phenytoin ← Seizure duration > 10min → On phenytoin

1. IV phenytoin (15-18 mg/kg)
- Usual adult dose - 1000 mg
- Dilute to 10 mg/ml in normal saline
- 20 min infusion with ECG monitoring
- Measure serum levels at 2h & 24h
- Aim for 10-20 mg/ml (40-80 mmol/L)

2. Alternative = IV fosphenytoin 22.5 mg/kg
- Dilute to 10 mg/ml in normal saline.
- Rate <100 mg/minute

1. IV phenobarbital (10 mg/kg)
- Rate = 100 mg/minute
- Monitor RR & BP

2. Send phenytoin level, correct deficit:

Additional phenytoin(mg/kg)=
0.7 × required phenytoin level(mg/l)
− current phenytoin level(mg/l)

Seizure duration > 30 minutes

General anaesthetic & transfer to ITU within 60–90 mins after initial therapy instituted.
Anaesthetic agents of choice = propofol, midazolam or thiopental
Further investigations to establish cause e.g. CT/MRI head, CSF:
EEG monitoring
Consider ICP monitoring, especially in children
Continue maintenance anti-epileptic therapy & previous AED

Note: If failure to respond—could this be pseudostatus?

Fig. 3.1 Management of status epilepticus.

Further reading

Meierkord H, Boon P, Engelsen B, et al. (2010). EFNS guideline on the management of status epilepticus in adults. *Eur. J. Neurol.*, **17**, 348–55.

Acute neuromuscular weakness

Acute flaccid paralysis may be due to disorders of:
- nerve;
- muscle;
- neuromuscular junction.

In the early stages of an acute myelopathy due to trauma, an intraspinal haemorrhage or myelitis due to inflammatory or infectious causes, clinical signs may resemble those of a peripheral rather than a central disorder.

Clinical features

- The tempo of progression will give a clue to aetiology. For example, sudden-onset paraparesis is most likely to be due to a vascular insult to the spinal cord such as anterior spinal artery (ASA) thrombosis.
- Most of the neuromuscular causes tend to have a subacute course, progressing over a few days.
- An exception are the periodic paralyses (both hyperkalaemic and hypokalaemic) which may be recurrent. Key finding is depressed or absent reflexes which will also be found in weakness due to secondary hypokalaemia. In the periodic paralyses attacks may last for minutes or hours in hyperKPP and hours/days in hypoKPP.
- Significant sensory deficit is unusual in GBS, whereas a pure motor deficit without sensory loss is unusual in vasculitic neuropathy.
- Sensory level and sphincter dysfunction implies a spinal cord disorder. Spinal cord compression without pain and a sensory level is unusual.
- Back pain may be a feature of GBS.
- Autonomic dysfunction occurs in GBS, but pupillary dilatation and hypersalivation are found in botulism. Persistent hypertension and tachycardia in association with pure motor weakness occurs in porphyria.

Differential diagnosis

See Table 3.2.

Table 3.2 Differential diagnosis of acute neuromuscular weakness

Disorder	Clinical features	Investigations
Peripheral nerve disorders		
Guillain–Barré syndrome	Subacute onset but may be sudden; few sensory signs; no sphincter involvement. Vascular autonomic dysfunction; no sensory level	NCT shows slowing but may be normal. CSF protein ↑; few cells, 10–20 mm³
Vasculitic neuropathy	Patchy motor and sensory loss; pain and dysaesthesia. Underlying primary vasculitic or rheumatological syndrome	NCT may reveal clinically asymptomatic lesions. Nerve ± muscle biopsy
Acute intermittent porphyria	Distal motor neuropathy hypertension, and tachycardia	Blood and urine analysis
Diphtheria	Oropharyngeal weakness at onset. Pharyngeal membrane	NCT—axonal neuropathy; serology
Heavy metal poisoning, e.g. lead	Motor neuropathy, blue gum line, Mees lines, abdominal pain	Serum lead level
Neuromuscular junction disorders		
Myasthenia gravis	Fluctuating muscle weakness, ocular, bulbar, respiratory involvement. Reflexes intact	Tensilon test, ACh receptor antibodies. EMG studies show decrement. Single fibre—jitter
Lambert–Eaton syndrome	Variable muscle weakness. Ocular muscles spared. Underlying carcinoma	Voltage-gated calcium-channel antibodies. EMG shows potentiation
Botulism	Muscle weakness; ophthalmoplegia with pupillary and autonomic changes	Isolation of organism from wound; serology

Table 3.2 (Contd.)

Disorder	Clinical features	Investigations
Muscle disorders		
Inflammatory myopathy	Muscle pain and weakness, usually proximal. Rhabdomyolysis	CPK ↑, EMG myopathic; muscle biopsy
Hypokalaemic periodic paralysis	Autosomal dominant. Duration: hours to days. Triggers: rest after exercise, carbohydrate meal, stress	Short exercise EMG; mutation in *CACNA1S* gene
Hyperkalaemic periodic paralysis	Autosomal dominant. Duration: minutes to hours. Triggers: rest after exercise, K^+-containing foods	Short exercise EMG; mutation in *SCN4A* gene
Anterior horn cell disorder		
Due to poliovirus or other enteroviruses	Acute lower motor neuron syndrome	Stool culture; CSF PCR
Myelopathic disorders		
Acute transverse myelitis	Initially, flaccid rather than spastic. Sphincter involvement, sensory level. May be first episode of demyelination or viral, e.g. herpes varicella zoster	MRI spine ± brain; CSF for oligoclonal bands; PCR
Anterior spinal artery syndrome	Acute flaccid paralysis with sensory level. Sparing of posterior columns	MRI thoracic spine; cardiac, thrombophilia, vasculitic screen. Consider spinal AV malformation (usually thoracolumbar)
Functional disorders	Bizarre gait, Hoover's sign, non-organic sensory level, e.g. anterior not posterior chest.	MRI and CSF to exclude organic disorder

Guillain–Barré syndrome (GBS)

Epidemiology

Most common cause of acute neuromuscular paralysis. Annual incidence: 1–2/100 000. Occurs sporadically but epidemics occur in Northern China (AMAN).

Pathophysiology

Two-thirds preceded by a GI or URT infection. Most common are:

- *Campylobacter jejuni;*
- cytomegalovirus (CMV);
- Epstein–Barr virus;
- *Haemophilus influenzae;*
- *Mycoplasma pneumoniae.*

75% cases due to an acute inflammatory demyelinating neuropathy (AIDP) with cellular and antibody mechanisms playing a role. In cases preceded by *C. jejuni* infection, molecular mimicry results in ganglioside antibodies (GM1). Significance of antibodies more apparent in the Miller Fisher variant (GQ1b antibody) and acute motor axonal neuropathy (AMAN) with the GD1a antibody.

Clinical features

- Onset is with progressive, usually ascending, weakness with or without paraesthesia. By definition nadir is reached in 4 weeks.
- Severe back pain may occasionally be a feature.
- Cranial nerve involvement involves the facial and bulbar musculature.
- Tendon reflexes are gradually lost.
- Up to 25% have respiratory muscle weakness that may require ventilation.
- Autonomic involvement (cardiac arrhythmia, hypertension, hypotension).

Regional variants

- Miller Fisher syndrome (ophthalmoplegia, ataxia, and areflexia) strongly associated with the GQ1b antibody.
- Pharyngo-cervico-brachial pattern.
- Acute oropharyngeal palsy (similar to diphtheria).
- Flaccid paraparesis variant.
- Pure sensory variant.
- Acute pandysautonomia.

Investigations

- Blood tests to exclude conditions that mimic GBS (☐ see 'Acute neuromuscular weakness', pp. 56–8) including K^+, porphyria.
- Check immunoglobulin levels as patients with IgA deficiency may develop anaphylaxis with IV immunoglobulin.
- CSF examination: usually ↑ protein level but may be normal in the first week. WCC is usually normal (< 5 cells/mm³) (cytoalbuminaemic dissociation). If ↑ consider HIV infection (seroconversion), Lyme disease, or malignant infiltration (e.g. lymphoma).

- Antibody measurements have little role to play in diagnosis but may have a prognostic role (GD1a).
- NCT may be normal in the early stages (see Chapter 8).
  - Focal conduction block is a diagnostic hallmark but occurs proximally and may be difficult to demonstrate.
  - 'F' waves may be prolonged indicative of a proximal demyelination.
  - Acute axonal degeneration occurs in AMAN or AMSAN but in AIDP may be due to secondary axonal damage associated with a poor outcome in terms of residual deficit.

Management

Disease-modifying treatment

- Intravenous immunoglobulin (IV Ig) has become the treatment of choice. Similar efficacy to plasma exchange (PE). Dose: 0.4 g/kg/day for 5 days.
- PE effective compared with supportive treatment alone. Four exchanges sufficient for moderate to severe disease. In mild disease (able to stand but not run), two exchanges may be adequate.
- Combining PE and IV Ig does not confer additional benefit.
- Although there are no data, in patients who show no response after 2 weeks (especially if there is still evidence of conduction block):
  - consider repeat course IV Ig *or*
  - consider PE.
- If there is a relapse after a course of IV Ig, a repeat course may be reasonable.
- Corticosteroids have not been shown to be useful in GBS.

General supportive management

Warn ITU and anaesthetist about a patient with GBS in hospital.

- Respiratory: failure to recognize this insidious complication is one cause of mortality. Regular monitoring of vital capacity (VC), not peak flow, is essential. If this falls below 20 mL/kg (1.5 L for an average adult), transfer to the ITU. By the time O_2 saturation or the PO_2 falls, it is too late.
- Swallowing: need SALT assessment. If compromised consider NG tube or PEG.
- Cardiac: brady- and tachyarrhythmias as well as fluctuations in blood pressure occur as a result of autonomic involvement. ECG monitoring essential on severely affected patients at least until they are recovering.
- Thromboembolic: all patients should be on low molecular weight heparin + TED stocking for DVT prevention.
- Neuropathic pain is common: treat with gabapentin, carbamazepine, or analgesics such as tramadol. Amitriptyline should be avoided especially in the early stages because of its potential cardiac side effects.
- Depression needs to be anticipated and treated if necessary.
- Bowel functioning needs regulation—constipation occurs due to immobility and drug side effects.
- Physiotherapy: essential in the early stages to prevent contractures and later during rehabilitation.

Outcome

Mortality is 5%. At 1 year 15% unable to walk unaided. Poor outcome associated with:

- older age;
- preceding diarrhoeal illness;
- severity and rapid rate of deterioration;
- electrically inexcitable nerves, and muscle wasting.

Further reading

van Doorn PA, Ruts L, Jacobs BC (2008). Clinical features, pathogenesis and treatment of Guillain–Barré syndrome. *Lancet Neurol.*, **7**, 939–50.

Acute headache (thunderclap headache)

- 2% of visits to A&E department are due to headache.
- In patients with 'worst ever' headache and a normal neurological examination, 12% may have a subarachnoid haemorrhage (SAH). If neurological exam is abnormal, this becomes 25%. The diagnosis of SAH is missed initially in up to 32%.

'Thunderclap headache' may be defined as an abrupt-onset, often a 'worst ever', headache that is maximal in seconds but may develop in minutes.

Differential diagnoses

Vascular causes
- SAH.
- Carotid and vertebral artery dissection.
- Cerebral venous thrombosis.
- Arterial hypertension.

Non-vascular causes
- Meningoencephalitis.
- Intermittent hydrocephalus (colloid cyst of the third ventricle).
- Spontaneous intracranial hypotension.

Primary headache syndromes
- Coital cephalgia (headache associated with sexual activity). Note: first ever episode—exclude SAH.
- Crash migraine.
- Benign cough and exertional headache.
- Ice-pick or idiopathic stabbing headache.
- Exploding head syndrome.

Clinical features

The 'red flags' in a patient with such a presentation include:
- worst ever headache;
- onset with exertion (20% of SAH occur with exertion, e.g. sexual intercourse);
- impaired alertness or conscious level, neck stiffness, progressive neurological deterioration;
- abnormal neurological examination (third or sixth nerve palsy, papilloedema, subhyaloid haemorrhage, hemiparesis, or diplegia (anterior communicating aneurysm)).

A first episode of headache cannot be classified as tension-type headache (IHS criteria for diagnosis requires at least 9 similar episodes) or migraine (4 previous episodes required for diagnosis) without aura.

Investigations

All patients should have a CT scan and, if that is negative, a lumbar puncture. CT scans become less sensitive to the detection of blood with time:

- day 1   95%
- day 3   74%
- day 7   50%
- day 14   30%
- day 21   almost 0%.

Therefore 5% of scans in patients with SAH are normal initially. Technical factor: thin cuts (< 10 mm) are more sensitive than thicker cuts; if the haemoglobin is < 10g/L, blood appears isodense. Expertise in reading CT scans is essential.

If the CT scan is negative, an LP should be performed provided that there are no contraindications such as signs of ↑ICP.

- Always measure OP—elevated in 60% of SAH, and in cerebral venous thrombosis.
- Sample should be centrifuged immediately and the CSF compared with plain water in a glass tube against a white background.
- In SAH, usually > 100 000 RBC + 1–2 WBC per 1000 RBC. If there are a lot more white cells consider meningitis complicated by a traumatic tap.
- Alternatively, a few days after a SAH, a meningitic reaction may occur. In SAH protein is usually elevated.
- Xanthochromia (resulting from breakdown of haemoglobin to oxyhaemoglobin (pink) and bilirubin (yellow)) may take at least 12 hours to develop; hence the recommendations to delay LP until 12 hours after ictus unless meningitis is a strong possibility. This may disappear after 14 days.
- Although spectrophotometry is more sensitive than visual inspection in looking for xanthochromia, it is not widely available.
- Other causes of xanthochromia: jaundice, elevated CSF protein (> 1.5g/L), malignant melanoma, and rifampicin.
- If CT positive or there is persistently bloody CSF and/or xanthochromia by visual inspection, CT angiogram or formal cerebral angiography + neurosurgical opinion.

SAH versus traumatic tap

- OP elevated in SAH.
- Use three-tube test against a white background for xanthochromia.
- WBC—in SAH, 1 per 1000 RBC. After 3–5 days, polymorphs and lymphocytes.

Subarachnoid haemorrhage (SAH)

SAH occurs in 1/10 000 of the population per year in the UK.

Clinical presentation

Clinical severity varies widely.

- Headache—worst ever headache; 'hit on the back of the head'. May occur during strenuous activity such as sexual intercourse. Associated with vomiting.
- Coma.
- Sudden death.

Examination may reveal:

- typical signs of meningism (neck stiffness, photophobia, positive Kernig's sign);
- presence of subhyaloid haemorrhages on fundoscopy;
- signs of ↑ICP (bradycardia, hypertension);
- (late) papilloedema.

See Tables 3.3 and 3.4 for grading systems for SAH.

Causes

- Berry aneurysm.
- Traumatic and infectious aneurysms.
- Clotting disorder, e.g. warfarin.
- Dural AVM.

Diagnosis

- CT scan positive in 95% in first 24 hours. If negative proceed to:
  - LP—measuring opening pressure and looking for evidence of blood and/or xanthochromia;
  - check clotting screen.
- If CT scan positive or LP positive → CT angiogram or digital subtraction angiography (formal catheter angiography) (📖 see Chapter 7).

Management

See Fig. 3.2 for flowchart.

Cerebral vasospasm

- Focal cerebral ischaemia as a result of cerebral artery vasospasm is the greatest cause of neurological morbidity.
- Vasospasm is maximal from 5 to 10 days post-SAH.

Standard prevention and treatment

- Calcium antagonist nimodipine 60 mg 4-hourly has been shown to decrease the rate of development of vasospasm-induced ischaemic deficits from > 25% to < 20%.
- Hydration with normal saline.

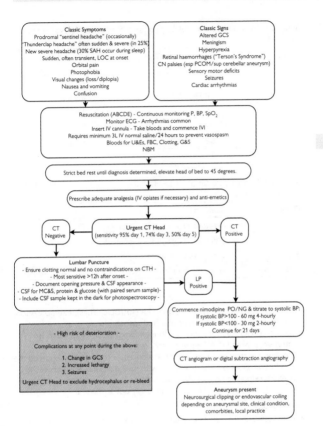

Classic Symptoms
Prodromal "sentinel headache" (occasionally)
"Thunderclap headache" often sudden & severe (in 25%)
New severe headache (30% SAH occur during sleep)
Sudden, often transient, LOC at onset
Orbital pain
Photophobia
Visual changes (loss/diplopia)
Nausea and vomiting
Confusion

Classic Signs
Altered GCS
Meningism
Hyperpyrexia
Retinal haemorrhages ("Terson's Syndrome")
CN palsies (esp PCOM/sup cerebellar aneurysm)
Sensory motor deficits
Seizures
Cardiac arrhythmias

Resuscitation (ABCDE) - Continuous monitoring P, BP, SpO₂
Monitor ECG - Arrhythmias common
Insert IV cannula - Take bloods and commence IVI
Requires minimum 3L IV normal saline/24 hours to prevent vasospasm
Bloods for U&Es, FBC, Clotting, G&S
NBM

Strict bed rest until diagnosis determined, elevate head of bed to 45 degrees.

Prescribe adequate analgesia (IV opiates if necessary) and anti-emetics

Urgent CT Head
(sensitivity 95% day 1, 74% day 3, 50% day 5)

CT Negative

CT Positive

Lumbar Puncture
- Ensure clotting normal and no contraindications on CTH -
- Most sensitive >12h after onset -
- Document opening pressure & CSF appearance -
- CSF for MC&S, protein & glucose (with paired serum sample) -
- Include CSF sample kept in the dark for photospectroscopy -

LP Positive

Commence nimodipine PO/NG & titrate to systolic BP:
If systolic BP>100 - 60 mg 4-hourly
If systolic BP<100 - 30 mg 2-hourly
Continue for 21 days

- **High risk of deterioration** -

Complications at any point during the above:

1. Change in GCS
2. Increased lethargy
3. Seizures

Urgent CT Head to exclude hydrocephalus or re-bleed

CT angiogram or digital subtraction angiography

Aneurysm present
Neurosurgical clipping or endovascular coiling
depending on aneurysmal site, clinical condition,
comorbities, local practice

Fig. 3.2 Management flowchart for SAH.

Table 3.3 World Federation of Neurological Surgeons (WFNS) grading system for SAH

Grade	Glasgow Coma Scale (GCS) score	Motor deficit
1	15	Absent
2	14–13	Absent
3	14–13	Present
4	12–7	Present or absent
5	6–3	Present or absent

Table 3.4 Fisher classification of SAH on the basis of the blood load on the brain CT scan

Grade	Blood on CT
1	No blood detected (SAH diagnosed on LP)
2	Diffuse/vertical layers < 1 mm thick
3	Localized clot or layers > 1 mm thick
4	Intracerebral or intraventricular clot with diffuse or no SAH

- 'Triple H' therapy = hypertension (with inotropic drugs), haemodilution, and hypervolaemia; used in established vasospasm.
- Use of colloid solutions such as albumin, dextran, or hexastarch (to improve flow and rheology viscosity).
- Chemical (papaverine) or balloon angioplasties to physically open up the cerebral arteries are also used, but with mixed results. Appears most useful around the time of endovascular (coil) or neurosurgical (clip) interventions, but the effects are probably not sustained.

Investigations
- Many units utilize transcranial Doppler to monitor cerebral arterial flow as a surrogate marker of vasospasm.
- Xenon-CT and diffusion–perfusion MRI are also used when available to study deficits in regional cerebral perfusion.

Securing the aneurysm to prevent rebleeding
Timing of the definitive treatment of cerebral aneurysms (coiling or clipping) will depend on:
- patient's general and neurological condition;
- extent of angiographically defined vasospasm;
- the ethos of the neurosurgical unit as to what degree the patients are treated 'early' or 'late'.

However, emergency treatment is only advocated in those with large ICHs secondary to middle cerebral artery aneurysms.

Hydrocephalus

📖 See Chapter 7, 'Hydrocephalus', pp. 470–2.

Outcome and prognosis

- Angiogram-negative SAH. Following SAH, cerebral angiography is negative in 15–20% of cases, typically associated with prepontine (perimesencephalic) blood on CT. Has a typically benign course. Patient may have headaches for several weeks but no further haemorrhages. Small risk for development of hydrocephalus.
- Patients with SAH due to an aneurysm:
  - 30% die, usually out of hospital;
  - 30% recover completely;
  - 30% recover with some disability.

Further reading

Kassell NF, Torner JC, Haley EC Jr, Jane JA, Adams HP, Kongable GL (1990). The International Cooperative Study on the Timing of Aneurysm Surgery. Part 1: Overall management results. *J. Neurosurg.*, **73**, 18–36.

Kassell NF, Torner JC, Jane JA, Haley EC Jr, Adams HP (1990). The International Cooperative Study on the Timing of Aneurysm Surgery. Part 2: Surgical results. *J. Neurosurg.*, **73**, 37–47.

Molyneux A, Kerr R, Stratton I, et al. (2002). International Subarachnoid Aneurysm Trial (ISAT) of neurosurgical clipping versus endovascular coiling in 2143 patients with ruptured intracranial aneurysms: a randomised trial. *Lancet*, **360**, 1267–74.

Imaging of SAH: examples

See Fig. 3.3 for acute subarachnoid haemorrhage with acute hyperdense blood within the basal cisterns, Sylvian fissures, and anterior interhemispheric fissure. A small amount of sulcal blood is also shown (*small black arrow*). Note the mild degree of communicating hydrocephalus.

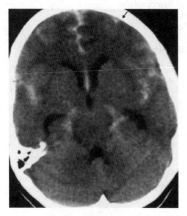

Fig. 3.3 Subarachnoid haemorrhage (SAH) (non-enhanced CT).

See Fig. 3.4 for acute SAH in the suprachiasmatic cistern and fourth ventricle with a focal haematoma in the inferior aspect of the anterior interhemispheric fissure at the site of the anterior communicating artery (ACom). Note the surrounding bilateral inferior frontal parenchymal low attenuation representing early ischaemia. Catheter angiography confirmed the presence of an irregular small aneurysm (*black arrow*) arising from the junction of the A1 and A2 segments of the left anterior cerebral artery (*open black arrow*). There is marked vasospasm and slower flow in the proximal left anterior cerebral artery (*black arrowheads*) with reduced opacification of the distal vessels in the ACA territory.

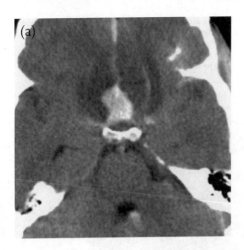

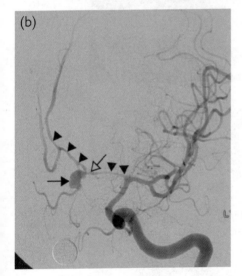

Fig. 3.4 Subarachnoid haemorrhage (SAH); anterior communicating artery aneurysm. (a) Non-enhanced CT; (b) digital subtraction angiography.

See Fig. 3.5 for extensive acute subarachnoid haemorrhage which is shown within the anterior interhemispheric fissure, fourth ventricle, and Sylvian fissures, prominently on the right. Communicating hydrocephalus. The distribution is suggestive of a right MCA aneurysm which is shown on subsequent MRI as a rounded signal flow void (*black arrow*).

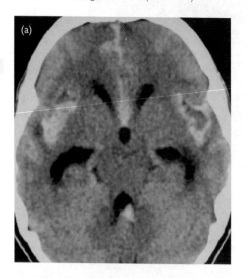

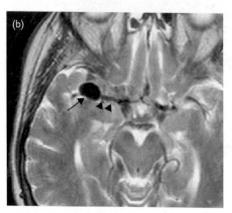

Fig. 3.5 Right middle cerebral artery (MCA) aneurysm and acute SAH.
(a) Non-enhanced CT; (b) axial T₂-weighted; (c) 3-dimensional TOF MRA of the circle of Willis; and (d) MRA maximum intensity projection (MIP) MRI.

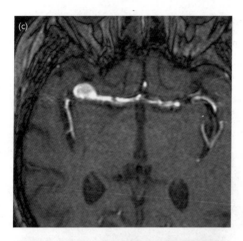

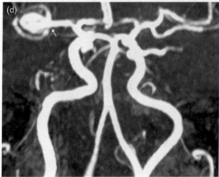

Fig. 3.5 Right middle cerebral artery (MCA) aneurysm and acute SAH. (c) MRA and (d) rotated MIP image demonstrate the aneurysm arising at the bifurcation of the right MCA. The linear flow void in (b) (*black arrowheads*) represents the M1 segment of the right MCA.

Figure 3.6 shows an ill-defined hyperdensity within the right Sylvian fissure proximally (*open white arrowheads*) in keeping with acute SAH. The fundus of the large PCom artery aneurysm (*white arrowheads*) is directed postero-laterally and the neck arises from the communicating segment of the right internal carotid artery (*white arrows*). This is confirmed on digital subtraction angiogram following selective catheterization of the right internal carotid artery. In (b) the aneurysm (*open black arrowheads*) arises via a relatively narrow neck (*black arrow*) from the communicating segment of the right ICA. Note contrast within the right posterior cerebral artery (*closed black arrowheads*) indicating the presence of a prominent persistent posterior communicating artery.

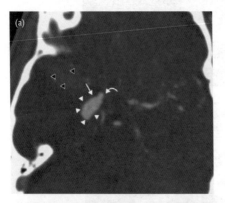

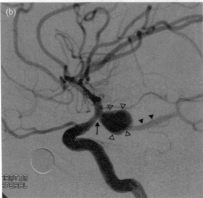

Fig. 3.6 Right posterior communicating artery (PCom) aneurysm and SAH. (a) Axial multiplanar reformation (MPR) from CT angiogram; (b), (c), (d) digital subtraction angiogram and coil embolization.

Figures 3.6 (c) and (d) depict the post-endovascular coil embolization of the aneurysm with the coil ball in (c) (*black arrowheads*) subtracted from the image in (d). The aneurysm is completely excluded and the posterior communicating artery is preserved with continued flow within the posterior cerebral artery (*black arrowheads* in (d)).

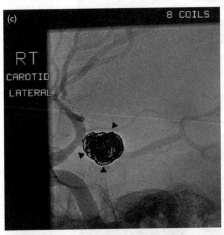

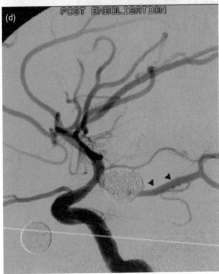

Fig. 3.6 (c), (d) Post-endovascular coil embolization of the aneurysm.

Figure 3.7 shows hyperdense subarachnoid blood within the left cerebellar pontine angle extending into the fourth ventricle. The CT angiogram demonstrates a small rounded aneurysm arising at the origin of the left PICA (*black arrow*).

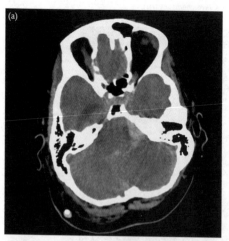

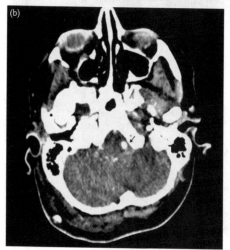

Fig. 3.7 SAH: left posterior inferior cerebellar artery (PICA) aneurysm.
(a) Non-enhanced CT; (b) axial image from CT angiogram.

Acute focal neurological syndromes

In patients who present with acute focal neurological deficit, the history and examination should point to the site of pathology and the possible pathological mechanism(s).

Clinical notes

Onset of symptoms

- Sudden onset of focal neurological dysfunction without warning suggests a vascular aetiology.
- Slow progression ('march') of symptoms over a few seconds suggests an ictal phenomenon.
- Progression over minutes or hours points to a migrainous diathesis.
- Exceptions to these rules occur since occasionally a stroke may progress in a stepwise manner over hours or days.
- Gradual development of focal neurological deficit over days or weeks and months indicates a space-occupying lesion such as a tumour.

Duration of symptoms

The only factor distinguishing a TIA from a stroke is that the duration of TIA is < 24 hours, although most episodes last only a few minutes.

Nature of symptoms

- Cerebrovascular events cause negative symptoms and signs, i.e. loss of sensory, motor, language, or visual function.
- Ictal events generally cause positive phenomena such as tingling in an arm or leg.
- Migraine may cause both positive and negative symptoms and signs—tingling marching up the arm and dysphasia.
- Space-occupying lesions will result in a progressive loss of function or may trigger positive ictal symptoms.

Additional symptoms and signs

- Associated throbbing unilateral headache during or after the development of neurological symptoms points to migraine, but headache occurs in 15% of patients with TIAs, 25% of patients with acute ischaemic stroke, and all cases of SAH.
- Carotid and vertebral artery dissection may both cause focal neurological deficits in association with head, face, neck, or ocular pain.
- In an elderly patient with monocular visual loss temporal arteritis must be excluded.
- Subdural haematoma may present with an acute onset with or without headache.
- Partial seizures may progress rapidly to generalized tonic–clonic seizures.
- 2% of patients presenting with an acute stroke may have a seizure, either partial or generalized, at onset.
- Meningoencephalitis may present with symptoms and signs such as headache, neck stiffness, and photophobia, as well as focal signs due to an associated vasculitis.

Loss of consciousness

- TIA and ischaemic stroke patients very rarely present with loss of consciousness.
- If this does occur, the most likely causes are SAH, a large brainstem stroke, or a massive hemispheric intracerebral haemorrhage.
- Large hemispheric ischaemic strokes may progress to coma after a few days (secondary haemorrhage).
- Following a seizure, some patients may present with Todd's paresis.

Causes of acute focal neurological symptoms and signs

- Transient ischaemic attack (TIA)/stroke.
- Migraine aura.
- Partial (focal) seizure.
- Intracranial structural lesions:
  - tumour;
  - subdural haematoma;
  - AVM;
  - giant aneurysm.
- Multiple sclerosis and inflammatory CNS disorders.
- Metabolic disorders:
  - hypoglycaemia;
  - hypo- and hypercalcaemia;
  - Wernicke's encephalopathy.
- Meningoencephalitis:
  - cerebral abscess;
  - associated vasculitis;
  - specific organisms, e.g. herpes simplex and temporal lobes, *Listeria monocytogenes* and brainstem involvement.
- Other disorders:
  - myasthenia gravis;
  - hyperventilation and panic attacks;
  - somatization disorders.

Management of acute ischaemic stroke

See Table 3.5 for NIH Stroke Scale and Fig. 3.8 for flowchart.

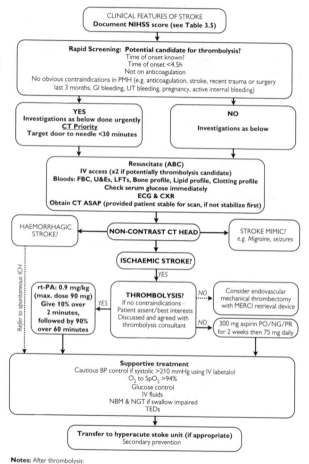

CLINICAL FEATURES OF STROKE
Document NIHSS score (see Table 3.5)

Rapid Screening: Potential candidate for thrombolysis?
Time of onset known?
Time of onset <4.5h
Not on anticoagulation
No obvious contraindications in PMH (e.g. anticoagulation, stroke, recent trauma or surgery last 3 months, GI bleeding, UT bleeding, pregnancy, active internal bleeding)

YES
Investigations as below done urgently
CT Priority
Target door to needle <30 minutes

NO
Investigations as below

Resuscitate (ABC)
IV access (x2 if potentially thrombolysis candidate)
Bloods: FBC, U&Es, LFTs, Bone profile, Lipid profile, Clotting profile
Check serum glucose immediately
ECG & CXR
Obtain CT ASAP (provided patient stable for scan, if not stabilize first)

HAEMORRHAGIC STROKE? ← **NON-CONTRAST CT HEAD** → STROKE MIMIC? e.g. *Migraine, seizures*

Refer to spontaneous ICH

ISCHAEMIC STROKE?

↓ YES

rt-PA: 0.9 mg/kg
(max. dose 90 mg)
**Give 10% over
2 minutes,
followed by 90%
over 60 minutes**

←YES— **THROMBOLYSIS?**
If no contraindications -
Patient assent/best interests
Discussed and agreed with
thrombolysis consultant

—NO→ Consider endovascular mechanical thrombectomy with MERCI retrieval device

—NO→ 300 mg aspirin PO/NG/PR for 2 weeks then 75 mg daily

Supportive treatment
Cautious BP control if systolic >210 mmHg using IV labetalol
O_2 to SpO_2 >94%
Glucose control
IV fluids
NBM & NGT if swallow impaired
TEDs

Transfer to hyperacute stoke unit (if appropriate)
Secondary prevention

Notes: After thrombolysis:
• Do not catheterize or insert NG tube for 24 hrs
• BP should be <185/110
• Follow up CT after 24 hrs
• After 24 hrs start aspirin if no haemorrhage on post-thrombolysis CT
• Angio oedema, anaphylaxis rare complication. More common in patients on ACE inhibitors

Fig. 3.8 Flowchart for management of acute ischaemic stroke.

Table 3.5 National Institutes of Health Stroke Scale (NIHSS)

N I H
STROKE
SCALE

Patient Identification. ___ ___–___ ___–___ ___   Pt. Date of Birth ___/___/___

Hospital _____ (___–___)   Date of Exam ___/___/___

Interval: [ ] Baseline [ ] 2 hours post treatment [ ] 24 hours post onset of symptoms ±20 minutes [ ] 7–10 days [ ] 3 months [ ]
Other _____ (___–___)

Time: ___:___ ___ [ ]am [ ]pm   Person Administering Scale _____

Administer stroke scale items in the order listed. Record performance in each category after each subscale exam. Do not go back and change scores. Follow directions provided for each exam technique. Scores should reflect what the patient does, not what the clinician thinks the patient can do. The clinician should record answers while administering the exam and work quickly. Except where indicated, the patient should not be coached (i.e., repeated requests to patient to make a special effort).

Instructions	Scale Definition	Score
1a. Level of Consciousness: The investigator must choose a response if a full evaluation is prevented by such obstacles as an endotracheal tube, language barrier, orotracheal trauma/bandages. A 3 is scored only if the patient makes no movement (other than reflexive posturing) in response to noxious stimulation.	0 = Alert; keenly responsive. 1 = Not alert; but arousable by minor stimulation to obey, answer, or respond. 2 = Not alert; requires repeated stimulation to attend, or is obtunded and requires strong or painful stimulation to make movements (not stereotyped). 3 = Responds only with reflex motor or autonomic effects or totally unresponsive, flaccid, and areflexic.	
1b. LOC Questions: The patient is asked the month and his/her age. The answer must be correct - there is no partial credit for being close. Aphasic and stuporous patients who do not comprehend the questions will score 2. Patients unable to speak because of endotracheal intubation, orotracheal trauma, severe dysarthria from any cause, language barrier, or any other problem not secondary to aphasia are given a 1. It is important that only the initial answer be graded and that the examiner not "help" the patient with verbal or non-verbal cues.	0 = Answers both questions correctly. 1 = Answers one question correctly. 2 = Answers neither question correctly.	
1c. LOC Commands: The patient is asked to open and close the eyes and then to grip and release the non-paretic hand. Substitute another one step command if the hands cannot be used. Credit is given if an unequivocal attempt is made but not completed due to weakness. If the patient does not respond to command, the task should be demonstrated to him or her (pantomime), and the result scored (i.e., follows none, one or two commands). Patients with trauma, amputation, or other physical impediments should be given suitable one-step commands. Only the first attempt is scored.	0 = Performs both tasks correctly. 1 = Performs one task correctly. 2 = Performs neither task correctly.	
2. Best Gaze: Only horizontal eye movements will be tested. Voluntary or reflexive (oculocephalic) eye movements will be scored, but caloric testing is not done. If the patient has a conjugate deviation of the eyes that can be overcome by voluntary or reflexive activity, the score will be 1. If a patient has an isolated peripheral nerve paresis (CN III, IV or VI), score a 1. Gaze is testable in all aphasic patients. Patients with ocular trauma, bandages, pre-existing blindness, or other disorder of visual acuity or fields should be tested with reflexive movements, and a choice made by the investigator. Establishing eye contact and then moving about the patient from side to side will occasionally clarify the presence of a partial gaze palsy.	0 = Normal. 1 = Partial gaze palsy; gaze is abnormal in one or both eyes, but forced deviation or total gaze paresis is not present. 2 = Forced deviation, or total gaze paresis not overcome by the oculocephalic maneuver.	
3. Visual: Visual fields (upper and lower quadrants) are tested by confrontation, using finger counting or visual threat, as appropriate. Patients may be encouraged, but if they look at the side of the moving fingers appropriately, this can be scored as normal. If there is unilateral blindness or enucleation, visual fields in the remaining eye are scored. Score 1 only if a clear-cut asymmetry, including quadrantanopia, is found. If patient is blind from any cause, score 3. Double simultaneous stimulation is performed at this point. If there is extinction, patient receives a 1, and the results are used to respond to item 11.	0 = No visual loss. 1 = Partial hemianopia. 2 = Complete hemianopia. 3 = Bilateral hemianopia (blind including cortical blindness).	
4. Facial Palsy: Ask – or use pantomime to encourage – the patient to show teeth or raise eyebrows and close eyes. Score symmetry of grimace in response to noxious stimuli in the poorly responsive or non-comprehending patient. If facial trauma/bandages, orotracheal tube, tape or other physical barriers obscure the face, these should be removed to the extent possible.	0 = Normal symmetrical movements. 1 = Minor paralysis (flattened nasolabial fold, asymmetry on smiling). 2 = Partial paralysis (total or near-total paralysis of lower face). 3 = Complete paralysis of one or both sides (absence of facial movement in the upper and lower face).	
5. Motor Arm: The limb is placed in the appropriate position: extend the arms (palms down) 90 degrees (if sitting) or 45 degrees (if supine). Drift is scored if the arm falls before 10 seconds. The aphasic patient is encouraged using urgency in the voice and pantomime, but not noxious stimulation. Each limb is tested in turn, beginning with the non-paretic arm. Only in the case of amputation or joint fusion at the shoulder, the examiner should record the score as untestable (UN), and clearly write the explanation for this choice.	0 = No drift; limb holds 90 (or 45) degrees for full 10 seconds. 1 = Drift; limb holds 90 (or 45) degrees, but drifts down before full 10 seconds; does not hit bed or other support. 2 = Some effort against gravity; limb cannot get to or maintain (if cued) 90 (or 45) degrees, drifts down to bed, but has some effort against gravity. 3 = No effort against gravity; limb falls. 4 = No movement. UN = Amputation or joint fusion, explain: _____ 5a. Left Arm 5b. Right Arm	___ ___ ___

(Continued)

Table 3.5 (Contd.)

Instructions	Scale Definition	Score
6. Motor Leg: The limb is placed in the appropriate position; hold the leg at 30 degrees (always tested supine). Drift is scored if the leg falls before 5 seconds. The aphasic patient is encouraged using urgency in the voice and pantomine, but not noxious stimulation. Each limb is tested in turn, beginning with the non-paretic leg. Only in the case of amputation or joint fusion at the hip, the examiner should record the score as untestable (UN), and clearly write the explanation for this choice.	0 = No drift; leg holds 30-degree position for full 5 seconds. 1 = Drift; leg falls by the end of the 5-second period but does not hit bed. 2 = Some effort against gravity; leg falls to bed by 5 seconds, but has some effort against gravity. 3 = No effort against gravity; leg falls to bed immediately. 4 = No movement. UN = Amputation or joint fusion, explain: _____ 6a. Left Leg 6b. Right Leg	
7. Limb Ataxia: This item is aimed at finding evidence of a unilateral cerebellar lesion. Test with eyes open. In case of visual defect, ensure testing is done in intact visual field. The finger-nose-finger and heel-shin tests are performed on both sides, and ataxia is scored only if present out of proportion to weakness. Ataxia is absent in the patient who cannot understand or is paralyzed. Only in the case of amputation or joint fusion, the examiner should record the score as untestable (UN), and clearly write the explanation for this choice. In case of blindness, test by having the patient touch nose from extended arm position.	0 = Absent. 1 = Present in one limb. 2 = Present in two limbs. UN = Amputation or joint fusion, explain: _____	
8. Sensory: Sensation or grimace to pinprick when tested, or withdrawal from noxious stimulus in the obtunded or aphasic patient. Only sensory loss attributed to stroke is scored as abnormal and the examiner should test as many body areas (arms [not hands], legs, trunk, face) as needed to accurately check for sensory loss. A score of 2, "severe or total sensory loss," should only be given when a severe or total loss of sensation can be clearly demonstrated. Stuporous and aphasic patients will, therefore, probably score 1 or 0. The patient with brainstem stroke who has bilateral loss of sensation is scored 2. If the patient does not respond and is quadriplegic, score 2. Patients in a coma (item 1a=3) are automatically given a 2 on this item.	0 = Normal; no sensory loss. 1 = Mild-to-moderate sensory loss; patient feels pinprick is less sharp or is dull on the affected side; or there is a loss of superficial pain with pinprick, but patient is aware of being touched. 2 = Severe to total sensory loss; patient is not aware of being touched in the face, arm, and leg.	
9. Best Language: A great deal of information about comprehension will be obtained during the preceding sections of the examination. For this scale item, the patient is asked to describe what is happening in the attached picture, to name the items on the attached naming sheet and to read from the attached list of sentences. Comprehension is judged from responses here, as well as to all of the commands in the preceding general neurological exam. If visual loss interferes with the tests, ask the patient to identify objects placed in the hand, repeat, and produce speech. The intubated patient should be asked to write. The patient in a coma (item 1a=3) will automatically score 3 on this item. The examiner must choose a score for the patient with stupor or limited cooperation, but a score of 3 should be used only if the patient is mute and follows no one-step commands.	0 = No aphasia; normal. 1 = Mild-to-moderate aphasia; some obvious loss of fluency or facility of comprehension, without significant limitation on ideas expressed or form of expression. Reduction of speech and/or comprehension, however, makes conversation about provided materials difficult or impossible. For example, in conversation about provided materials, examiner can identify picture or naming card content from patient's response. 2 = Severe aphasia; all communication is through fragmentary expression; great need for inference, questioning, and guessing by the listener. Range of information that can be exchanged is limited; listener carries burden of communication. Examiner cannot identify materials provided from patient response. 3 = Mute, global aphasia; no usable speech or auditory comprehension.	
10. Dysarthria: If patient is thought to be normal, an adequate sample of speech must be obtained by asking patient to read or repeat words from the attached list. If the patient has severe aphasia, the clarity of articulation of spontaneous speech can be rated. Only if the patient is intubated or has other physical barriers to producing speech, the examiner should record the score as untestable (UN), and clearly write an explanation for this choice. Do not tell the patient why he or she is being tested.	0 = Normal. 1 = Mild-to-moderate dysarthria; patient slurs at least some words and, at worst, can be understood with some difficulty. 2 = Severe dysarthria; patient's speech is so slurred as to be unintelligible in the absence of or out of proportion to any dysphasia, or is mute/anarthric. UN = Intubated or other physical barrier, explain:_____	
11. Extinction and Inattention (formerly Neglect): Sufficient information to identify neglect may be obtained during the prior testing. If the patient has a severe visual loss preventing visual double simultaneous stimulation, and the cutaneous stimuli are normal, the score is normal. If the patient has aphasia but does appear to attend to both sides, the score is normal. The presence of visual spatial neglect or anosagnosia may also be taken as evidence of abnormality. Since the abnormality is scored only if present, the item is never untestable.	0 = No abnormality. 1 = Visual, tactile, auditory, spatial, or personal inattention or extinction to bilateral simultaneous stimulation in one of the sensory modalities. 2 = Profound hemi-inattention or extinction to more than one modality; does not recognize own hand or orients to only one side of space.	

Reproduced from National Institute of Neurological Disorders and Stroke (<http://www.nihstrokescale.org>), with permission. <http://www.nihstrokescale.org/docs/HospitalStrokeScale.pdf>

Contraindications to use of thrombolysis in acute ischaemic stroke

- Age < 18 and > 80 years
- Symptoms onset > 4.5 hours or unclear time of onset (patients waking up from sleep cannot be considered unless they went to sleep within the last 4.5 hours and well at the time)
- Neurological deficit minor/rapidly resolving (NIHSS < 5)
- Evidence of intracranial haemorrhage
- Very severe stroke (NIHSS > 25) or CT > 1/3 MCA territory ischaemic changes
- Seizure activity at stroke onset
- SAH suspected
- Evidence of internal bleeding
- Stroke, head trauma, major surgery in last 3 months
- Prior stroke and diabetes
- History of intracranial haemorrhage
- History of CNS damage (neoplasm, aneurysm)
- History of intracranial or spinal surgery ever
- AVM or aneurysm
- Known bleeding diathesis
- GI or urinary tract bleeding in last 3 weeks
- Recent GI ulcer in last 3 months
- Oesophageal varices
- Severe liver disease
- Endocarditis or pericarditis
- Acute pancreatitis
- Pregnant or recent delivery (10 days)
- Recent puncture of non-compressible vessel (10 days)
- Lumbar puncture (in last 7 days)
- Recent CPR (< 10 days)
- History of haemorrhagic diabetic retinopathy

Further reading

Al-Mahdy H (2009). Management of acute stroke. *Br. J. Hosp. Med.*, **70**, 572–7.
Intercollegiate Stroke Working Party (2012). *National clinical guideline for stroke*, 4th edition. London: Royal College of Physicians.
McArthur KS, Quinn TJ, Dawson J, Walters M (2011). Diagnosis and management of transient ischaemic attack and ischaemic stroke in the acute phase. *BMJ*, **342**, 812–817.
NICE (2008). *Stroke: diagnosis and initial management of stroke and transient ischaemic attack.* NICE Clinical Guideline 68.

Spontaneous intracranial haemorrhage (ICH)

- Spontaneous ICH is a common cause of morbidity.
- 20% of strokes are caused by cerebral haemorrhage (75% ICH and 25% SAH).
- Risk factors for ICH are similar to those with ischaemic stroke:
  - age;
  - male gender;
  - hypertension;
  - smoking;
  - diabetes;
  - excess alcohol.

Aetiology

- Haemorrhage is due to rupture of small vessels and microaneurysms in perforating vessels.
- Underlying vascular conditions should be considered:
  - AVM;
  - aneurysm;
  - cavernoma;
  - amyloid angiopathy;
  - cerebral venous thrombosis.
- Haemostatic factors:
  - anticoagulant drugs;
  - antiplatelet drugs;
  - coagulation disorders;
  - thrombolytic therapy.
- Other aetiologies:
  - drug abuse (cocaine);
  - moyamoya syndrome;
  - haemorrhage into a tumour (metastatic malignant melanoma, renal, thyroid, and lung carcinoma, choriocarcinoma, oligodendroglioma, and ependymoma).
- Clues to the aetiology may come from the site:
  - basal ganglia in hypertensive bleeds;
  - Sylvian fissure in MCA aneurysms;
  - lobar bleeds in amyloid angiopathy.

Clinical features

- Sudden ictus as a stroke.
- ± signs and symptoms of ↑ICP—severe headache and vomiting.
- Seizures and meningism.

Imaging features

See 📖 'Imaging of ICH: examples', pp. 86–9.
- CT scan is sensitive diagnostically.
- MRI may help to differentiate hypertensive haemorrhage from other causes.

Management

- Standard medical support.
  - Stop antiplatelet drugs, reverse anticoagulation.
- Surgical evacuation of the haematoma depends on location, age, and premorbid performance status of the patient. Recent STICH trials suggest no benefit for surgery versus conservative management in the early stages. Infratentorial haematomas are special cases—may warrant surgical intervention for evacuation or shunt insertion for hydrocephalus.

Further reading

Gupta RK, Jamjoom AA, Nikkar-Esfahani A, Jamjoom DZ (2010). Spontaneous intracerebral haemorrhage: a clinical review. *Br. J. Hosp. Med.*, **71**, 499–504.

Imaging of ICH: examples

Figure 3.9 shows acute right frontoparietal intraparenchymal haematoma with high-density elements anteriorly and slightly lower attenuation components posteriorly (*white arrowheads*), indicating less acute blood. Note the small rim of surrounding low attenuation and associated mass effect with ipsilateral sulcal effacement. Figure 3.10 shows a typical ganglionic haematoma with acute haemorrhage involving the right lentiform nucleus.

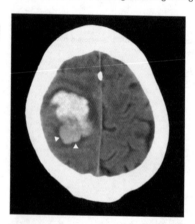

Fig. 3.9 Acute primary intracerebral haematoma (non-enhanced CT).

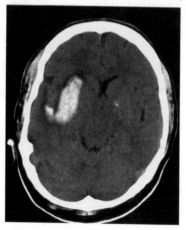

Fig. 3.10 Primary hypertensive haemorrhage (non-enhanced CT).

Figure 3.11 (a) shows a large area of ill-defined hyperdensity with little associated mass effect (*black arrows*). (b) Following contrast, multiple serpiginous enhancing structures are demonstrated in the centre of the hyperdense area, with surrounding parenchyma in keeping with the nidus of an AVM. (c) Right occipital AVM with multiple focal and serpiginous flow voids (*white arrowheads*). There is little associated mass effect. Note the large draining vein entering the vein of Galen (*white arrow*).

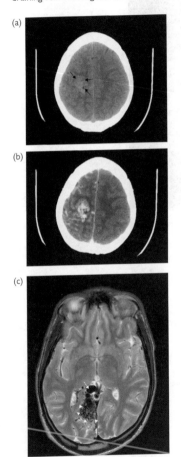

Fig. 3.11 Arteriovenous malformation: (a) non-enhanced CT; (b) contrast-enhanced CT; (c) T$_2$-weighted MRI.

Figure 3.12 was obtained from an elderly patient. Bilateral posteriorly distributed peripheral haemosiderin staining indicates previous lobar haemorrhage (*white arrows*), with multiple widely distributed foci of haemosiderin in both cerebral hemispheres (*black arrowheads*).

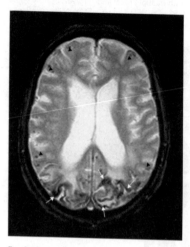

Fig. 3.12 Amyloid angiopathy (axial gradient echo T$_2$* MRI).

Figure 3.13 shows a large right inferomedial parietal cavernoma with a hypointense ring of haemosiderin surrounding more recent haemorrhage (predominantly extracellular methaemoglobin). Note the absence of surrounding white matter signal change, suggesting no recent extralesional haemorrhage.

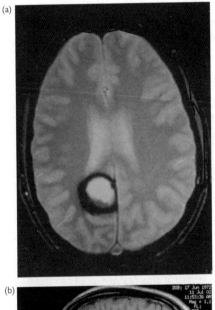

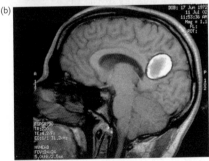

Fig. 3.13 Cavernous angioma: (a) axial gradient echo T_2^* and (b) sagittal T_1W MRI.

Delirium

Delirium is defined as a non-specific organic brain syndrome or acute brain dysfunction or acute brain failure within the setting of physical illness—medical or surgical.

Epidemiology

Common in general medicine, especially in the elderly.

Pathophysiology

Not well understood, but evidence for cholinergic underactivity and dopaminergic overactivity. ↑ activity in the hypothalamic–pituitary axis with ↑ cortisol levels.

Aetiology

Predisposing factors

- Old age (↓ cognitive reserve).
- Premorbid cognitive impairment (↓ cognitive reserve).
- Sensory (visual or auditory) impairment.
- Advanced physical disease.
- Malnutrition.

Precipitating factors

- Metabolic derangement.
- Hypoxia.
- Infection.
- Dehydration.
- Constipation (e.g. opiate induced).
- Pain.
- Drugs:
  - opioids;
  - benzodiazepines—paradoxical reaction in elderly;
  - anticholinergic side effect of drugs (e.g. oxybutinin);
  - antihistamines:
    — anti-emetics (e.g. cyclizine, cinnarizine, prochlorperazine)
    — sleeping tablets (e.g. promethazine)
    — anti-allergics (e.g. cetirizine, chlorphenamine);
  - antidepressants (e.g. tricyclics);
  - corticosteroids.

Clinical features

Acute onset with diurnal fluctuation of:
- Activity
  - Psychomotor—↑ arousal, distractibility, restlessness, and wandering. However, ↓ activity is as common, but is under-recognized and diagnosed as depressed or tired.
  - Sleep–wake cycle disturbance.
- Behaviour
  - Emotions: anxiety, fear, anger, mood changes (depression > mania).
  - Psychosis: hallucinations (usually visual) or delusions.
- Cognition
  - Fluctuating conscious level (GCS).
  - Attention assessed by asking patient to count backwards from 20 to 1 or to give the months of the year backwards or use digit span (􀂊 see Chapter 1, 'Bedside cognitive testing, including language', pp. 24–28).
  - Memory.
  - Orientation (may be relatively spared).

Look for signs of infection, dehydration, constipation.
Look at drug chart carefully.

Investigations

- First line:
  - blood tests—FBC, ESR, CRP, U&E, LFT, Ca, PO_4, glucose, blood cultures;
  - urine: dipstick, MSU;
  - CXR.
- Second line:
  - CT/MRI;
  - US abdomen;
  - LP;
  - EEG (in case of complex partial status).

Management

- Non-pharmacological:
  - treat infections;
  - rationalize drug input;
  - optimize hydration;
  - ensure adequate pain control;
  - remove unnecessary cannulae and catheters;
  - minimize changes to surroundings (e.g. change of bed or ward);
  - optimize sensory input (e.g. hearing aid battery);
  - normalize sleep–wake cycles by discouraging sleep during the day by providing stimulation; consider sleeping tablets for the short term;
  - non-confrontational approach, but these patients are challenging.
- Pharmacological—indications for treatment:
  - uncontrollable agitation despite non-pharmacological interventions;
  - danger to self, other patients, or staff;
  - in order to perform investigations or other treatments.

Medication

- Typical antipsychotics, e.g. haloperidol (< 3 mg/day).
- Atypical antipsychotics, e.g. olanzapine (PO or IM), risperidone (PO), or quetiapine (PO).
- Benzodiazepines (for alcohol withdrawal): short-acting, e.g. lorazepam (PO, IM, IV), midazolam (PO, IM, IV); longer-acting, e.g. chlordiazepoxide (PO), diazepam (PO, PR, IV), or clonazepam (PO).
- Currently no evidence for the use of cholinesterase inhibitors.
  Note: Concerns that atypical antipsychotics:
- ↑ risk of stroke in those with dementia and the elderly—still controversial;
- ↓ extrapyramidal side effects;
- ↓ hypotension side effects;
- ↑ expensive than the typical antipsychotics.

Further reading

Inouye, SK, Westendorp RGJ, Saczynski JS (2013). Delirium in elderly people. *The Lancet*, early online publication 28 August 2013.

Head injury (HI)

- Trauma is a leading cause of death in adults < 45 years.
- Head injury accounts for > 50% of these deaths.
- Alcohol is a significant factor in > 50% of these deaths.
- Mortality for patients undergoing neurosurgery for post-trauma complications is 40%.
- In the UK, 1500 per 100 000 attend A&E with HI, 300 per 100 000 are admitted, 15 per 100 000 are transferred to a neurosurgical unit, and 9 per 100 000 die every year.

Pathophysiology

- Diffuse or primary brain injury applies to structural and functional damage sustained at the time of injury.
- Mass lesions include haematomas (extradural, subdural, intracerebral) or intracerebral contusions that affect the frontal and temporal lobes at the site of injury (coup) or opposite the injury (contre-coup).
- Secondary insults relate to subsequent events to which the injured brain is acutely susceptible—hypoxia, hypoperfusion, hyperthermia, ↑ ICP, and metabolic derangements.

Assessment

1. Initial assessment according to ATLS protocols. Avoid hypoxia (O_2 sat. < 90%) and hypotension (systolic BP < 90 mmHg).
2. Assessment of conscious level using the Glasgow Coma Scale (see Table 3.6).
3. If GCS not depressed, detailed assessment of limb power, sensory assessment, cranial nerve function including pupillary responses, corneal reflexes, gag and cough reflexes.
4. Observe respiratory pattern and rate.
5. Check pulse and BP.
6. Check for scalp lacerations, rhinorrhoea, otorrhoea, haemotympanum, and extracranial injuries. Bruising associated with base of skull injuries includes Battle's sign and racoon eyes.
7. If possible determine retrograde and anterograde amnesia.

Head injuries are strongly associated with cervical injury.

Table 3.6 Glasgow Coma Scale (GCS)*

Score	Eye opening	Motor response	Verbal response
1	None	None	None
2	To pain	Extension	Sounds
3	To speech	Abnormal flexion	Words
4	Spontaneously	Flexion	Confused speech
5		Localizes	Orientated
6		Obeys commands	

*Note that the minimum GCS score is 3.

Classification

Severity
- Mild, GCS 13–15 after resuscitation.
- Moderate, GCS 9–12.
- Severe, GCS 3–8.

Post-traumatic amnesia
- Very mild, < 5min.
- Mild, 5–60min.
- Moderate, 1–24 hours.
- Severe, 1–7 days.
- Very severe, 1–4 weeks.
- Extremely severe, > 4 weeks.

Management
📖 See also Chapter 7.

Indications for urgent CT
- Depression of conscious level after resuscitation.
- Focal neurological signs.
- Epileptic seizure.
- CSF rhinorrhoea or otorrhoea.
- Basal skull fracture.
- Potential penetrating injury.
- Difficulty in assessment due to alcohol and drugs.
- Uncertain diagnosis.

Primary phase management
1. Regular neurological observation to detect any deterioration.
2. Sedation, intubation, and ventilation indicated for:
   - patients in coma with GCS < 9 or deteriorating GCS;
   - poor airway protection;
   - abnormal respiratory pattern;
   - PaO_2 < 9 kPa on air or < 13 kPa on O_2; $PaCO_2$ > 6 kPa or < 3kPa on O_2;
   - confused and/or agitated patients before CT;
   - significant maxillofacial injuries or oropharyngeal haemorrhage.

3. Mannitol 20% 1 g/kg: 200 mL for average adult may help lower ICP.
4. Corticosteroids have no place in the management of head injuries.
5. Referral to a neurosurgical centre and image transfer if possible of: all moderate to severe HI, abnormal CT scan, depressed GCS with normal CT scan, all penetrating injuries, uncertain CT findings due to lack of expertise.

Physiological parameters for transfer

- Assume ICP to be 30 mmHg and maintain cerebral perfusion pressure (CPP) (mean arterial pressure – ICP) at > 70 mmHg (with inotropes if necessary).
- Maintain PaO_2 > 15 kPa and $PaCO_2$ at 4–4.5 kPa.

Secondary phase management
Respiratory management

Aim for target arterial CO_2 of 4–4.5 kPa. If prolonged ventilation, consider tracheostomy.

ICP

Aim for an ICP < 25 mmHg and CPP > 70 mmHg. ICP is monitored via an intraventricular or intracerebral bolt placed close to the most affected region.

- Stage 1:
  - nurse head up tilt 10–15°;
  - SaO_2 > 97%;
  - PaO_2 > 11 kPa;
  - $PaCO_2$ at 4.5 kPa;
  - $SjvO_2$ > 55%;
  - temperature < 37°C.
- Stage 2:
  - mannitol, inotropes as necessary;
  - ↓ $PaCO_2$ to 4.0 kPa;
  - maintain $SjvO_2$ > 55%;
  - maintain temperature < 35–36°C (note: role of hypothermia is controversial);
  - consider external ventricular drain.
- Stage 3:
  - temperature 33°C;
  - consider decompressive craniectomy.
- Stage 4:
  - thiopental.

Management of specific head injuries

Space-occupying lesions

- Expanding mass lesions due to extradural and subdural haematomas need to be detected early.
- Initially, cerebral hemisphere compression causes contralateral focal signs, followed by deteriorating conscious level (GCS), and finally herniation of the ipsilateral uncus through the tentorial hiatus causes an ipsilateral third nerve palsy.
- Continued expansion leads to bilateral herniation and brainstem compression.
- Present with decerebrate posturing and Cushing's response (bradycardia and hypertension) followed by hypotension and diabetes insipidus.
- Rarely, a mass lesion causes ipsilateral hemiparesis through brainstem shift impacting the contralateral free edge of the tentorium (Kernohan's notch).

Extradural haematoma (EDH)

- Classically after a HI (e.g. cricket ball): instant LOC, followed by a lucid interval and later by a progressive decline in GCS.
- Haemorrhage is arterial (usually posterior branch of middle meningeal artery is torn at site of skull fracture).
- Bleeding is extradural and strips the dura mater from the inner aspect of the skull, compressing the brain.

Imaging
CT
- Biconvex high-density extra-axial mass.
- Some have low-attenuation components, 'swirl sign' indicative of hyperacute bleeding.
- Does not cross suture lines.
- 20% can develop or enlarge after a delay of 36 hours.
- 50% associated with other lesions, e.g. contre-coup contusions, SDH, and SAH.

Management
- True neurosurgical emergency: if necessary resuscitate during transfer.
- Surgical procedure: burr hole over pterion (to ensure that further haemorrhage escapes instead of expanding the clot further) followed by craniotomy and evacuation of the haematoma.

Outcome
- Depends on preoperative status.
- Patients with bilateral fixed dilated pupils may still recover if surgery is immediate.
- If preoperative GCS ≥ 8, 90–100% recovery. If GCS < 8, mortality rate 30%; good outcome 50–60%.

Acute subdural haematoma (ASDH)

- Occurs after high impact injury, e.g. fall from a height or RTA.
- Highest mortality rate among post-traumatic mass lesions.
- Immediate LOC with progressive decline in GCS.
- Haemorrhage is arterial and venous from contused cerebral cortex, cerebral arteries, and veins.
- Haemorrhage occurs between dura and brain with additional brain damage.

Imaging

- CT: crescentic hyperdense mass. May cross sutures and extend into the interhemispheric fissure and over tentorium. Hyperacute or active bleeding can be low density.
- Anaemia and coagulopathy can cause isodense acute haemorrhages.

Management

- Emergency trauma craniotomy with a large flap to expose entire haematoma and affected cortex for evacuation and haemostasis.
- Cerebral swelling is common and may require frontal or temporal lobectomy for decompression and bone flap removal.
- Patients usually require postoperative ventilation and ICP monitoring.

Outcome

Depends on:
- conscious level;
- extent of underlying brain injury;
- degree of secondary swelling.

Mortality, 50–70%. Good outcome in 20–40%.

Chronic subdural haematoma

- Late sequela of minor/moderate HI, usually in the elderly.
- A history of a low-velocity HI 4–8 weeks previously is often forgotten or ignored.
- There is a gradual evolution of:
  • headaches;
  • cognitive decline;
  • ataxia;
  • hemiparesis;
  • impaired conscious level.

Imaging

CT: low density or isodense mass that may be loculated.

Management

- Consider dexamethasone 2 mg TDS if treatment non-surgical.
- Cortical compression, midline shift, and contralateral hydrocephalus (due to obstruction of third ventricle) indicate need for surgery.
- Burr-hole drainage ± subdural drain.
- Reoperation required in 10–15% and further surgery in 5%.
- Complications, usually in the elderly: subdural empyema, < 1%.

Intracerebral haematoma

- Develops from major contusions or vascular injury.
- Management depends on clinical condition and extent of mass effect.
- Surgical evacuation via craniotomy is indicated when focal signs are evident or ↓ GCS.

Other complications

- Cortical contusions due to impact of the brain against corrugated bone or dura. Most common sites are the anterior-inferior temporal and frontal lobes.
- Parasagittal and dorsal brainstem lesions less common.
- May be multiple and bilateral.
- Frequently associated with ASDH and EDH.
- These may develop into mass lesions as the contusions mature.
- 25% develop diffuse brain swelling.
- Craniotomy with evacuation and/or lobectomy may be necessary to manage mass effect.

Traumatic SAH

- Most common cause of SAH and indicative of a severe brain injury.
- Blood is usually in the sulci adjacent to the contusions and SDH rather than in the basal cisterns.
- Vasospasm risk is low, but nimodipine 60 mg 4-hourly PO/via NG for 10 days is recommended.
- Hydrocephalus is rare.

Penetrating head injuries

- History of injury may be unclear or the patient may be unaware of a penetration.
- Mortality from gunshot wounds 50–70%.
- Should be suspected if:
    - intracranial air is seen on CT;
    - evidence of indriven bone.
  There is a particular risk of:
- infection (meningitis, cerebritis, and abscess);
- cortical injury;
- ICH;
- neurovascular injury (carotid artery, sagittal sinus);
- injury to the optic nerve.

Angiography is mandatory for deep penetrating injuries.

Management

- Close any CSF fistulae.
- ↑ risk of infection: use prophylactic antibiotics.
- ↓ epilepsy rate by removing bone spicules.
- Depressed fractures are locked in place and a circumferential craniectomy is performed.

- Haematoma, contused brain tissue, and implanted bone are removed.
- Elevation and debridement indicated for depression of > 1 cm with dural breach within 24 hours of injury.
- However, contraindicated when delayed, eloquent areas of the brain affected, or venous sinus involvement.

Diffuse axonal injury

- Results from shearing of axons within brain matter in a closed brain injury.
- Usually with immediate LOC and is a common cause of post-traumatic persistent coma.
- Risk of diffuse brain swelling.

Imaging

- CT:
  - normal initially in 50–80%;
  - later development of petechial haemorrhages.
- MRI more sensitive:
  - multiple hyperintense lesions on T_2W imaging and FLAIR, especially in corpus callosum and at the grey–white matter interface;
  - hypointense on T_2^* if haemorrhagic.
- Maintain a low threshold for re-imaging as appearances evolve.

Management

- Sedation, intubation, and ventilation.
- ICP monitoring and control.

Basal skull fractures

- Most are undisplaced and do not require surgery.
- Displaced fractures may compress cranial nerves (e.g. optic nerve) and require decompression.
- Unstable maxillofacial fractures require elective fixation.
- CSF leaks usually cease spontaneously within 7–10 days.
- Continued leakage requires surgical closure.
- Antibiotic prophylaxis not required for CSF leaks or base-of-skull fractures.
- Avoid NG tube in base-of-skull fractures; use orogastric tubes.

Seizures

- Occur commonly in the context of HI, especially if there is a depressed skull fracture.
- Treat with phenytoin, which can be given IV/orally/via NG tube.

Infection

- Antibiotics are only prescribed in the presence of infection—not as prophylaxis.
- Aspiration pneumonia and MRSA are common complications.

Delayed complications
- Vascular:
  - chronic subdural haematoma;
  - carotid dissection;
  - traumatic aneurysms;
  - carotid–cavernous fistula.
- Infection:
  - cerebral abscess;
  - meningitis;
  - subdural empyema.
- Epilepsy
- Cranial nerve deficits:
  - olfactory;
  - trigeminal;
  - facial;
  - vestibulo-cochlear (e.g. BPPV).
- Psychological: behavioural disturbance, depression.

Imaging of head injuries: examples

Figure 3.14 shows blunt trauma to the right frontal region with extracranial soft tissue swelling (*open white arrowheads*) and right frontal fracture (*closed white arrow*). There is an extensive underlying parenchymal contusion comprising low-attenuation components (*closed white arrowheads*) and central haemorrhagic change (*open white arrows*). There is an associated mass effect with ipsilateral sulcal and ventricular effacement and minor distortion of the midline. Note also the small right frontal extradural haematoma (*black arrow*).

Figure 3.15 shows blunt trauma to the left temporoparietal region (*white arrows*) with sudden cranial deceleration and angular rotation resulting in shear–strain forces causing large haemorrhagic contre-coup contusions in the inferior aspects of both frontal and right temporal lobes (*open white arrowheads*). Note also smaller foci of parenchymal haemorrhage in the occipital lobe bilaterally (*closed white arrowheads*), intraventricular and subarachnoid blood (*black arrows*), and an extensive tentorial subdural haematoma (*black arrowheads*).

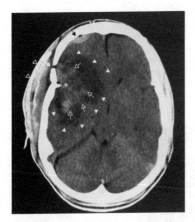

Fig. 3.14 Direct impact (non-enhanced CT).

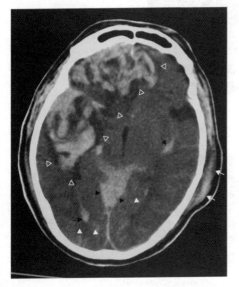

Fig. 3.15 Indirect impact (non-enhanced CT).

Large acute subdural haematoma with crescentic configuration overlying left cerebral convexity with minor extension into interhemispheric fissure is shown in Fig. 3.16 (*white arrowheads*). There is marked associated mass effect with ipsilateral sulcal and ventricular effacement and severe midline shift. Note the indirect site of impact over right parietal bone (*white arrow*). In contrast, note CSF clefts (*black arrowheads*) associated with bifrontal extradural haematoma in (b) which has a biconvex configuration. Frontal horns of the lateral ventricles are grossly effaced.

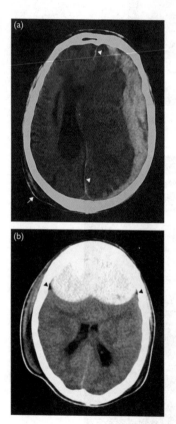

Fig. 3.16 Acute extra-axial haematoma (non-enhanced CT).

The large subdural haematoma over the left cerebral convexity and extending into the interhemispheric fissure shown in Fig. 3.17(a) is hyperdense in keeping with an acute haematoma. Figure 3.17(b) shows a subacute right-sided subdural haematoma with isodense to mildly hyperdense material overlying the right cerebral convexity (*white asterisk*) resulting in effacement and obscuration of ipsilateral cerebral sulci compared with the contralateral side (*black arrowheads*) and midline distortion.

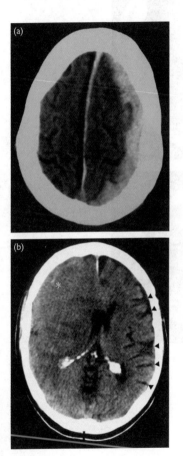

Fig. 3.17 Subdural haematoma: (a) and (b) non-enhanced CT.

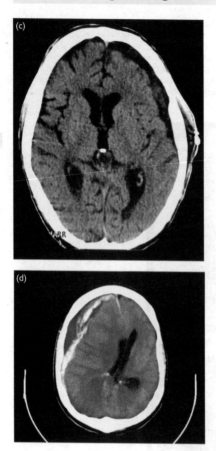

Fig. 3.17 Subdural haematoma: (c) and (d) non-enhanced CT.

The left frontal chronic subdural haematoma shown in Fig. 3.17(c) is predominantly hypodense but also demonstrates some mass effect with effacement of sulci in the underlying left frontal lobe. There is also a minor alteration in the configuration of the left frontal horn due to mass effect. Figure 3.17(d) shows a hyperacute right frontal subdural haematoma with mass effect. The hyperdense components represent acute haemorrhage; the low-attenuation material reflects active bleeding and unclotted oxygenated blood.

Figure 3.18 shows a severe shear–strain injury resulting in multiple foci of acute petechial haemorrhage involving the splenium and posterior aspects of the corpus callosum and frontal parenchyma predominantly at the grey–white matter interface.

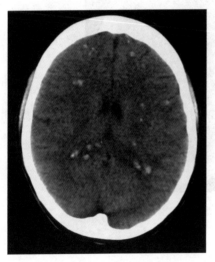

Fig. 3.18 Diffuse axonal injury (DAI): non-enhanced CT.

In Fig. 3.19 there is a reversal of the normal grey–white matter pattern with low-density change involving the cortex with generalized cerebral swelling indicative of hypoxic/anoxic brain injury.

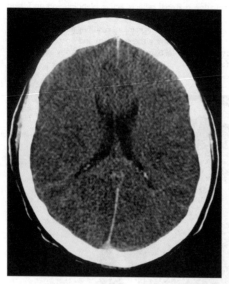

Fig. 3.19 Severe secondary brain injury: non-enhanced CT.

Spinal injuries

- These are often associated with multiple injuries and head trauma.
- Early detection and immobilization are vital to avoid secondary insults.
- Spinal level is defined by the affected vertebral level and the most cephalad cord segment involved.
- Completeness: the prognosis and management are dictated by whether the lesion is complete or not. Incomplete lesions (including sacral sparing, i.e. sensation and control of anal sphincter) may recover to a variable extent and may benefit from decompression.
- Spinal shock refers to both the haemodynamic effects of cord injury and the flaccid phase (first 1–2 weeks after cord injury).

Spinal stability

- Instability is defined as the loss of ability of the spine to maintain normal anatomical alignment under normal physiological loads. Instability refers to the increased likelihood of further spinal damage.
- Spinal stability is classifed according to the Denis three-column model of the spine:
  - anterior column = the anterior half of the vertebral body and annulus fibrosus and anterior longitudinal ligament (ALL);
  - middle column = the posterior half of the vertebral body and annulus fibrosus and posterior longitudinal ligament (PLL);
  - posterior column = pedicles, laminae, spinous processes, and ligaments.

  The spine is unstable if ≥ 2 columns are disrupted.

Acute cord injury

Management
1. Resuscitation and airway protection.
2. Immobilization of the neck and log rolling during assessment and resuscitation.
3. Treatment of life-threatening injuries and bleeding.
4. Urinary catheter.
5. Full neurological examination to determine level and completeness lesion.
6. Palpate spine for any 'step'.
7. Note any autonomic dysfunction, e.g. ileus, priapism.
8. IV methylprednisolone may improve outcome when administered within 8 hours of injury (30 mg/kg over 15 min bolus and maintenance 5.4 mg/kg/hour for 23 hours).

C1 and C2 fracture

C1 and C2 are rings. Fracture in two places is typical.

Atlanto-occipital dislocation
Distance between the anterior margin of the foramen magnum (basion) and dens > 12.5 cm. Usually fatal.

C1 fracture (Jefferson)

Caused by disruption of the C1 ring due to compression or a burst fracture.

Clinical features

Rarely have a neurological deficit as the spinal canal is wide and fragments burst outwards.

Imaging

- Open-mouth view X-ray: lateral displacement of C1 lateral masses relative to C2 lateral masses (overhang on C2 ≥ 7 mm).
- Lateral X-ray: fractures of anterior and posterior arch of C1.

Management

- This is an unstable fracture.
- Requires halo immobilization for 3 months (rigid orthosis using a ring (halo) attached to outer table of skull by four screws attached by vertical side bars joining a rigid jacket strapped to the chest).

C2 fractures

Odontoid peg fractures

Frequently associated with multiple injuries with high force impact.

Classification

- Type 1: upper dens fracture (10%).
- Type 2: base of neck of peg (60%).
- Type 3: transverse fracture through C2 vertebral body (30%).

Clinical features

Neurological deficit in 20% of type 2 fractures. Unusual in type 3 fractures.

Imaging

High-resolution CT from occiput to C3; MRI cervical cord.

Management

- All unstable fractures.
- Majority treated by halo immobilization. Surgical treatment with fixation is indicated in the following:
  - displacement of fracture > 4 mm;
  - persistent movement in halo;
  - non-union including fibrous union after 3 months;
  - comminuted type 2 fracture.

Hangman's fracture

Usually caused by high impact axial loading injury. Due to bilateral fractures of pars articularis of C2.

Clinical features

- Majority are neurologically intact.
- Complain of neck pain and a sensation of instability.
- May walk into A&E holding head!

Imaging
- Usually apparent on lateral cervical spine X-ray.
- MRI is indicated if neurological signs are present.

Management
- Minimally displaced fractures are treated in a SOMI (sterno-occipito-mandibular immobilizer) brace if compliant or halo jacket.
- If fractures displaced > 4 mm, halo is mandatory.

Indications for surgical treatment
- Displacement not reduced with judicious neck extension.
- Persistent movement in halo.
- Associated C2/3 disc disruption.
- Non-union after halo treatment for 3 months.

Subaxial (C3–C7) fractures
- Commonly associated with head injuries and severe neurological deficit.
- Flexion injuries are more severe.
- Fractures through vertebral body, wedge fractures, teardrop fractures (anterior portion of vertebral body), and avulsion fragments.

Clinical features
- Neck pain.
- Radiculopathy.
- Myelopathy.
- Tetraplegia.

Imaging
- AP and lateral cervical X-ray reveal majority of fractures.
- Flexion/extension lateral cervical spine views only to exclude occult instability and only in patients who are fully conscious.
- Increased anterior soft tissue shadow: (C1–4 normal = half vertebral body; C5–7 normal = whole vertebral body) if > requires further investigation with CT or MRI.
- MRI necessary in all patients with abnormal neurological signs.

Management
- Complete neurological deficit: further management aimed at avoiding secondary damage and maximizing rehabilitation.
- Unstable fractures treated with halo or internal fixation to allow early mobilization and avoid respiratory complications.
- Incomplete neurological injury with cord compression requires decompression and fixation (internal or external halo).
- Unstable injury without a deficit or stable deficit managed with a halo if minor displacement; otherwise internal fixation and fusion.

Cervical facet dislocation
- Hyperflexion injury resulting in superior facet 'jumping' inferior facet and becoming trapped in dislocation by rim of facet.
- Flexion alone results in bilateral facet dislocation accompanied by disc and ligament disruption.
- Flexion with rotation leads to unilateral facet dislocation.

Clinical features
- Usually severe cord injury.
- Unilateral facet dislocation: 25% are intact neurologically; 25% incomplete cord injury; 40% root injury; 10% complete cord injury.

Imaging
Lateral cervical spine X-ray shows anterior transposition of upper vertebra by 25% vertebral body width in unifacet dislocation and 50% vertebral body width in bilateral facet dislocations.

Management
- Skull traction with muscle relaxant, e.g. diazepam, commencing at 3 times upper vertebral levels in pounds, increasing by 4–10 pounds every 15 minutes until relocated using image intensifer. Cease at 10 pounds per vertebral level or if there is any evidence of overdistraction (any disc height > 10 mm).
- Open reduction if traction fails.
- Majority require internal fixation with interspinous wiring, lateral mass plates, and bone graft to maintain position.

Thoracolumbar fractures
- Caused by high force and associated with multiple trauma.
- Comprise wedge fractures (anterior ± posterior column), burst fractures (anterior and middle column), or fracture dislocations (all columns).
- Unstable if wedge > 75% vertebral height or three adjacent vertebrae wedged.

Clinical features
High proportion have a significant neurological deficit.

Imaging
Plain films followed by high-resolution CT or MRI.

Management
- Complete neurological deficit. Avoid secondary complications and maximize rehabilitation. If unstable, fractures are treated with prolonged bed rest or internal fixation to allow early rehabilitation.
- Incomplete neurological injury with cord compression requires early decompression and internal fixation.
- Unstable injury with no or stable deficit managed with bed rest, corset, or internal fixation. All others require internal fixation and fusion.

Rehabilitation of spinal cord injury
Survivors of spinal cord injury require expert management to avoid the complications of:
- DVT;
- bed sores;
- infections (e.g. UTI);
- respiratory failure;
- contractures;
- osteoporosis;
- psychological problems.

Imaging spinal injuries: examples

Figure 3.20 shows a slightly displaced fracture through the body of C2 in the coronal plane ((a) *white arrowheads*; (b) *black arrowheads*). There is slight anterior subluxation of C2 upon C3.

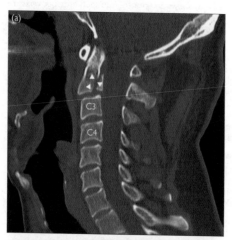

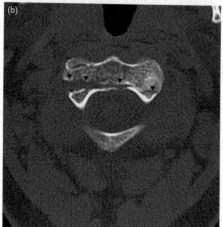

Fig. 3.20 Coronal fracture of body of C2 hangman's fracture: (a) CT sagittal MPR; (b) axial CT.

Figure 3.21 shows severe spinal injury with Grade 2 spondylolisthesis (anterior subluxation) of C4 upon C5, C4/5 intervertebral discal injury with hyperintensity and posterior bulge into vertebral canal (*closed white arrows*), and posterior ligamentous injury (*black arrow*). There is a shallow epidural haematoma posterior to the C4 vertebral body (*open white arrow*) which has elevated and posteriorly displaced the dura (*black arrowheads*). The spinal cord is distorted and displaced, although no cord contusion is evident at this stage. Note the shallow haematoma in the pre-vertebral soft tissue compartment (*open white arrowheads*).

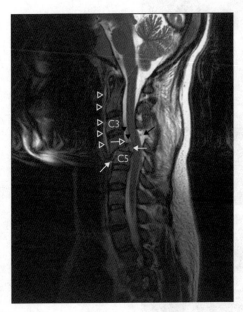

Fig. 3.21 Bilateral cervical facet subluxation: sagittal T₂W MRI.

Figure 3.22 shows Grade 2 spondylolisthesis of C6 upon C7 with large disc protrusion ((a) *white arrow*), epidural haematoma ((b) *open white arrowheads*), and rupture of the posterior ligamentous structures ((a) *open black arrow*). Discontinuity of the anterior longitudinal ligament indicates probable injury ((b) *closed white arrow*). The spinal cord is compressed and intramedullary signal change, in keeping with oedema, extends from C6 to T1 ((a) *closed black arrow*). Note the absence of intramedullary hyper-intensity on T_1W imaging or hypointensity on T_2W imaging, which would indicate spinal cord haemorrhage.

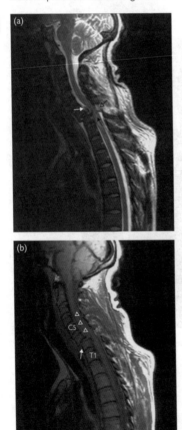

Fig. 3.22 Bilateral facet dislocation: (a) sagittal T_2W and (b) sagittal T_1W MRI.

Dynamic plain X-rays demonstrate marked instability at the atlanto-axial joint as a result of a fracture through the odontoid peg (Fig. 3.23). On flexion, there is marked anterior subluxation of the C1 ring and fracture fragment of C2 (*dotted line*) in relation to the inferior portion of C2 (*dashed line*) with consequent reduction in the calibre of the vertebral canal at this level.

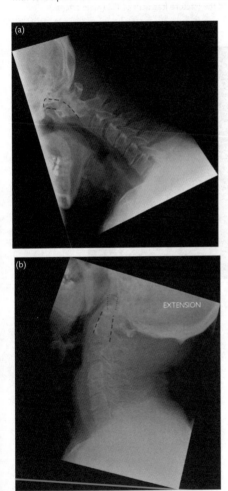

Fig. 3.23 Type 2 odontoid peg fracture: (a) flexion and (b) extension plain X-rays.

Further evaluation with MRI (Fig. 3.23(c)) confirms a fracture through C2 with possible interposition of soft tissue between the fractured fragments (*white arrow*). Intramedullary signal change and spinal cord volume loss (*black arrow*) are in keeping with myelomalacia and long-standing instability and intermittent spinal cord compression. Note the anterior arch of C1 (*white arrowhead*) and the fracture fragment of C2 (*white asterisk*).

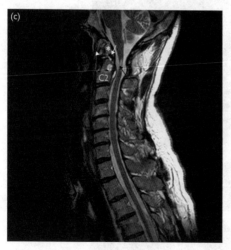

Fig. 3.23 (c) Sagittal T$_2$W MRI.

Meningitis

See Table 3.7 for risk factors for causative organisms, Table 3.8 for LP findings in meningitis, and Table 3.9 for specific therapies. See Fig. 3.24 for management flowchart for meningitis.

Incidence and microbiology

Annual incidence around 2–3/100 000 with peaks in infants and adolescence. Vaccination against *Haemophilus influenzae* type b and group C meningococcus has had significant impact.

Clinical features

Presenting features typically with headache, fever, photophobia, neck stiffness. In addition:
- cranial nerve palsies (III, IV, VI, VII);
- focal neurological deficits;
- seizures (20–30%)—usually in *S.pneumoniae* and *Haemophilus influenzae* meningitis;
- ↑ ICP (altered conscious level, hypertension, bradycardia, abnormal respiratory pattern, papilloedema (late));
- purpura or petechial haemorrhages (non-blanching with glass test)—*Neisseria meningitidis*;
- septic shock: *N.meningitidis*;
- tuberculous meningitis may be more insidious with gradual development of fever, weight loss, headache with progression to focal deficit, altered consciousness;
- look for evidence of immunosuppression as may be the first presentation of HIV or lymphoproliferative disorder (e.g. oral candidiasis, lymphadenopathy).

Table 3.7 Risk factors for potential causative organisms

Patient subgroup/features	Likely causative organism(s)
Age > 50 years	Listeria monocytogenes
Pregnancy, childbirth	Listeria monocytogenes
Diabetes mellitus	Streptococcus pneumoniae
Presence of seizures	Streptococcus pneumoniae, Haemophilus influenzae
Skull fracture, middle or inner ear fistula, alcoholism	Streptococcus pneumoniae
Penetrating skull trauma, CSF shunts	Staphylococcus, Gram-negative bacilli
From TB endemic country/PMH of TB/ insidious onset with weight loss, fevers, and focal deficits	Tuberculosis
Splenic dysfunction (splenectomy/sickle cell disease)	Streptococcus pneumoniae
T-lymphocyte dysfunction (HIV, chemotherapy, malignancy)	Listeria monocytogenes
Immunosuppression (HIV, neutropenia)	Fungal (cryptococcus), TB, pseudomonas.

Investigations

- Blood culture as latex agglutination bacterial antigen tests or PCR can be performed and may remain positive even after antibiotics.
- CXR for evidence of TB.
- CT scan does *not* exclude raised ICP (see 📖 Chapter 9, 'CNS infections', pp. 588–91).
- Lumbar puncture is contraindicated if:
  - signs of ↑ ICP;
  - ↓ GCS;
  - coagulopathy;
  - focal symptoms, signs, or seizures (unless CT scan normal);
  - cardiovascular compromise;
  - infection of skin at LP site.

See Table 3.8 for lumbar puncture and blood findings in different forms of meningitis.

Management

Choice of antibiotic

Choice of antibiotic depends on age of patient and any other associated features, e.g. immunocompromised. CT or LP should not delay first dose of antibiotic. In adults likely organisms are:

- *S.pneumoniae*;
- *N.meningitidis*;
- if > 50 years, *L.monocytogenes*.

Drug recommendation before identification of organism

- Meningitis with *typical* meningococcal rash:
  - IV 2.4 g benzylpenicillin 4-hourly or IV cefotaxime 2 g 6-hourly (8 g total). If history of penicillin allergy, IV chloramphenicol 50 mg/kg/day given in four divided doses.
- Meningitis without typical rash:
  - IV cefotaxime 2 g 6-hourly or IV ceftriaxone 2 g 12-hourly (total 4 g) *plus*
  - IV vancomycin (in suspected *S.pneumoniae* until sensitivities are known in case of resistance) 1 g 12-hourly *plus*
  - IV ampicillin 2 g 4-hourly if > 50 years to cover listeria.

Table 3.8 LP findings in meningitis

Condition	CSF pressure (mmH₂O)	WBC (/L)	Protein (g/L)	Glucose (mmol/L)
Normal	50–200	> 5 lymphocytes	0.2–0.45	75% blood glucose
Bacterial meningitis	↑	100–60 000, mainly neutrophils	0.5–5	< 40% blood glucose
Tuberculous meningitis	↑	10–500, neutrophils in early disease, lymphocytes later	0.5–5	↓ < 40% of blood glucose
Fungal meningitis	↑	25–500, mainly lymphocytes	0.5–5	↓
Viral meningitis	Normal or ↑	↑ lymphocytes	0.5–2	Normal

- If clear history of betalactam anaphylaxis:
  - chloramphenicol 25 mg/kg 6-hourly *plus*
  - vancomycin 500 mg 6-hourly;
  - if > 50 years add cotrimoxazole to cover listeria.

Therapy after identification from CSF or blood
- N.meningitidis:
  - 2.4 g benzylpenicillin IV 4-hourly or ampicillin 2 g 4-hourly;
  - if history of allergy to betalactams, chloramphenicol 25 mg/kg IV 6-hourly.
- S.pneumoniae:
  - ceftriaxone or cefotaxime;
  - add vancomycin or rifampicin 600 mg 12-hourly if patient from penicillin-resistant area.
- H.influenzae: cefotaxime or ceftriaxone.
- L.monocytogenes: ampicillin 2g 4-hourly + gentamicin 5 mg/kg divided into 8-hourly doses;
- tuberculosis meningitis: isoniazid 5–10 mg/kg 24-hourly + rifampicin 8–15 mg/kg 24-hourly + pyrazinamide 20–30 mg/kg 24-hourly + pyridoxine 25 mg.

↑ ICP

A medical emergency. Patient should be managed on ITU. Give mannitol 0.25 g/kg IV over 10 minutes. May require sedation, intubation, and ventilation to reduce PCO_2 and controlled hypothermia.

Seizures

Should be treated initially with lorazepam 4 mg IV, followed by phenytoin 18 mg/kg as a loading dose under ECG monitoring followed by maintenance dose IV. If seizures continue, treat as for status epilepticus.

Corticosteroids

Shown to reduce morbidity in adults specifically in S.pneumoniae and tuberculous meningitis. Data do not include meningococcal meningitis but it is reasonable to consider at least until organism isolated—10 mg dexamethasone 6-hourly IV for 4 days with first dose given with first antibiotic dose.

Table 3.9 Specific therapies once organisms identified from blood/CSF

Organism	Specific therapy
N.meningitidis	Benzylpenicillin 2.4 g IV (4-hourly) or ampicillin 2 g (4-hourly) *If betalactam allergy give chloramphenicol 25 mg/kg (6-hourly)
S.pneumoniae	Ceftriaxone or cefotaxime Add vancomycin or rifampicin (600 mg 12-hourly) if from penicillin-resistant area
H.influenzae	Cefotaxime or ceftriaxone
L.monocytogenes	Ampicillin 2 g (4-hourly) + gentamycin 5 mg/kg (divided into 8-hourly doses)
Tuberculosis	Isoniazid 5–10 mg/kg 24-hourly + rifampicin 8–15 mg/kg 24-hourly + pyrazinamide 20–30 mg/kg 24-hourly + ethambutol 15 mg/kg + pyridoxine 10–25 mg. > 50 kg standard dose = rifampicin 600 mg, isoniazid 300 mg, pyrazinamide 2 g, ethambutol 15 mg/kg, pyridoxine 10–25 mg; < 50 kg = rifampicin 450 mg, isoniazid 300 mg, pyrazinamide 1.5 g, ethambutol and pyridoxine as above.

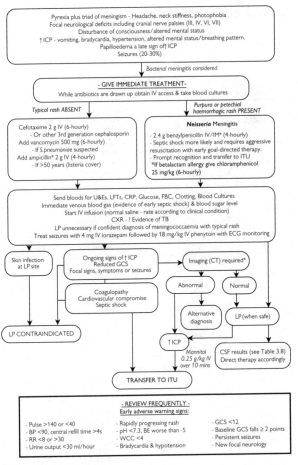

Fig. 3.24 Meningitis management flowchart.

Further reading

Chaudhuri A, Martinez-Martin P, Kennedy PG (2008). EFNS guidelines on community acquired bacterial meningitis: report of an EFNS Task Force on acute bacterial meningitis in older children and adults. *Eur. J. Neurol.*, **15**, 649–55.

Spinal cord disorders

See Fig. 3.25 for anatomy, signs/symptoms, and pathology of various spinal cord lesions and Fig. 3.26 for diagnosis flowchart.

Lesion	Anatomy	Signs/Symptoms	Example pathology
Complete*		All tracts are interrupted at the site of the lesion causing pyramidal, sensory and autonomic dysfunction below the level of the lesion. Clinically pinprick most useful in localizing.	Trauma Tumour (metastatic)
Brown-Séquard syndrome*		1. Ipsilateral pyramidal weakness 2. Ipsilateral dorsal column loss (proprioception) 3. Contralateral spinothalamic loss (pain, temperature)	MS Cord compression
Central cord syndrome*		1. Early suspended (cape-like) pain and temp loss with preservation of dorsal columns 2. Forward extension = pyramidal weakness 3. Lateral extension = ipsilateral Horner's	Syrinx Intramedullary cord tumour
Anterior cord syndrome*		1. Areflexic, flaccid paraparesis 2. Sphincter disturbance 3. Pain and temperature loss with dorsal column (proprioception and light touch) preservation	Anterior spinal artery occlusion
Anterior horn cell syndrome		1. Diffuse weakness, atrophy, and fasciculations 2. Reduced tone 3. Sensory symptoms absent	Spinal muscular atrophy syndromes
Combined anterior horn cell pyramidal tract syndrome		1. LMN signs (fasciculations, atrophy, weakness ± pseudobulbar) 2. UMN signs (↑ plantars, spasticity ±bulbar) 3. Preservation of sphincters	Amyotrophic lateral sclerosis
Posterolateral column syndrome		1. Dorsal column loss (proprioception, vibration) 2. UMN signs (↑ reflexes, ↑ plantars, weakness) 3. Preservation of pain and temperature	Subacute combined degeneration of the spinal cord
Posterior column syndrome		1. Dorsal column loss (proprioception, vibration) 2. ± Lancinating pains (often lower limb) 3. ± Lhermitte's sign	Tabes dorsalis
Conus medullaris*	Sacral cord and autonomic output	1. Early sphincter loss, sacral sensory change 2. Minor motor involvement	Post-viral myelitis
Cauda equina*	Cauda equina spinal roots	1. Flaccid lower limb weakness 2. Followed by sphincter involvement	Disc compression

* Cause of acute spinal cord syndrome.

Fig. 3.25 Signs/symptoms of spinal cord lesions.

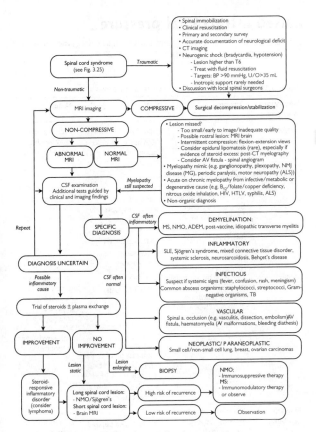

Fig. 3.26 Spinal cord compression diagnosis flowchart.

Raised intracranial pressure

See Table 3.10 for the anatomy and signs of herniation syndromes, and Fig. 3.27 for management flowchart.

Table 3.10 Common cerebral herniation syndromes

Herniation syndrome	Anatomy	Signs	Notes
Cingulate	Cingulate gyrus herniates under the falx	Typically asymptomatic ACA at risk of kinking, causing bilateral frontal infarcts	Warning sign of impending central herniation
Central	Diencephalon forced through tentorial incisura. Pituitary may be sheared causing DI. PCA may be compressed causing infarction	Early ↓ GCS Midbrain signs (dilated minimal/ unreactive pupils and Cheyne–Stokes) poor prognostic sign Bilateral Babinski Decorticate/ decerebrate	Usually due to more chronic causes (e.g. tumour) compared with uncal
Uncal	Uncus or hippocampal gyrus is forced over edge of tentorium	Early confusion Early CN III palsy Late (but rapid) coma Contralateral weakness Ipsilateral weakness in Kernohan's notch phenomena (compression of contralateral cerebral peduncle and CN VI— false localizing signs) Decorticate rare	Often due to rapidly expanding haematoma. Impaired consciousness a late sign with rapid deterioration
Upward cerebellar	Cerebellar vermis ascends above tentorium. May cause compression of SCA, great vein of Galen, and cerebral aqueduct, leading to hydrocephalus	Ataxia Unequal fixed pupils (may be small) Bilateral Babinski. ↓ GCS. Central respirations	Associated with posterior fossa masses. May be exacerbated by ventricular damage
Tonsillar	Cerebellar tonsils 'cone' through foramen magnum	Ataxia CN VI palsy Bilateral Babinski ↓ GCS Central respirations	Rapidly fatal. Occurs with both supra- and infratentorial masses. Can occur post-LP

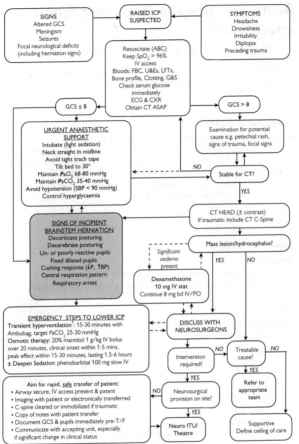

Fig. 3.27 Management flowchart for raised intracranial pressure.

[1]Note: prophylactic hyperventilation NOT recommended as it exacerbates cerebral ischaemia by causing vasoconstriction in an already compromised brain and has been associated with poorer outcome. Use transiently if signs of brainstem herniation appear.

Acute encephalitis (including limbic encephalitis)

- Limbic system = hippocampus, amygdala, hypothalamus, insular and cingulate cortex.
- Definition: cortical brain infection or inflammation, acute or subacute (days to months) with features which may include:
  - memory impairment;
  - seizures.

Differential diagnosis:

- Infections (see 🕮 Chapter 5, 'Viral encephalitis', pp. 370–2).
- Paraneoplastic syndromes, e.g. NMDA receptor encephalitis (see 'Anti-NMDA receptor encephalitis', pp. 132–3). See also 🕮 Chapter 5, 'Paraneoplastic syndromes: central nervous system', pp. 334–5.
- Autoimmune disorders (voltage gated K⁺ complex channel complex antibodies (usually associated with LG11)).
- Tumour, e.g. lymphoma.
- Vasculitis.
- Wernicke–Korsakoff syndrome.

Infectious causes

Aetiology
- Herpes simplex (HS) type 1 (70% in immunocompetent patients).
- Immunocompromised host: herpes simplex type 2, human herpes virus 6 and 7, enterovirus.

Clinical features
- Abrupt-onset confusion, memory impairment, seizures.
- Fever (may be absent).

Investigations
- CT/MRI:
  - Swelling, mass effect and high signal in mesial temporal structures.
- CSF:
  - ↑ WCC (lymphocytosis);
  - ↑ protein;
  - sugar usually normal;
  - CSF PCR for HS sensitivity and specificity 95%.

Treatment
- IV aciclovir (10 mg/kg tds) for 14–21 days—monitor renal function;
- treat seizures with IV phenytoin;
- If PCR negative—consider other causes, repeat CSF and PCR; if clinical picture convincing continue with aciclovir.

Voltage-gated potassium channel (VGKC) complex antibodies associated limbic encephalitis (LGI1 antibody)

- Note: VGKC antibodies (CASPR2 antibody) also associated with:
  - cramp fasciculation syndrome;
  - acquired neuromyotonia (Isaac's syndrome);
  - Morvan's syndrome (neuromyotonia, sleep disorders, autonomic dysfunction, cognitive changes).

Clinical features:
- Subacute amnestic syndrome.
- Confusion, behavioural disturbance.
- Seizures (brachio facial dystonic seizures).
- ↓ Na due to SIADH.

Investigations
- VGKC antibodies in serum and/or CSF.
- MRI: signal change in mesial temporal lobe structures.
- EEG: diffuse slowing with or without temporal spikes.
- CSF:
  - ↑ WCC (lymphocytosis);
  - ↑ protein (sometimes) matched oligoclonal bands.

Management
- Variable combinations of PE, IV Ig, corticosteroids. Recent open-label study showed immunological and clinical remission with PE (50 mL/kg), followed by IV Ig (2 g/kg) and IV methylprednisolone 1 g × 3 days. Maintenance with oral prednisolone 1 mg/kg with slow taper.

Further reading

Kennedy PG, Steiner I (2013). Recent issues in herpes simplex encephalitis. *J. Neurovirol.*, **19**(4), 346–50.

Schott J (2006). Limbic encephalitis: a clinician's guide. *Pract. Neurol.*, **6**, 143–53.

Wong SH, Saunders MD, Larner AJ, Das K, Hart IK (2010). An effective immunotherapy regimen for VGKC antibody positive limbic encephalitis. *J. Neurol. Neurosurg. Psychiatry*, **81**, 1167–9.

Anti-NMDA receptor encephalitis

Recently recognized syndrome affecting mainly women (80%). A multi-centre population-based study of encephalitis in UK found 4% caused by anti-NMDA receptor encephalitis. Consider diagnosis in any case, especially < 50 years, with rapid change in behaviour, psychosis, abnormal movements, seizures, autonomic instability, hypoventilation.

Clinical features

* Age: median 23 years (range 5–76 years).
* Prodromal viral-like syndrome common.
* Psychiatric symptoms:
  * anxiety, agitation;
  * delusional and paranoid ideation;
  * visual and/or auditory hallucination;
  * catatonia.
* Seizures.
* Memory loss.
* Movement disorders:
  * orofacial dyskinesias;
  * choreoathetoid movements;
  * complex abdominal pelvic movements;
  * dystonic posturing.
* Autonomic instability.
* Central hypoventilation.
* ↓ conscious level.

Investigations

* Blood: + NMDA receptor antibodies.
* CSF:
  * ↑ WCC (lymphocytosis);
  * Protein ↑ or normal;
  * Oligoclonal bands + or –;
  * NMDA receptor antibody +.
* EEG: slow-wave activity ± focal spikes—extreme delta brush sign.
* MRI: may be normal (up to 50%) or show abnormalities (FLAIR or ↑ T2) with enhancement of mesial temporal lobes, cerebral cortex, cerebellum, corpus callosum brainstem, basal ganglia.
* Tumour search with US, MRI, CT: ovarian teratoma (may be bilateral) in 60%. Consider transvaginal US. Other tumours: SCC lung, testicular teratoma.

Management

* May require ITU.
* Tumour resection—better prognosis.
* No controlled trial data. Treat with IV methylprednisolone + IV Ig and/or plasma exchange. Second-line treatment: cyclophosphamide and/or rituximab.

Prognosis
- Early detection of tumour—better outcome.
- Slow recovery.
- 75% recover; 25% severe deficits or death.
- Relapses may occur.

Further reading
Dalmau J, Lancaster E, Martinez-Hernandez E, Rosenfeld MR, Balice-Gordon R (2011). Clinical experience and laboratory investigations in patients with anti-NMDAR encephalitis. *Lancet Neurol.*, 10, 63–74.

Common clinical presentations

Loss of consciousness *136*
Acute vertigo *138*
Spastic paraparesis *142*
Ataxia *144*
Acute visual failure *148*
Coma *152*
Coma prognosis *156*
Excessive daytime sleepiness *158*
Tremor *162*
Tics *165*
Chorea and athetosis *166*
Myoclonus *168*
Dystonia *170*
Foot drop *172*
Unilateral hand weakness/paraesthesiae *174*

Loss of consciousness

A common problem.

- Eyewitness account (verbal or written) is essential. May need to contact eyewitnesses by telephone.
- Better to label an episode '?Cause' than diagnose epilepsy if not sure. Time will make the diagnosis clear. Avoid trials of anticonvulsants.
- Advise the patient about implications for driving. Tell patient it is their duty to inform the DVLA. See ℘ <http://www.gov.uk/current-medical-guidelines-dvla-guidance-for-professionals> for medical guidelines.

Aetiology

Neurological causes

- Epileptic seizures.*
- Raised ICP (tumour, especially posterior fossa lesions; hydrocephalus, e.g. due to colloid cyst).
- SAH.
- Sleep disorders (narcolepsy, cataplexy).
- Basilar artery migraine (rare).
- Cerebrovascular disease (rare, unless massive stroke or brainstem).

Neurally mediated syncope

- Neurocardiogenic (vasovagal) syncope.*
- Carotid sinus syncope.
- Situational syncope (cough, micturition).

Cardiac syncope

- Cardiac arrhythmias* (see also 📖 Chapter 6, 'Neurological symptoms: cardiac disease', pp. 396–9).
- Structural cardiopulmonary disease (aortic stenosis, hypertrophic obstructive cardiomyopathy (HOCM), pulmonary embolus).

Orthostatic or postural hypotension

- Drugs*, e.g. vasodilators, antidepressants, L-dopa preparations.
- Autonomic neuropathy (GBS, diabetes, amyloid).
- Autonomic failure (MSA, PD).
- Addison's disease.

Metabolic disorders

- Hypoglycaemia.
- Hyperventilation-induced alkalosis.

Psychiatric disorders

- Psychogenic non-epileptic attacks.*

* Most common causes.

Diagnosis
See Table 4.1. The eyewitness account will help make the diagnosis.

Investigations
Consider the following:
- Blood: Hb (anaemia), glucose (especially in diabetics or if preprandial), K^+, Ca^{2+}.
- ECG and 24-hour tape (may need to be repeated). Must be reported by experienced personnel. If necessary, a prolonged cardiomemo (reveal device); echocardiogram for cardiac syncope.
- Note: long QT (corrected QT > 450 ms); short QT (corrected < 350 ms).
- Tilt table testing. Sensitive for syncopal tendencies.
- EEG by itself does not diagnose epilepsy. 50% false-negative rate for interictal EEG in patients with epilepsy. Reduced to 30% by repeating and 20% with sleep-deprived EEG. False-positive EEG in up to 2% healthy young adults.
- Ictal video–EEG–telemetry most sensitive and specific test for epilepsy. Note: frontal lobe epileptic seizures may appear normal even on ictal EEG.
- Imaging (preferably with MRI) for focal seizures, focal signs, or signs and symptoms of ↑ ICP.

Table 4.1 Features differentiating vasovagal syncope from epileptic seizures

	Seizure	Syncope
Trigger	Rare—flashing lights, hyperventilation	Common (blood, needles, hot environment, standing, pain)
Prodrome	Common—auras	Very common—nausea, lightheadedness, tinnitus, greying vision
Onset	Sudden	Gradual
Duration	1–3min	1–30sec
Convulsive jerks	Common—prolonged	Common—brief
Incontinence	Common	Uncommon
Tongue biting	Common	Rare
Post-event confusion	Common	Rare
Colour	Pale, cyanotic (tonic–clonic seizures)	Very pale

Further reading
NICE (2010). *Transient loss of consciousness ('blackouts') management in adults and young people.* NICE Clinical Guideline 109.

Acute vertigo

Vertigo is the illusion of rotation caused by asymmetry of neural activity between the right and left vestibular nuclei. Bilateral damage does not cause vertigo. It is essential to determine whether the vertigo is central or peripheral since cerebellar infarction/haemorrhage can be life-threatening and requires neurosurgical intervention.

Acute vertigo with no other signs or symptoms is unlikely to be due to vertebrobasilar ischaemia.

Aetiology

- Mechanical: benign paroxysmal positional vertigo (BPPV) due to otoliths moving in the posterior semicircular most commonly and the horizontal semicircular canals less often (see 🕮 Chapter 5, 'Benign paroxysmal positional vertigo (BPPV)', pp. 344–7). First episode of Ménière's.
- Infectious (viral): acute vestibular neuritis; affects lateral semicircular canal function.
- Vascular:
  - Infarction within the territory of the anterior vestibular artery, a branch of the internal auditory artery, which in turn branches from the anterior inferior cerebellar artery (AICA). Clinical presentation is similar to that of vestibular neuritis but usually occurs in older patients with risk factors for stroke, such as diabetes, hypertension, and cardiac disease (e.g. atrial fibrillation).
  - *Brainstem stroke accompanied by other signs*
    — Horner's syndrome.
    — Dysarthria.
    — Incoordination.
    — Diplopia.
    — Numbness of the face.
  - Inferior cerebellar artery infarction can present with only vertigo, nystagmus, and postural instability.
- Multiple sclerosis: can produce an evolving vestibular syndrome with a plaque around the 8th nerve root entry zone but other signs present.
- First attack of Ménière's syndrome.
- Migrainous vertigo in a migraneur with headache and vertigo not necessarily occurring together. Diagnosis of exclusion.

Clinical features

Clinical presentation is with acute-onset vertigo, nausea, and vomiting.

In BPPV, the vertigo lasts for seconds; in Ménière's for minutes/hours; in migraine for hours.

Spontaneous nystagmus

- Peripheral origin is indicated by the following characteristics:
  - Horizontal with a torsional component.
  - Does not change direction with a change in gaze.
  - Bidirectional nystagmus implies central pathology.
  - Slow phase towards affected ear; fast phase towards unaffected ear.

- Visual fixation ↓ the nystagmus, and removing fixation ↑ it. At bedside, if Fresnel lenses not available, use an ophthalmoscope focused on the optic disc or the retinal blood vessels with the other eye covered. The nystagmus should be evident in the primary position. Note that the direction of the nystagmus is inverted when viewed through the ophthalmoscope.
- Central nystagmus is often purely horizontal or vertical and changes in direction with changes in the position of the gaze (i.e. bi- or multidirectional).
- Purely vertical and purely torsional nystagmus are usually also of central origin.
- Horizontal–torsional nystagmus may occur in both peripheral and central disorders.
- Visual fixation has little effect on nystagmus of central origin.

The head impulse test

A bedside test of the horizontal vestibulo-ocular reflex (see Fig. 4.1).
- Indicates absent lateral semicircular canal function on affected side.
- If a catch-up saccade occurs in one direction and not the other, this indicates ipsilateral peripheral vestibular lesion within the labyrinth or the 8th nerve including the root entry zone in the brainstem.

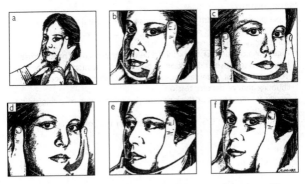

Fig. 4.1 The head impulse test. The examiner turns the patient's head as rapidly as possible about 15° to one side and observes the ability of the patient to keep fixating on a distant target. The patient illustrated has a right peripheral lesion with a severe loss of right lateral semicircular canal function. While the examiner turns the patient's head towards the normal left side (top row), the patient is able to keep fixating on target. In contrast, when the examiner turns the patient's head to the right, the vestibulo-ocular reflex fails and the patient cannot keep fixating on target (e) so that she needs to make a voluntary rapid eye movement, i.e. a saccade, back to target (f) after the head impulse has finished; this can easily be observed by the examiner. It is essential that the head is turned as rapidly as possible; otherwise smooth pursuit eye movements will compensate for the head turn. Reproduced with permission from G.M. Halmagyi (2005). Diagnosis and management of vertigo. *Clin. Med.* 5, 159–65. Royal College of Physicians.

Fukuda or Unterberger's test

Marching on the spot with eyes closed and arms out. Positive test—patient veers to side of the lesion. Cerebellar lesion patients unable to stand unaided to do test. Does not discriminate between central and peripheral causes.

Other signs

- Patients with a peripheral lesion can typically stand but veer/tilt to the side of the lesion. Those with a central lesion are often unable to stand without support.
- If signs not typically peripheral, assume central and investigate.

Recurrent attacks of acute vertigo

May be due to one of the following:

- Ménière's disease.
- Migraine.
- Posterior circulation TIAs (rare); brief crescendo of attacks heralding stroke. Some may be associated with diplopia, dysarthria, or facial numbness.
- Episodic ataxia.

Differential diagnosis

See Table 4.2.

Management

- If peripheral, treat with vestibular sedatives, e.g. betahistine 8–16 mg tds. Symptoms always resolve in a few days due to vestibular compensatory mechanisms.
- If central, consider CT to exclude a cerebellar infarction/haemorrhage. MRI more sensitive at detection of posterior fossa infarcts. Some develop cerebral oedema, resulting in hydrocephalus, and need urgent shunting and/or decompression.
- Significant number of posterior circulation infarcts due to cardiogenic embolism.
  • ECG, 24-hour ECG, transthoracic and/or transoesophageal echo.

Table 4.2 Differential diagnoses of acute vertigo

Cause	History	Examination	Investigation
Benign paroxysmal positional vertigo (BPPV)	Onset after head injury, infections	Vertigo on change in head position (e.g. bending down)	Perform Epley manoeuvre (see Fig. 5.21) Looking upwards, turning in bed Normal neurolocal exam except + Hallpike's test (see Fig. 5.20)
Acute vestibular neuritis	Develops over hours and resolves in days; viral infection	Spontaneous 'peripheral' nystagmus, positive head impulse test	Unilateral caloric hypoexcitability, audiogram normal. MRI normal
Labyrinthine infarction	Abrupt onset; previous vascular disease	As for vestibular neuritis	As for neuritis; MRI-silent infarcts
Perilymph fistula	Abrupt onset; associated head trauma, barotrauma, coughing or sneezing; may be associated with chronic otitis and cholesteatoma	As for neuritis; possible perforation of tympanic membrane. Positive fistula test (vertigo and nystagmus induced by pressure in the external canal)	As for labyrinthitis; CT temporal bone may show erosion from cholesteatoma
Brainstem and cerebellar infarction	Abrupt onset; history of vascular disease; other neurological symptoms	Spontaneous central nystagmus; head impulse test positive only if root entry zone involved; focal neurological signs	Unilateral caloric hypoexcitability if anterior inferior cerebellar artery involved. MRI shows infarction in medulla, pons, or cerebellum

Note: Ménière's syndrome can initially present with acute vertigo but it rarely lasts more than 4 or 5 hours (other symptoms: low-frequency tinnitus, hearing loss, and a sense of fullness in the ears).

Further reading

Bronstein A, Lempert T (2007). *Dizziness: a practical approach to diagnosis and management.* Cambridge: Cambridge University Press.

Spastic paraparesis

Bilateral upper motor neuron signs in the legs. A common presentation caused by a variety of disorders.

Clinical features

- Gait is effortful and stiff, 'walking through mud'.
- Check for a sensory level—anterior and posterior.
- In degenerative conditions the abdominal reflexes remain, e.g. MND.
- Patients presenting with a short history, associated back pain, and bladder and bowel symptoms (urgency, incontinence)—emergency assessment necessary (cord compression).
- Lesions at lower end of spinal cord above L1 and involving cauda equina (e.g. dural AVM) will have a mixture of upper and lower motor neuron signs (e.g. extensor plantars and absent ankle jerks).

Aetiology

See Table 4.3. In cases of undiagnosed spastic paraparesis consider a trial of L-dopa for dopa-responsive dystonia.

Table 4.3 Causes of spastic paraparesis

Cause	Comment
Structural causes	
Parasagittal lesion	E.g. meningioma or dominant anterior cerebral artery infarction affecting medial areas of both frontal lobes
Spinal disease	Note: sensory level may be lower than expected
Degenerative disease	Cervical or thoracic disc disease
Syringomyelia	Typically affecting spinothalamic fibres with sparing of posterior column fibres; anterior horn cell damage causes wasting of hand muscles if syrinx in cervical/thoracic region
Tumours	Intradural and extradural e.g. meningioma
Inflammatory disorders	
Demyelination e.g. MS	Investigations: MRI brain, cord, oligoclonal bands in CSF, VER
Sarcoidosis	Investigations: MRI with gadolinium; blood and CSF ACE; 24 hr urinary calcium; CXR, gallium or PET scan; histology e.g. skin, liver, muscle, or lymph node
Sjögren's, SLE	ENA, ANA, dsDNA
Neuromyelitis optica (NMO)	NMO antibody (aquaporin-4)

Table 4.3 (Contd.)

Cause	Comment
Vascular disorders	
Anterior spinal artery syndrome	Level T10, sparing posterior columns. Investigation MRI
Vascular malformations: cavernomas dural AV fistulae glomus intramedullary AV fistula	MRI (FIESTA sequence + experienced neuroradiologist) looking for flow voids + medullary signal change Spinal angiography for definitive diagnosis + treatment
Genetic disorders	
Adrenoleucodystrophy	Investigations: VLCFA; MRI; synacthen test
Hereditary spastic paraparesis	Diagnosis: family history; genetic testing
Infections	
HIV vacuolar myelopathy	Investigations: HIV test; CD4; viral load
Syphilis	Investigations: blood and CSF VDRL, TPHA
HTLV-1	Investigations: blood and CSF HTLV-1
Metabolic disorders	
B_{12} deficiency	Investigations: B_{12}, homocysteine, methylmalonic acid
Copper deficiency	Malabsorption, post-gastrectomy, use of copper chelating agents; copper levels
Degenerative disorders	
Cerebral palsy (spastic diplegia)	Birth history; non-progressive
Motor neuron disease (primary lateral sclerosis)	Investigations: MRI brain, cord; EMG/NCT/CMCT; CSF

Further reading

Wong SH, Boggild M, Enevoldson TP, Fletcher NA (2008). Myelopathy but normal MRI: what to do next. *Pract. Neurol.*, **8**, 90–102.

Ataxia

Ataxia implies incoordination and results from disorders of:
- cerebellum and its associated pathways;
- loss of proprioceptive sensory input in peripheral nerve disorders and in spinal cord lesions affecting the posterior columns (sensory ataxia).

Cerebellar disease

Signs of cerebellar disease

- Gait ataxia—wide-based, reeling. May be more apparent when turning or stopping suddenly. When mild, only tandem gait may be impaired.
- Dysmetria—an inability to perform acute finger-to-nose movements accurately with past pointing or a similar inability on heel/shin testing.
- Dysdiadokinesia—inability to perform rapid alternating movements.
- Tremor—intention or 'hunting' tremor (kinetic). Postural (static) tremors may also occur.
- Loss of rhythm—rapid tapping on the back of the hand or tapping the heel on the opposite knee.
- Hypotonia.
- Dysarthria—with slurred speech and a scanning dysarthria as words are broken up into syllables; impaired modulation of volume.
- Eye movements—broken up pursuit movements; overshooting or undershooting targets on saccadic eye movements (saccadic dysmetria). Macrosaccadic square-wave jerks in primary position (sudden short-duration movements laterally with rapid correction).
- Nystagmus—coarse nystagmus with the fast phase in the direction of the lesion; multidirectional nystagmus.
- Hyporeflexia.

Differential diagnoses of acquired cerebellar ataxia

- Toxic: alcohol.
- Drugs:
  - phenytoin;
  - lithium.
- Vascular:
  - ischaemic stroke;
  - haemorrhage.
- Inflammatory: demyelination (MS, ADEM).
- Neoplastic:
  - metastases (breast, bronchus);
  - primary brain tumours (in children, pilocytic astrocytoma and medulloblastoma);
  - paraneoplastic syndrome, associated with: small cell lung cancer (anti-Hu, anti-PCA2, ANNA 3), ovarian cancer (anti-Yo), breast cancer (anti-Yo and Ri), testicular cancer (anti-Ta/Ma2), Hodgkin's lymphoma (anti-Tr), neuroblastoma (anti-Hu), and thymoma (anti-CRMP5/CV2).

- Infectious/post-infectious:
  - viral cerebellitis (measles);
  - SSPE;
  - HIV;
  - Miller Fisher syndrome (ataxia, areflexia, ophthalmoplegia + GQ1b antibody).
- Prion: sporadic or variant CJD.
- Structural:
  - Arnold–Chiari malformation;
  - AVM;
  - basilar invagination (Paget's disease).
- Degenerative: cerebellar variant of MSA.
- Nutritional or GI related:
  - vitamin E deficiency—malabsorption (cystic fibrosis, bowel resection), chronic liver disease;
  - thiamine (B_1 deficiency), e.g. in Wernicke's encephalopathy;
  - coeliac disease (with myoclonus).
- Endocrine: T_4.

Differential diagnoses of hereditary cerebellar ataxias
- In general the autosomal dominant ataxias (ADCAs) and other autosomal disorders that may have ataxia as an additional feature, such as Huntington's disease, dentatorubral pallidoluysian atrophy (DRPLA), Gerstmann–Sträussler–Scheinker (GSS), tend to present at age > 25 years (i.e. late onset).
- Autosomal recessive ataxias, inborn errors of metabolism, mitochondrial disorders, and episodic ataxias present at age < 25 years.

Autosomal dominant cerebellar ataxias
At least 25 spinocerebellar ataxia genes. Ataxia in combination with any of the following—pyramidal, peripheral nerve, ophthalmoplegia, dementia. Absence of a family history does not exclude the possibility of diagnosis.
- SCA 2—slow saccades, upper limb areflexia.
- SCA 3—dystonia, parkinsonism, facial myokymia, bulging eyes.
- SCA 6—'pure cerebellar syndrome'.
- SCA 7—pigmentary macular dystrophy.

Recessive ataxias
See Table 4.4.

Inborn errors of metabolism
- Hexoaminidase A or B deficiency.
- Adrenoleucodystrophy.
- Wilson's disease.

Episodic ataxias
See Table 5.22.

Mitochondrial disorders with ataxia
• NARP (neuropathy–ataxia–retinitis pigmentosa).
• MELAS (mitochondrial encephalopathy with lactic acidosis and stroke-like episodes).
• MERRF (myoclonic epilepsy with ragged red fibres).

Sensory ataxia

Clinical features
Any marked loss of proprioception will result in sensory ataxia.
• Signs of a neuropathy with loss of joint position sense.
• Pseudoathetosis of fingers when arms outstretched and eyes closed.
• Upper limb position sense loss is tested by attempting to bring both horizontally outstretched index fingers together in the midline with eyes closed.
• Heel/shin testing deteriorates with eye closure.
• Positive Romberg's sign.

Differential diagnoses of sensory ataxia
• CIDP.
• Paraproteinaemic neuropathy (IgM).
• Refsum's disease (due to defect in phytanic acid metabolism. Other features include deafness, retinitis pigmentosa). A rarer defect of pristanate metabolism presents in a similar fashion (Massion Vernier disease).
• Sensory ganglionitis (paraneoplastic, Sjögren's syndrome, idiopathic).
• Friedreich's ataxia has a significant peripheral nerve component.
• Spinal cord disorders (affecting posterior columns):
  • cervical spondylosis;
  • demyelination (MS).
  • B_{12} and copper deficiency.

Further reading
Ataxia UK (2009). Management of the ataxias: guidelines on best clinical practice. ♪ <http://www.ataxia.org.uk>.
Klockgether T (2010). Sporadic ataxia with adult onset: classification and diagnostic criteria. *Lancet Neurol.*, **9**, 94–104.

Table 4.4 Differential diagnoses of autosomal recessive cerebellar ataxias

Disease	Age of onset (range) yrs	Clinical/laboratory features	Genetics
Friedreich's ataxia	5–15 (0–60)	Kyphoscoliosis, pes cavus, lower limb areflexia, ↑ plantars, axonal neuropathy, cardiomyopathy, impaired GTT	Frataxin gene, chr 9q13
Ataxia telangiectasia	1–6 (0–20)	↓IgG and IgA (↑ infections), skin and conjunctival telangiectasia, oculomotor apraxia chorea, dystonia, hypogonadism, absent lower limb reflexes	ATM, chr 11q22.3
Ataxia with oculomotor apraxia type 1	2–6 (2–18)	Common in Japan, Portugal. Oculomotor apraxia, chorea, cognitive impairment, areflexia, severe axonal neuropathy, ↓ albumin, ↑ cholesterol, ↑ LDL, ↓ HDL	Apratataxin, chr 9p13.3
Abetalipo-proteinaemia	2–17	Friedreich's phenotype + steatorrhea, retinitis pigmentosa, distal amyotrophy, acanthocytes, absent VLDL/LDL, ↓ cholesterol, ↓ vitamin A, E, K	Microsomal triglyceride transfer protein (MTP), chr 4q22
Ataxia with vitamin E deficiency (AVED)	2–20 (2–52)	Friedreich's phenotype + head titubation, no cardiomyopathy or ↓ GTT, vitamin E ↓	α-tocopherol protein, chr 8q13
ARSACS (autosomal recessive spastic ataxia of Charlevoix-Saguenay)	1–5	Ataxia, spasticity, pyramidal syndrome, neuropathy, retinal hypermyelination (Optical Coherence Tomography (OCT))	chr 13q11 SACS gene (sacsin)

Acute visual failure

Monocular transient visual loss

- Amaurosis fugax due to emboli from carotid vessels or heart.
  - Sudden onset lasting 5–15 minutes. Described as a curtain being pulled downwards in front of the eye. Loss may be quadrantic or total and may be accompanied by contralateral limb signs due to ipsilateral hemispheric ischaemia.
- Closed-angle glaucoma—accompanied by halos around lights and may not always be associated with redness and pain.
- Transient visual obscurations (TVOs) are grey-outs precipitated by postural change or straining. Causes:
  - chronic papilloedema due to ↑ICP;
  - hypotension and hypoperfusion.
  - TVO that are gaze-evoked suggest orbital tumours.
- Retinal migraine is rare and results from transient vasospasm that responds to calcium-channel blockers.

Bilateral transient visual loss

- Usually due to transient visual cortical dysfunction.
- In patients < 40 years old this is most commonly due to migraine.
- Other causes include thromboembolism, hypotension, or hyperviscosity.
- In children may occur post-trauma or as part of the benign occipital epilepsy syndrome in childhood.

Non-progressive unilateral sudden visual loss

- Usually due to ischaemia of the optic nerve or retina.
- Anterior ischaemic optic neuropathy (AION) presents with infarction of the optic disc and is due to atherosclerosis or temporal arteritis.
- Optic nerve infarction due to embolism is rare.
- Retrobulbar optic nerve infarction (or posterior ischaemic optic neuropathy) occurs in the setting of cerebral hypoperfusion perioperatively.
- Central retinal artery or branch occlusion is due to emboli or arteriosclerosis. Field defects may be altitudinal, quadrantic, or total. A cherry-red spot at the macula is pathognomonic.
- Central retinal vein occlusion occurs in hypertensives, diabetics, or those with a thrombophilia. A haemorrhagic retinopathy results in a dense central scotoma with preserved peripheral vision.

- Idiopathic central serous chorioretinopathy results from leakage of fluid into the subretinal space. Symptoms include a positive scotoma (black or grey spot in the visual field), metamorphosia (distortion of images), or micropsia. Fluorescein angiography is necessary for diagnosis.
- Retinal and vitreous haemorrhage.

Non-progressive bilateral sudden visual loss

- Usually a result of an infarct in the visual radiation causing a homonymous hemianopia.
- Bilateral occipital infarcts can result in tubular or checkerboard visual fields or total cortical blindness.
- Anton's syndrome due to bilateral parieto-occipital infarcts causes cortical blindness accompanied by denial and confabulation.
- Leber's hereditary optic neuropathy:
  - maternally transmitted mitochondrial disorder;
  - mutations have been identified at positions 11778, 3460, 15257, and 14484;
  - presentation is in young men with a rapid permanent loss of central vision;
  - in the acute phase typical findings include circumpapillary telangiectatic microangiopathy, pseudopapilloedema, an absence of fluorescein leakage, and marked arteriolar narrowing.

Visual loss of sudden onset with progression (unilateral)

Usually due to acute optic neuritis (see Table 4.5 for diagnosis). Most common cause is demyelination.

Typical symptoms

- Periocular pain and pain on eye movement.
- Progressive visual loss over a few days.
- Phosphenes or photopsias (spontaneous flashes of light) on movement.
- Spontaneous improvement in vision.
- Uthoff's phenomenon—temporary decrease in VA with increased body temperature after a bath or exercise.
- Fading of vision and Pulfrich's phenomenon (misperception of the trajectory of moving objects).

Typical signs

- ↓ VA, colour vision, contrast sensitivity.
- Variety of field defects including centrocaecal scotoma.
- Relative afferent pupillary defect (RAPD).
- Optic disc may be normal or swollen.
- Associated uveitis or retinal perivenous sheathing.

Table 4.5 Differential diagnosis of acute optic neuritis

Diagnosis	Clinical features	Investigations
Corticosteroid responsive optic neuropathy (CROI)		
Sarcoidosis SLE Autoimmune optic neuropathy Behçet's disease Neuromyelitis optica	Progressive severe visual loss, often bilateral, isolated or part of a multisystem disorder. More common in Africans and Afro-Caribbeans. Relapse on steroid withdrawal.	Gadolinium-enhanced MRI brain and orbits, CSF, ANA, ACE, 24 hr urinary calcium, CXR, gallium scan, tissue biopsy NMO antibody
Other inflammatory causes		
Post-infectious Post-vaccinial ADEM Neuro-retinitis	Bilateral, childhood, good prognosis, swollen disc, macular star, spontaneous recovery	*Bartonella*, *Borrelia*, syphilis serology
Compressive optic neuropathy		
Tumours e.g. meningioma, glioma, pituitary adenoma Metastases Thyroid ophthalmopathy	Painless, optic atrophy at presentation	MRI, biopsy
Aneurysms	Painful	
Sinus mucocoeles	Painful	
Infectious optic neuropathy		
Syphilis TB Lyme disease Viral optic neuritis (HIV)	Progressive visual loss, disc oedema, vitreous cellular reaction	Serology, CSF, CXR, tuberculin test
Toxic and nutritional optic neuropathy		
Vitamin B$_{12}$ deficiency Tobacco–alcohol ambylopia Methanol intoxication Ethambutol	Bilateral, symmetrical Poor prognosis	B$_{12}$, homocysteine, methylmalonic acid
Cuban and Tanzanian epidemic opticomyelopathy		?Dietary

Coma

Coma is the state of unrousable unconsciousness. The Glasgow Coma Scale (GCS) (see 📖 Chapter 3, 'Head injury (HI)', pp. 94–6) defines coma as:
- failure to open eyes in response to verbal command (E2);
- motor response no better than weak flexion (M4);
- incomprehensible sounds in response to pain (V2).

Neuroanatomy and neuropathology

Consciousness, which is the state of awareness of self and environment with the ability to respond appropriately to stimuli, results from:
- arousal (ascending reticular activating system (RAS));
- awareness (cerebral cortex).

Coma results from damage to the RAS in the brainstem or extensive bilateral cortical damage.

Aetiology

- Head injury.
- Medical causes of coma:
  - cerebrovascular disease (50%);
  - hypoxic–ischaemic injury (20%);
  - metabolic and infective (30%).

General assessment of coma

History
Crucial to contact family, attending ambulance personnel. Obtain PMH, travel, drug details.

General examination
- Temperature (↑ or ↓).
- Pulse and BP (septicaemia, Addison's disease).
- Skin lesions (rash, needle marks, bruises, pigmentation).
- Respiration:
  - slow shallow breaths—drug intoxication;
  - deep rapid respiration—metabolic acidosis;
  - periodic respiration—cardiac failure, brainstem lesion;
  - rapid shallow respiration—brainstem lesion.
- Breath odour (alcohol, ketones, hepatic, or renal failure).
- Abdominal examination (hepatosplenomegaly in liver or lymphoproliferative disease, polycystic kidneys).
- Otoscopy (blood).

Neurological assessment

- Check for meningism (meningitis, SAH).
- Fundoscopy:
  - papilloedema;
  - subhyaloid haemorrhages (SAH);

- retinopathy (diabetes, hypertension, infection (e.g. choroidal tubercle), HIV).
- Level of consciousness (GCS). Note: if facial injuries or tracheostomy, verbal response is unassessable.

Neurological examination: motor and sensory system

Look for asymmetry, evidence of significant cortical (decorticate) or brainstem (decerebrate) damage.

- Observe for seizure activity (focal or general: implies cortical damage).
- Tone.
- Posture.
- Reflexes, plantar responses.
- Response to pain:
  - using a pen, press nailbed of finger and toe;
  - apply supraorbital pressure in case of damage to spinothalamic damage in limbs. Flexor response = cortical or upper brainstem injury; extensor response = brainstem injury.

Neurological examination: brainstem function

- Pupillary responses with an appropriate bright light (not the ophthalmoscope).
  - Unilateral fixed dilated pupil (CN III palsy due to tentorial herniation or PCom artery aneurysm).
  - Bilateral fixed dilated pupils: severe brainstem damage or atropine-like drugs used in resuscitation.
  - Midpoint, fixed = midbrain lesion.
  - Small pinpoint = pontine lesion (also opiates).
  - Small reactive pupils = diencephalic (thalamus) lesion.
  - Horner's syndrome = hypothalamus, brainstem, or internal carotid artery lesion.
- Eye deviation.
  - Conjugate lateral deviation caused by ipsilateral frontal lesion or brainstem (PPRF) lesion.
  - Dysconjugate eyes due to CN III, IV, or VI palsy or brainstem lesion.
  - Skew deviation in brainstem lesions.
- Spontaneous eye movements.
  - Repetitive horizontal deviations (ping-pong gaze) = brainstem lesion.
  - Retractory nystagmus (eyes jerk back into orbits) = midbrain lesion.
  - Downward ocular bobbing = pontine lesion.
- Reflex eye movements (see Fig. 4.2).
  - Oculocephalic manoeuvre. Head moved side to side—normally eyes deviate to opposite side. If brainstem affected eyes remain fixed.
  - Oculovestibular test. First check that tympanic membrane is intact. Instil 50–200 mL ice cold water into EAM: normal tonic response = eyes deviate to side of instillation with nystagmus and quick phase away from side of instillation. Dysconjugate or absent response = brainstem lesion.
- Corneal reflex.

Classification of coma

Coma without focal signs or meningism
- Hypoxic–ischaemic injury.
- Metabolic.
- Toxic.
- Post-ictal.

Coma with meningism
- Meningoencephalitis.
- SAH.

Coma with focal signs
- Haemorrhage.
- Infarction.
- Abscess.
- Tumour.
- Hypoglycaemia can cause focal signs.

Investigations
- Metabolic screen.
- CT scan or MRI if possible, especially in coma with meningism or focal signs.
- Normal CT does not exclude ↑ ICP.
- EEG (see 🕮 Chapter 8, 'EEG and diffuse cerebral dysfunction', pp. 538–9).
- If no contraindications, consider LP.

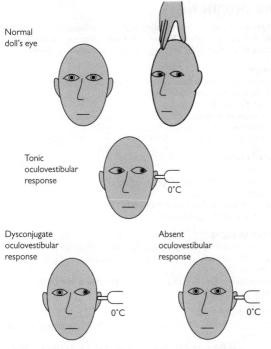

Normal
doll's eye

Tonic
oculovestibular
response

0°C

Dysconjugate
oculovestibular
response

0°C

Absent
oculovestibular
response

0°C

Fig. 4.2 Reflex eye movements. Reprinted from D. Bates (2004). *Medicine*, **32**(10), 69–74, with permission from Elsevier.

Coma prognosis

Neurologists are often asked to prognosticate on comatose patients in ITU in order that decisions about further active treatment can be made. The prognosis can be affected by aetiology, depth, and duration of coma.

Aetiology
- Drug overdose patients have a good prognosis despite significant impairment of brainstem function.
- Likelihood of good recovery:
  - metabolic or infection, 25%;
  - hypoxic–ischaemic injury, 10%;
  - cerebrovascular disease or SAH, 5%.

Depth of coma
Within 6 hours:
- if eye opening, 20% chance of good recovery compared with 10% if no eye opening;
- no motor response, 3%; if flexion or better, 15%;
- no noise, 8%; groaning, 30%.

Duration of coma
The chance of making a good recovery decreases with time:
- by day 3, 7% will make a moderate or good recovery;
- after day 14, 2%;
- patients who remain in a coma for > 7–15 days, will either die or remain in a vegetative state.

Prognostic signs
The data for prognostic signs in coma are poor. No single clinical sign can act as a predictor.
- At 24 hours, in the absence of both oculovestibular and corneal reflexes and extension to pain, in the absence of sedative drugs, the chance of a good recovery is < 3%.
- Intact pupillary and corneal responses and localization to pain at 24 hours indicates a 40% chance of good recovery.
- In one series 93% (of 70 patients), who did not have withdrawal or better on motor examination at 3 days, had no recovery or developed a persistent vegetative state; 7% had some recovery but were left with severe long term disability. Conversely, out of 26 patients with withdrawal or better and orientating spontaneous eye movements, 77% showed moderate to good recovery at 1 year.[1]

Further reading

Posner JB, Saper CB, Schiff N, Plum F (2007). *Plum and Posner's Diagnosis of Stupor and Coma* (4th edn). New York: Oxford University Press.

Wijdicks EF, Hildra A, Young GB, et al. (2006). Practice parameter: prediction of outcome in comatose survivors after cardiopulmonary resuscitation (an evidence-based review): report of the Quality Standards Subcommittee of the American Academy of Neurology. *Neurology*, **67**, 203–10.

Reference

1. Levy DE, Caronna JJ, Singer BH, Lapinski RH, Frydman H, Plum F (1985). Predicting outcome from hypoxic–ischaemic coma. *JAMA*, **253**, 1420–6.

Excessive daytime sleepiness

- The Epworth sleepiness scale (Box 4.1) is a useful tool in the clinic to assess the common complaint of sleepiness.
- Anyone with sleepiness causing problems with work and driving or an Epworth score of > 12 despite having > 7 hours sleep each night should be investigated.

Causes of persistent sleepiness

- Lack of sleep:
  - inadequate time in bed;
  - sleep disruption (e.g. babies);
  - shift work.
- Sleep disruption:
  - obstructive sleep apnoea/hypopnoea syndrome (OSAHS);
  - periodic limb movement disorder.
- Sleepiness with normal sleep:
  - narcolepsy;
  - idiopathic hypersomnolence;
  - neurological causes, e.g. tumours of hypothalamus, pineal, or upper brainstem, bilateral paramedian thalamic infarcts, head injury, MS; drugs;
  - psychological, e.g. depression, seasonal affective disorder (SAD).

Causes of intermittent sleepiness

- Kleine–Levin syndrome (episodic disorder associated with bulimia, hypersexuality).
- Catamenial hypersomnia.

Box 4.1 Epworth Sleepiness Scale

Name:

Date:

Your age: (years)

Your sex: Male/Female

How likely are you to doze off or fall asleep in the situations described below, in contrast to feeling just tired?

This refers to your usual way of life in recent times.

Even if you haven't done some of these things recently, try to work out how they would have affected you.

Use the following **scale** to choose the most appropriate number for each situation:
- 0, would never doze
- 1, slight chance of dozing
- 2, moderate chance of dozing
- 3, high chance of dozing

Situation	Chance of dozing
Sitting and reading...	–
Watching TV...	–
Sitting inactive in a public place (e.g. a theatre or a meeting)..	–
As a passenger in a car for an hour without a break..	–
Lying down to rest in the afternoon when circumstances permit..	–
Sitting and talking to someone................................	–
Sitting quietly after a lunch without alcohol...........	–
In a car, while stopped for a few minutes in the traffic...	–
Total...	–

Score
- 0–10, normal range
- 10–12, borderline
- > 12/24, abnormal

Reproduced from Johns, MW (1991). *Sleep*, **14**, 540–5, with permission from the American Academy of Sleep Medicine.

Obstructive sleep apnoea/hypopnoea syndrome (OSAHS)

- Most common cause of sleepiness most often found in middle-aged and elderly men.
- Incidence: 20–50/100 000.
- Risk factors:
  - 50% are obese (collar size > 17 inches);
  - retrognathia—results from excessive relaxation of the upper airway muscles during sleep.
- Sleep fragmentation is due to repeated cycles of apnoea and arousal.
- Result is a sixfold increased risk of RTA but also hypertension, cardiac arrhythmias, and heart failure.
- Investigations include an overnight study of breathing pattern and oximetry. A limited study does not exclude the diagnosis, and polysomnography may be necessary.
- Management includes:
  - weight loss;
  - reduction of alcohol intake;
  - most will require continuous positive airway pressure (CPAP).

Narcolepsy

- Classical tetrad:
  - sleepiness;
  - hypnagogic hallucinations;
  - sleep paralysis;
  - cataplexy.
- Onset in teens or twenties. Incidence: 0.2/100 000.
- Cause may be related to a reduction in hypocretin production from the hypothalamus.
- Sleepiness is characterized by irresistible sleep attacks in inappropriate situations, such as whilst eating.
- Cataplexy is due to a sudden loss of muscular tone, falling to the ground, or head drop. Facial twitching may occur. Episodes last for a few seconds but may be as long as 10 minutes. There is no loss of awareness. Triggers include emotional outbursts such as laughing.
- 85% of Caucasians are HLA DR2 DQw1 +ve. (However, this is present in 22–40% of the normal population and lacks diagnostic specificity.)
- Multiple sleep latency test (MSLT) is the most useful investigation.

Treatment
- Sleepiness:
  - modafinil (200–400 mg/day);
  - methylphenidate (10–100 mg/day);
  - selegiline (2.5–10 mg/day);
  - dexamfetamine (5–60 mg/day).
- Cataplexy sleep paralysis, and hypnagogic hallucinations respond to fluoxetine 20–40 mg/day, clomipramine 20–200 mg/day.

Periodic limb movement disorder

- Common—30% over 65 years.
- Recurrent limb movements every 20–40 seconds during non-REM sleep.
- Associated with daytime sleepiness.
- May be associated with other sleep disorders such as restless legs syndrome (RLS), narcolepsy, obstructive sleep apnoea.
- Treatment as for RLS (dopamine agonists, L-dopa).

Further reading

Reading PJ (2010). Sleep disorders in neurology. *Pract. Neurol.*, **10**, 300–9.

Stores G (2007). Clinical diagnosis and misdiagnosis of sleep disorders. *J. Neurol. Neurosurg. Psychiatry*, **78**, 1293–7.

Tremor

- Defined as a rhythmical involuntary oscillatory movement of a body part.
- Normal physiological tremor 5–12 Hz (↑ anxiety, caffeine, T4↑).

Phenomenological classification

- Rest tremor.
- Action tremor—produced by voluntary contraction of muscle.
  - Postural tremor: present while maintaining posture against gravity.
  - Kinetic tremor—occurs during voluntary movement.
  - Intention tremor—occurs with target-directed movement with increase in amplitude at termination of movement (cerebellar).
  - Task-specific tremor, e.g. writing tremor.
  - Isometric tremor, e.g. orthostatic tremor.

Essential tremor (ET)

- Sporadic or autosomal dominant:
  - gene ETM1 on chr 3q13 and ETM2 on chr 2p22-25;
  - DAT scan used to discriminate between ET and parkinsonian tremor.

Clinical features

- 50% + FH.
- Bilateral.
- Symmetrical.
- Postural or kinetic tremor of hands (e.g. tea cup).
- Associated with head tremor and/or voice tremor.
- 50% respond to alcohol.
- Slowly progressive.

Differential diagnosis

- Dystonic tremor (asymmetric, irregular).
- Parkinson's disease.
- Hyperthyroidism.
- Neuropathic tremor.

Management

- Propranolol up to 320 mg/day.
- Primidone up to 250 mg tds (side effects common).
- Topiramate (up to 400 mg/day).
- Gabapentin (mixed results).
- Stereotactic surgery (lesional or deep brain stimulation) to VIM nucleus of thalamus should be considered in severe cases.

Dystonic tremor

Presentation
- Jerky irregular action tremor.
- Task-specific, e.g. writer's cramp with jerky spasms.

Management
- Botulinum toxin under EMG guidance.
- Anticholinergic drugs.
- Propranolol and primidone.

Task-specific tremor
- Localized essential tremor, e.g. primary writing tremor.
- Affects writers, musicians, sports persons (golfers, dart players).
- Consider:
  • botulinum toxin;
  • beta-blockers;
  • anticholinergics.

Holmes' tremor (rubral, midbrain, thalamic tremor)
- Irregular low-frequency tremor at rest, posture, and intention.
- Involves proximal and distal arm muscles.
- Site of lesion thalamus to midbrain.
- Causes:
  • stroke;
  • AVM;
  • tumour;
  • demyelination.
- May respond to L-dopa or dopamine. Surgery as for ET.

Primary orthostatic tremor
- Presentation with unsteadiness on standing.
- Improves with walking.
- May be associated with cerebellar degeneration.
- Frequency 14–18 Hz.
- Tremor palpated or auscultated over calf muscles (helicopter rotor blades).
- Responds to clonazepam.

Neuropathic tremor
Usually with demyelinating neuropathy:
- AIDP;
- CIDP;
- IgM paraproteinaemic neuropathy;
- HMSN I;
- porphyria (paroxysmal tremor).

Characteristically, an action tremor similar to ET. PET studies indicate cerebellar activity.

Drug-induced tremor
- Alcohol.
- Salbutamol.
- Lithium.
- Steroids.
- Ciclosporin.
- Sodium valproate.

Palatal tremor (low frequency 1–2 Hz)

Site of pathology is the Guillain–Mollaret triangle formed by the red nucleus, olives, and dentate nucleus.
- Essential (associated with clicking heard by patient which is due to contraction of the tensor veli palatini in the Eustachian tube).
- Symptomatic:
  - tumour;
  - Whipple's disease;
  - neuroferritinopathy;
  - demyelination.

Psychogenic tremor
- May be sudden onset.
- Unusual combinations of rest and postural/intention tremor.
- Decrease in amplitude and frequency with distraction.
- 'Entrainment'—change in frequency during voluntary contraction or movements of contralateral hand.
- External loading ↑ amplitude, whereas PD and ET ↓.
- Coactivation—resistance to passive movement with change in tone and tremor.
- Past history or other features of somatization or conversion disorder.

Further reading

Barker R, Burn D (2004). Tremor. *Adv. Clin. Neurosci. Rehabil.*, **4**(1), 13–14.
Burn D (2003). Approach to the patient with a movement disorder. *Adv. Clin. Neurosci. Rehabil.*, 3(2), 27–8.

Tics

- Rapid stereotypic involuntary movements.
- Can be voluntarily suppressed but suppression leads to build-up of internal tension.
- Triggered by stress or boredom.
- Male preponderance (3:1).
- Peak age of onset around 7 years.
- Causes:
  • Gilles de la Tourette syndrome;
  • neuroacanthocytosis;
  • neuroleptics;
  • common in Asperger's patients;
  • head trauma.

Patients present with the following:
- Motor tics:
  • eye winks;
  • eye blinks;
  • grimaces;
  • head tosses;
  • sniffs;
  • throat clearing.
- Vocal tics:
  • foul utterances (coprolalia);
  • repeating sounds or words (echolalia).

Resolution usually occurs at the end of adolescence.

Treatment
- When mild, no treatment.
- If socially disabling:
  • clonazepam;
  • neuroleptics but side effect of tardive dyskinesia;
  • reserpine;
  • tetrabenazine.

Chorea and athetosis

- Chorea: continuous flow of irregular, brief, jerky, flowing movements.
- Athetosis—slower flowing movements.
- May be incorporated into semi-purposeful movements.

Causes

- Hereditary:
  - Huntington's disease;
  - benign hereditary chorea;
  - neuroacanthocytosis (chorea, dystonia, lip and tongue biting, orofacial dyskinesia, ↑ CK, neuropathy with amyotrophy, parkinsonism, dementia);
  - Wilson's disease;
  - SCA;
  - ataxia telangiectasia;
  - mitochondrial disease (Leigh's disease).
- Infection:
  - Sydenham's chorea (post-streptococcal);
  - HIV;
  - SSPE;
  - vCJD.
- Vascular (often hemichorea):
  - infarction;
  - polycythaemia.
- Metabolic:
  - hyper- and hypoglycaemia;
  - hyperthyroidism;
  - hypocalcaemia.
- Immunological:
  - SLE;
  - anti-phospholipid syndrome;
  - pregnancy—chorea gravidarum.
- Drug-induced:
  - anti-Parkinsonian drugs;
  - dopamine antagonists drugs, e.g. phenothiazines;
  - oral contraceptive (previous history of Sydenham's chorea);
  - amphetamines, cocaine.

Treatment

- Neuroleptics, e.g. sulpiride, risperidone, olanzapine.
- Tetrabenazine (side effect, depression).

Myoclonus

Sudden shock-like involuntary movement:
- Positive myoclonus: brief muscle contraction.
- Negative myoclonus: pause in muscle activity (asterixis).

Classification

- Distribution:
  - generalized;
  - focal;
  - multifocal;
  - segmental.
- Clinical presentation:
  - spontaneous;
  - action;
  - reflex (auditory, visual, or to touch).
- Site of origin:
  - cortical;
  - brainstem;
  - spinal cord.

Aetiology

Physiological
- Hypnic jerks.
- Hiccup.

Epileptic
- Focal epilepsy:
  - EPC.
- Myoclonic epilepsies:
  - progressive myoclonic epilepsy (Unverricht–Lundborg disease).

Encephalopathies
- Metabolic (liver, renal failure).
- Infections:
  - prion diseases;
  - HIV;
  - SSPE;
  - post-anoxic.
- Drugs, e.g. tricyclics, L-dopa.

Degenerative conditions
- Alzheimer's disease.
- MSA.
- Corticobasal degeneration.
- Cerebellar degeneration—Ramsay Hunt syndrome (e.g. coeliac disease).

Hereditary
- Huntington's disease.
- Mitochondrial disorders.
- Myoclonic dystonia (DYT 11).

- Storage disorders:
  - Lafora body disease;
  - sialidosis;
  - ceroid lipofuscinosis (Batten's disease, Kuf's disease);
  - lipidosis (Tay–Sachs disease, Krabbe's disease).

Focal lesions
Brain or spinal cord.

Cortical myoclonus

- Myoclonic jerks triggered by movement or stimulus-sensitive.
- Distal muscles most affected.
- EEG may be diagnostic:
  - cortical discharges time-locked to myoclonic jerks;
  - giant cortical somatosensory evoked potentials.

Brainstem myoclonus

- Bilateral synchronous jerking with adduction of arms, flexion of elbows, flexion of trunk and head.
- Stimulus-induced: tap nose, lip, or head, or loud noise.

Aetiology
- Paraneoplastic.
- Brainstem encephalitis.
- MS.
- Encephalomyelitis with rigidity.

Spinal myoclonus

Two types:
- Rhythmic, repetitive, bilateral, jerking one or two adjacent parts. Persist during sleep.
- Propriospinal myoclonus:
  - usually trunk muscles—flexion;
  - prominent when lying down;
  - stimulus-sensitive.

Aetiology
- Inflammatory cord lesion.
- Tumour.
- Trauma.
- Functional.

Treatment of myoclonus

- Clonazepam—250 micrograms starting dose.
- Sodium valproate.
- Piracetam or levetiracetam.

Further reading

Barker R (2003). Myoclonus. *Adv. Clin. Neurosci. Rehabil.*, **3**(5), 20–2.

Dystonia

Syndrome caused by sustained muscle contraction resulting in twisting and repetitive movements or postures that are due to co-contraction of antagonistic muscles.

- Focal dystonia: one body part.
- Segmental dystonia: two or more adjacent body parts.

Classification

- Primary dystonias: dystonia and dystonic tremor only clinical manifestation.
  - DYT1 dystonia (see 📖 Chapter 5, 'Inherited movement disorders', pp. 362–3);
  - sporadic, usually adult onset.
- Dystonia plus syndromes:
  - dopa-responsive dystonia (DRD) (see 📖 Chapter 5, 'Inherited movement disorders', pp. 362–3);
  - myoclonic dystonia.
- Heredodegenerative syndromes:
  - Wilson's disease;
  - HD (see 📖 Chapter 5, 'Inherited movement disorders', pp. 362–3);
  - SCA (see 📖 Chapter 5, 'Hereditary ataxias', pp. 350–1);
  - Lubag (dystonia–parkinsonism);
  - early-onset PD (PARKIN 2) (see 📖 Chapter 5, 'Inherited movement disorders', pp. 362–3);
  - Hallervorden–Spatz disease;
  - neuroacanthocytosis (also chorea, orofacial dyskinesias, axonal neuropathy, CPK ↑, tongue biting, seizures, and cognitive decline);
  - Lesch–Nyhan syndrome.
- Degenerative syndromes:
  - MSA;
  - PSP;
  - CBD.
- Secondary dystonias:
  - perinatal trauma/hypoxia;
  - stroke;
  - focal lesions, especially putamen or rostral midbrain.

Investigations

- Exclude Wilson's disease:
  - serum copper and caeruloplasmin levels;
  - 24 hour urinary copper;
  - slit-lamp examination for Kayser–Fleischer rings.
- Onset < 25 years—check DYT1 gene.
- MRI especially in generalized or hemidystonia dystonia, additional neurological signs.
- Consider other genetic tests as above (e.g. HD, SCA).
- *Fresh* blood films for acanthocytes × 3 (neuroacanthocytosis).

Management

- Consider trial of L-dopa in any patient with onset < 40 years, especially childhood or adolescent, for DRD.
- Anticholinergic drugs, e.g. benzhexol up to 80 mg/day.
- If unhelpful, especially in generalized dystonia, consider:
  - tetrabenazine;
  - pimozide;
  - sulpiride.
- Thalamic (GPi) deep brain stimulation now an option.
- Focal dystonia—local botulinum toxin (cervical dystonia, blepharospasm, task-specific dystonias, laryngeal dystonia).

Further reading

Edwards M, Bhatia K (2004). Dystonia. *Adv. Clin. Neurosci. Rehabil.*, **4**(2), 20–4.

Jankovic J (2006). Treatment of dystonia. *Lancet Neurol.*, **5**, 864–72.

Phukan J, Albanese A, Gasser T, Warner T (2011). Primary dystonia and dystonia-plus syndromes: clinical characteristics, diagnosis and pathogenesis. *Lancet Neurol.*, **10**, 1074–84.

Foot drop

Common clinical presentation due to weakness of ankle dorsiflexor (tibialis anterior). Flail foot implies additional weakness of plantar flexors.

Neuroanatomical localization

Most common causes

- Common peroneal nerve (CPN) palsy innervated by L4, L5 (pressure at fibular head or within fibular tunnel).
- L5 radiculopathy.

Unusual causes

- Lesions in lumbosacral plexus (affecting L4, L5 roots or selective CPN fibres).
- Sciatic nerve preferentially selecting CPN fibres.
- Anterior horn cell disease.
- Myelopathy.
- Cortical lesion foot area.
- Distal myopathies (e.g. IBM).
- Dystonia (e.g. dopa-responsive dystonia).
- Myasthenia gravis.

Clinical features

History

- External pressure around fibular head, e.g. sitting cross-legged, sleeping awkwardly, prolonged bed rest, weight loss, kneeling for prolonged periods, during labour/surgery lithotomy position.
- Radicular back pain but not always present in disc prolapse (L5/S1).
- Trauma to lateral knee or popliteal fossa.
- Enquire about previous episodes involving other nerves, e.g. ulnar, brachial plexus suggesting HNPP, vasculitis.
- Foot drop occurring on exercise may suggest lumbar canal stenosis or occasionally spinal cord demyelination.

Examination

- Gait:
  - may reveal bilateral foot drop or spasticity;
  - attempt to stand on heels and toes—weakness of plantar flexion may be evident.
- Examine for ↑ tone, pyramidal weakness, brisk reflexes, extensor plantar response.
- Examine for other nerve lesions which may suggest a mononeuritis multiplex (vasculitis, HNPP).
- CPN lesion: weakness of dorsiflexion (tibialis anterior); extensor hallucis longus and foot evertors (peronei muscles); sensory loss in anterolateral leg and dorsum of foot (variable). Ankle jerk normal.
- Examine glutei, hamstrings, tibialis posterior, gastrocnemius, looking for evidence of multiple roots, lumbosacral plexus, or sciatic nerve involvement.

- Foot inversion supplied by tibialis posterior and also L4, L5 roots. Therefore if also weak implies root or common peroneal + tibial separately or sciatic nerve lesion.
- Absent ankle jerk suggests L5/S1 root, lumbosacral plexus, or sciatic nerve lesion.
- Palpate CPN around fibular head for tenderness and thickness (leprosy, CIDP, infiltration).
- Elicit Tinel's sign by tapping nerve around fibula.
- Palpate buttock, posterior thigh, and popliteal fossa for masses.
- Straight-leg raising (sciatic stretch test) causing pain consistent with root lesion.
- Look for fasciculation in upper/lower limbs or suggestion of mixed upper and lower motor neuron signs (MND).
- Weakness of other muscles to suggest myopathy, e.g. quadriceps, finger flexors (IBM).

Investigations

NCT/EMG

- May reveal lesion outside peroneal nerve territory, i.e. sciatic or plexus.
- Conduction block at fibula around fibular head.
- Other disorders—myopathy, MND.
- Degree of denervation helps predict recovery.

MRI

- Lumbar spine—disc prolapse, foraminal stenosis.
- Brain and whole spine if CNS signs.
- Lumbosacral plexus, sciatic nerve to popliteal fossa with gadolinium if dictated by NCT/EMG or localization not possible.

Blood tests

- FBC + ESR.
- U&E, glucose, LFT, Ca, PO_4.
- CPK.
- Vasculitis (ANA, dsDNA, ENA, ANCA).
- HNPP chromosome 17 deletion.

Other investigations as indicated

- CSF (cells, protein, cytology, oligoclonal bands).
- Nerve biopsy (vasculitis, infiltration, leprosy, CIDP, HNPP) and/or muscle biopsy.
- ACh receptor antibody.
- CXR.

Further reading

Stewart JD (2010). Focal peripheral neuropathies (4th edn). West Vancouver: JBJ Publishing.

Unilateral hand weakness/ paraesthesiae

Localization

- Peripheral nerve (median, ulnar, radial).
- Brachial plexus.
- Spinal root (radicular).
- Spinal cord.
- Cerebral cortex or thalamus.

Clinical features

History

- Thumb + index + middle + half ring = median; little + half ring = ulnar. Can be unreliable
- Thumb + index = C6; middle finger = C7. Associated with neck pain/ discomfort radiating down arm. Sensory symptoms may be triggered by specific neck movements/postures (e.g. neck flexion/extension).
- Spinal cord—pins and needles paraesthesiae more diffuse, affecting arm and hand; may be bilateral ± unilateral or bilateral leg symptoms. + Lhermitte's phenomenon suggests demyelination.
- Symptoms affecting ring + little finger extending just beyond wrist— ulnar. If symptoms extend to medial aspect of forearm suggests medial cutaneous nerve of forearm, either mononeuritis multiplex or brachial plexus lesion.
- Symptoms of pins and needles, aching, and pain radiating up the arm mainly at night is suggestive of carpal tunnel syndrome (CTS).
- Thoracic outlet syndrome (TOS):
  - presents insidiously;
  - usually unilateral;
  - thenar muscles with weakness, wasting of APB + some involvement of ulnar innervated muscles + sensory involvement of lower trunk of brachial plexus, i.e. ulnar, medial cutaneous nerve of forearm, and arm.
- Acute onset with shoulder pain—consider acute brachial neuritis (Parsonage–Turner syndrome). Although usually upper trunk involved, with weakness and wasting around shoulder, anterior interosseous nerve may be involved.

Examination

- Look for wasting:
  - First dorsal interosseous muscle (FDIO); hypothenar eminence—ulnar.
  - Abductor polllicis brevis (APB); thenar eminence (median nerve).

- Weakness:
  - Median nerve at wrist (CTS) weakness of APB + opponens pollicis brevis (OPB). Check flexor pollicus longus (FPL) = anterior interosseous nerve branch = high median nerve.
  - Ulnar nerve at elbow = weakness of FDIO + abductor digiti minimi (ADM) + flexor digitorum profundus (FDP) 4 and 5. Tested by flexing DIP against resistance. However, ulnar nerve lesions at elbow (most common site of lesion) do not always result in weakness of FDP due to selective fascicular damage.
  - Weakness of median and ulnar innervated hand muscles = T1 lesion. Anterior horn cell, root, or brachial plexus.
  - Sudden-onset paraesthesiae affecting whole or part of hand—consider cortical cause or if associated with dysaesthesia thalamic lesion (both much rarer than radicular or peripheral nerve lesions).
- Reflexes:
  - Absent/depressed biceps and/or supinator reflexes (C5/C6 root) lesions; absent triceps jerk (C7).
- Sensory testing:
  - Check median, ulnar, radial territories. Also lateral cutaneous nerves of arm and forearm; medial cutaneous nerves of arm and forearm (see diagram inside front cover). Notoriously unreliable!
  - Look for cortical sensory loss (sensory inattention, impaired two-point discrimination test, dysgraphaesthesia).
  - Palpate ulnar nerves at elbows in flexion and extension looking superficiality and prolapse. Tap this site with tendon hammer (ulnar nerve Tinel's sign). Tap flexor retinaculum with tendon hammer (median nerve Tinel's sign).

Investigations

- NCT/EMG
  - TOS: ↓ ulnar and medial cutaneous nerve SAP; ↓ median ± ulnar CMAP, ↑ ulnar F waves. EMG abnormal, especially APB.
- MRI cervical spine, e.g. cervical disc, syringomyelia.
- In suspected TOS, plain cervical X-ray may show elongated transverse process C7 (cervical rib). MRI does not reliably show fibrous band but helps exclude other structural causes.
- MRI brain if cortical or thalamic lesion suspected.
- Blood tests—check T4 (CTS), blood sugar.

Management

- CTS (see 📖 Chapter 5, 'Carpal tunnel syndrome', pp. 286–7).
- Ulnar neuropathy (see 📖 Chapter 5, 'Ulnar neuropathy', pp. 288–90).
- 'True' TOS—supraclavicular exploration. In 'non-specific' milder cases, conservative management with posture correction and stretching exercises relieves symptoms in 60–80%. Careful follow-up for development of true TOS.

Cerebrovascular disease: stroke 178
Management of stroke 182
Prevention of ischaemic stroke 184
Cerebral venous thrombosis 186
Images in cerebrovascular disease 188
Dementia: introduction 198
Alzheimer's disease (AD) 202
Frontotemporal dementia (FTD) 206
Other dementias 208
Creutzfeldt–Jakob disease (CJD) 210
Epilepsy: introduction 214
Management of epilepsy 218
Women and epilepsy 224
Seizures versus dissociative non-epileptic attack disorder (NEAD)
    or pseudoseizures 226
Headache: migraine—introduction and clinical features 228
Migraine: differential diagnosis, investigations, and IHS criteria 230
Management of acute migraine: the stepped care regimen 232
Management of migraine 234
Migraine and women 236
Primary short-lasting headaches 240
Cluster headache 242
Trigeminal neuralgia 244
Idiopathic intracranial hypertension (IIH) 246
Parkinsonism and Parkinson's disease: introduction 250
Clinical features of parkinsonism and PD 252
Differential diagnosis of PD and investigation 254
Drug-induced parkinsonism 257
Medical management of PD 258
Surgical treatment of PD 262
Management of other problems in PD 264
Multiple system atrophy (MSA) 266
Progressive supranuclear palsy (PSP) 268
Corticobasal degeneration (CBD) 269
Peripheral nerve disorders: introduction and clinical approach 270
Diagnosis of peripheral nerve disorders 272
Investigations in peripheral nerve disorders 274
Diabetic neuropathies 276
Chronic inflammatory demyelinating polyneuropathy (CIDP) 278
Multifocal motor neuropathy with conduction block (MMN-CB) 282
Vasculitic neuropathy 284

Neurological disorders

Carpal tunnel syndrome 286
Ulnar neuropathy 288
Muscle disorders: classification and features 292
Muscle disorders: investigations 294
Dermatomyositis, polymyositis, and inclusion body myositis 298
Channelopathies 302
Motor neuron disease: introduction and clinical features 306
Motor neuron disease: investigations and management 308
Multiple sclerosis: introduction and clinical features 310
Multiple sclerosis: investigations and diagnosis 312
Multiple sclerosis: management 318
Neuromyelitis optica 322
Myasthenia gravis: introduction, clinical features, and investigations 324
Myasthenia gravis: management 326
Myasthenia gravis due to MuSK antibodies 330
Paraneoplastic disorders: introduction 332
Paraneoplastic syndromes: central nervous system 334
Paraneoplastic syndromes: peripheral nervous system 336
Paraneoplastic syndromes: investigations and management 338
Vertigo, dizziness, and unsteadiness: introduction 340
Dizziness, unsteadiness, or 'off balance': neurological causes 342
Benign paroxysmal positional vertigo (BPPV) 344
Dizziness, unsteadiness, or 'off balance': non-neurological causes 348
Neurogenetic disorders: introduction 349
Hereditary ataxias 350
Genetic neuropathies 352
Inherited myopathies 356
Myotonic dystrophy (MD) 360
Inherited movement disorders 362
Inherited mitochondrial disorders 364
Inherited dementias 367
Hereditary metabolic diseases 368
Viral encephalitis 370
Neurology of HIV/AIDS: introduction 373
Neurological disorders due to HIV 374
Opportunistic infections associated with HIV 376
MRI images in infectious diseases 380
Somatization (or functional or conversion) disorders 384
Lumbar puncture 388
Intravenous immunoglobulin (IV Ig) 392
Diagnosis of brainstem death 394

Cerebrovascular disease: stroke

- Third most common cause of death worldwide and most common cause of neurological disability.
- Incidence 240/100 000/year.
- In UK, 110 000 people have their first stroke, 40 000 recurrent strokes.
- Defined by the rapid onset of focal neurological deficit due to infraction or haemorrhage lasting more than 24 hours.
- Transient ischaemic attack (TIA)—symptoms and signs resolve within 24 hours. This concept now outdated as MRI may show appropriate infarcted area despite rapid recovery.
- However, these definitions may change as newer treatments for reperfusion, such as thrombolysis given earlier, become routine.
- Early risk of stroke after TIA or minor stroke is high:
  - 7 day risk, 5%.
  - 14 day risk, 10%.
  - Thereafter, risk 5%/year with additional risk of MI 2–3%/year.

Aetiology

Ischaemic stroke (80%)

- Atherothromboembolism:
  - carotid and vertebral disease;
  - intracranial disease;
  - aortic arch atheroma.
- Cardioembolism.
- Small vessel disease (lacunar stroke).
- Arterial dissection.
- Inflammatory vascular disorders:
  - giant cell arteritis;
  - systemic vasculitides, e.g. SLE;
  - primary angiitis.
- Haematological disorders:
  - antiphospholipid antibody syndrome (APAS);
  - sickle cell disease;
  - thrombophilic states.
- Genetic disorders:
  - CADASIL;
  - mitochondrial disorders, e.g. MELAS.
- Infections:
  - meningitis, e.g. TB;
  - HIV.
- Others:
  - migraine;
  - COC, pregnancy.

Cerebral haemorrhage (15%)

Intracerebral haemorrhage

- Small vessel disease (hypertension).
- AVM.
- Cerebral amyloid angiopathy.

- Tumours.
- Cerebral venous thrombosis.
- Haematological disorders:
  - anticoagulants, antiplatelet drugs, and thrombolytic therapy;
  - coagulation disorders.
- Drug abuse, e.g. cocaine.
- Moyamoya syndrome.

Subarachnoid haemorrhage
- Aneurysm.
- Trauma.
- Dural AV fistula.
- AV malformation.

Risk factors
See Table 5.1.

Clinical features
Anterior circulation (carotid territory)
- Amaurosis fugax/retinal infarction (monocular visual loss).
- Hemiparesis.
- Hemisensory loss.
- Hemianopia (optic tract and radiation).
- Dysphasia.
- Sensory inattention.
- Visual inattention.

Posterior circulation (vertebrobasilar)
- Ataxia.
- Cranial nerve involvement:
  - diplopia;
  - facial sensory loss;
  - LMN facial palsy;
  - vertigo;
  - dysphagia;
  - dysarthria.

Table 5.1 Relative risk (RR) of stroke

Risk factors	RR
Age (> 75 versus 55–64 years)	5
Hypertension (160/95 versus 120/80)	7
Smoking	2
Diabetes	2
Ischaemic heart disease	3
Atrial fibrillation	5
Previous TIA	5

- Hemiparesis (may be bilateral).
- Hemisensory loss (may be bilateral).
- Hemianopia (occipital lobe).
- Cortical blindness—basilar artery occlusion.

Lacunar strokes
- Pure motor strokes (face, arm, and leg) in the posterior limb of internal capsule.
- Pure sensory stroke (thalamus).
- Ataxic hemiparesis (weakness and ataxia affecting the same side) due to a pontine lesion.
- Clumsy hand/dysarthria due to a lesion in the pons or internal capsule.

Paradoxical embolic stroke
Embolus from venous thromboembolism entering arterial circulation. Increasingly recognized cause of strokes especially in young:
- Caused by venous thrombosis, e.g. oral contraceptive pill, long plane journey or thrombophilic tendency.
- Cardioembolic stroke, e.g. posterior cerebral artery territory or small cortical infarct.
- Intracardiac shunt identified, e.g. patent foramen ovale (PFO), but this is present in 25% of population. Associated atrial septal aneurysm ↑ risk of stroke.

Investigations

Blood tests (first-line)
- FBC and ESR.
- Ca^{2+} (hypo- or hypercalcaemia may be a cause of focal deficit).
- U&E, creatinine, LFT.
- Glucose.
- Thyroid function.
- Cholesterol.
- Clotting screen.

Blood tests (second-line)
- Thrombophilia screen:
  • protein C, S, and antithrombin III defects;
  • factor V Leiden mutation 20210GA;
  • antiphospholipid antibody; cardiolipin antibody;
  • lupus anticoagulant;
  • IgM, IgG, beta 2 glycoprotein antibody.
- Blood cultures—bacterial endocarditis (BE).
- Homocysteine.
- Lactate.
- Cardiac enzymes.

Other investigations
- Urine analysis (diabetes, haematuria in BE or vasculitis, toxicology screen).
- ECG (AF, MI).
- Echocardiogram and TOE.

Imaging
- Should be performed within 24 hours to exclude haemorrhagic stroke and other causes, e.g. tumours.
- CT: reveals appropriate lesion in 50%.
- Susceptibility weighted imaging (SWI) more sensitive than CT for haemorrhage.
- T_2-weighted images show lesions in 90% by 24 hours.
- Multiple infarcts suggest cardioembolism or vasculitis.
- Diffusion-weighted images (DWIs) show changes within minutes. Useful to distinguish acute from chronic changes (e.g. lacunar infarct from perivascular spaces).
- Imaging of extracranial vessels should be performed in all patients with TIA or mild to moderate stroke:
  - carotid and vertebral ultrasonography;
  - MR or CT angiography (MRA/CTA).

Management of stroke

General management

- Admission to a stroke unit has been shown to reduce mortality by 30% and improve outcome.
- Blood pressure: cerebral autoregulation is disturbed after stroke. Optimal management uncertain but consider treatment if sustained BP > 220/120 in infarction and 185/115 in cerebral haemorrhage. Lower levels in the acute stage should not be treated unless coexistent with hypertensive encephalopathy, aortic dissection, acute MI, or LVF.
- Oxygenation: no data available but O_2 should be given if saturation < 92%.
- Control of blood glucose: hyperglycaemia in acute stroke associated with poor outcome. Maintain normal levels with insulin if necessary.
- Pyrexia is usually due to infection, which should be treated, but may be due to very large infarcts.
- Swallowing and nutrition: if abnormal swallow arrange SALT assessment. Consider NG or PEG tube feeding. Advice from dietician for nutritional support.
- Physiotherapy: early mobilization and rehabilitation to minimize physical deterioration, restore function, and develop strategies for coping with impairment.
- DVT prevention: routine prophylaxis not recommended. Consider LMWH if high risk, e.g. previous DVT. Graded compression stockings— no benefit.
- Seizures occur in 2%—focal or generalized. Conventional AED for recurrent events.
- Depression and neuropsychiatric complications such as emotional lability in 50%. Use TCAs or SSRIs.

Specific treatment of acute stroke

Acute ischaemic stroke

- Thrombolysis: time-dependent benefit up to 4.5 hours. Greatest benefit in first 90 minutes, ↓ subsequently. See 📖 Chapter 3, 'Management of acute ischaemic stroke', pp. 80–3.
  - Patient given TPA, aspirin delayed until after 24 hour post-thrombolysis scan has excluded haemorrhage.
- Antiplatelet drugs:
  - aspirin started within 48 hours ↓ mortality and recurrent stroke.
  - CT first to exclude haemorrhage. Loading dose 300 mg followed by 75 mg daily. If intolerant to aspirin, use clopidogrel.
- Anticoagulation:
  - immediate treatment with heparin reduces DVT and PE but associated with increased risk of cerebral haemorrhage and therefore not recommended.
  - AF or other cardioembolic cause—treat with aspirin and start oral anticoagulation after at least 2 weeks; if TIA and no significant lesion on MRI oral anticoagulation can start immediately;
  - at present no data on heparin in dissection.

Surgery
Malignant middle cerebral territory syndrome
- Occurs in 1–10% of patients with supratentorial hemispheric infarcts.
- Arises 2–5 days after stroke.
- 80% mortality rate.
- Best predictor is early CT hypodensity > 50% of cerebral hemisphere.
- Meta-analysis of three studies of decompressive surgery showed for a modified Rankin score (mRS) ≤ 4 an absolute risk reduction (ARR) of 51%; mRS ≤ 3, ARR 23%; survival irrespective of functional outcome, ARR 50%.
- Although only applicable to a small group of patients, benefits of surgery are clearly established.
- The following should be considered for decompression within 24 hours of presentation:
  - Age < 60 years
  - MCA territory infarct
  - NIHSS > 15
  - Reduced LOC to a score of 1 or more on the 1a criteria of NIHSS
  - Signs on CT > 50% MCA infarct or infarct volume > 145 cc on DWI MRI
- Posterior fossa craniectomy/decompression for large cerebellar infarcts.

Acute intracranial haemorrhage
- Stop anticoagulants and antiplatelet drugs. Correct coagulation deficits.
- Cerebellar haemorrhage may cause hydrocephalus due to aqueduct compression. Referral to neurosurgeon for decompression and/or shunting.
- The STICH trial found no benefit for early clot removal versus conservative management in outcome or mortality at 6 months. Suggestion of subgroup benefit with haematomas 1 cm or less from cortical surface.

Prevention of ischaemic stroke

Primary prevention

Atheroembolism

- Avoidance and treatment of risk factors:
  - hypertension;
  - diabetes;
  - smoking;
  - hypercholesterolaemia.
- Risk of stroke in patients with asymptomatic carotid stenosis is much less than in those with symptomatic stenosis—2% per annum versus 15% in first year.
- The Asymptomatic Carotid Surgery Trial (ACST) found a significant reduction in stroke risk after surgery, but 32 patients would have to be operated upon to prevent one stroke or death over 5 years. A high-risk subgroup who would benefit needs to be identified using specialized radiological techniques.
- Atrial fibrillation: non-rheumatic AF risk of stroke ↑ fivefold. ↑ if other risk factors present:
  - ↑ age;
  - hypertension;
  - impaired LV function;
  - valve disease;
  - diabetes.
  - High risk: 8–12% annual stroke risk if age > 75 years, diabetes, hypertension. Warfarin with target INR 2–3 reduces stroke risk by 60%. If warfarin contraindicated, use aspirin.
  - Low risk: 1% annual stroke risk. If age < 65 years and no other risk factors use aspirin.

Primary intracerebral haemorrhage
Hypertension major risk factor.

Secondary prevention

- Lifestyle changes, e.g. smoking, weight, alcohol reduction, ↑ physical activity.
- BP: PROGRESS trial showed ↓ in haemorrhagic and ischaemic stroke using perindopril and indapamide even if BP normal. Therefore all patients with TIA, stroke, or intracerebral haemorrhage should be started on medication. Medication dependent on co-morbidities. Combination of ACE inhibitor (or angiotensin II receptor antagonist) and calcium channel blocker (or diuretic in the elderly). Aim for BP 130/80. Caution in those with severe bilateral carotid or vertebrobasilar disease. Treatment may not be necessary if BP consistently < 130/70.
- Heart Protection Study (HPS) (simvastatin 40 mg) and Stroke Prevention by Aggressive Reduction in Cholesterol Levels (SPARCL) (atorvastatin 80 mg) suggest prescribing if cholesterol > 3.5 mmol/L or LDL cholesterol > 2.6 mmol/L. Caution in ICH since may ↑ risk of recurrent haemorrhage unless at risk of ischaemic stroke or MI.

- Antiplatelet drugs
  - Aspirin (75–300 mg) reduces risk of recurrent stroke, MI, and vascular death by 13%. If GI side effects add proton pump inhibitor.
  - Clopidogrel (75 mg) may be slightly more effective and should be used in those intolerant of aspirin. Side effects—diarrhoea, skin rash, thrombocytopenia.
  - Dipyridamole probably inferior to aspirin. Combination of aspirin 75 mg + dypiridamole modified release (200 mg bd) is more effective than aspirin alone. Side effect—headache which settles in 2 weeks. Combined preparation available but contains only 25 mg aspirin.
- Warfarin has no benefit for secondary prevention in patients in sinus rhythm.
- AF patients (including paroxymal AF, atrial flutter) should be anticoagulated after stroke. INR between 2 to 3. Novel anticoagulants—dabigatran, apixaban, rivaroxaban at least as effective and safe as warfarin.
- Surgical/endovascular treatment.
  - Carotid endarterectomy highly beneficial in those with > 70% stenosis; moderately beneficial for those with 50–69%.
  - Higher risk of stroke and therefore benefit in those with recent symptoms, ulcerated plaque, and hemisphere presentation rather than amaurosis fugax.
  - Early surgery in the first few weeks (3–6) after TIA or minor stroke becoming more common.
  - Operative mortality 1.1%; operative risk of stroke approximately 5%. Surgery to be done by unit with audited periop mortality and morbidity < 5%.
- Carotid endovascular treatment.
  - For most patients endarterectomy remains preferred choice.
  - Carotid artery stenting associated with increased risk of periprocedure stroke and death in patients > 70 years versus endarterectomy.
  - In < 70 years, stenting may be as effective as endarterectomy.
  - Stenting may be considered for patients not suitable for endarterectomy because of medical, anatomical, or technical issues.

Further reading

Ferro JM, Massaro AR, Mas JL (2010). Aetiological diagnosis of ischaemic stroke in young adults. *Lancet Neurol.*, **9**, 1085–96.

Hankey, GJ (2014). Secondary stroke prevention. *Lancet Neurol.*, **13**, 178–94.

Hankey GJ, Eikelboom J (2010). Antithrombotic drugs for patients with ischaemic stroke and TIA to prevent recurrent major vascular events. *Lancet Neurol.*, **9**, 273–84.

Sudlow C (2008). Preventing further vascular events after a stroke or TIA: an update on medical management. *Pract. Neurol.*, **8**, 141–57.

Cerebral venous thrombosis

Epidemiology
- Incidence 0.22/100 000.
- Most frequent in neonates. Women > men.
- Risk factors:
  - pregnancy and puerperium;
  - oral contraceptive pill;
  - ENT infections;
  - cancer;
  - prothrombotic states;
  - dural AV fistulae.

Clinical features
- ↑ ICP as idiopathic intracranial hypertension:
  - headache;
  - visual obscurations;
  - papilloedema;
  - CN VI palsy.
- Focal neurological deficit:
  - hemiparesis;
  - dysphasia;
  - seizures.
- Diffuse encephalopathy:
  - delirium;
  - coma;
  - seizures;
  - multifocal neurological deficits.
- Cavernous sinus syndrome:
  - CN III, IV, VI, V^1 palsy;
  - proptosis.

Investigations
- Imaging: CT + CT venogram or MRI + MR venogram. See 📖 'Cerebrovascular disease: stroke', pp. 178–81.
- Lumbar puncture not necessary if diagnosis definite after imaging:
  - after exclusion of mass lesion;
  - OP > 20 cm CSF.

Management
- Treat associated infection.
- Anticoagulation with heparin followed by warfarin for 6 months. Lifelong if prothrombotic conditions exist.
- If not responding, or deteriorating, consider local thrombolysis therapy.

- ↑ ICP:
  - repeated LP or external lumbar drain or lumboperitoneal shunt;
  - mannitol;
  - if not responding, or deteriorating consider sedation, ventilation, and decompression craniectomy.
- Seizures: IV phenytoin or valproate.

Further reading

Bousser MG, Ferro J (2007). Cerebral venous thrombosis: an update. *Lancet Neurol.*, **6**, 162–70.
Einhaupl K, Stam J, Bousser MG, et al. (2010). EFNS guideline on the treatment of cerebral venous and sinus thrombosis in adult patients. *Eur. J. Neurol.*, **17**, 1229–35.

Images in cerebrovascular disease

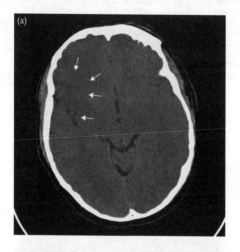

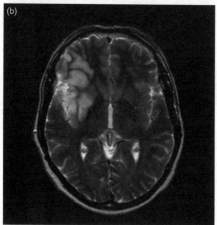

Fig. 5.1 Acute right MCA territory infarct: (a) non-enhanced CT; (b) T$_2$ axial MRI; (c) DWI; (d) ADC map.

Figure 5.1 (a) shows subtle low attenuation in the right inferior frontal gyrus, frontal operculum, insular cortex, and putamen (*white arrows*) consistent with acute ischaemia. (b) The T$_2$ sequence shows gyral expansion, with efface-ment of local CSF spaces and abnormal signal in the corresponding area.

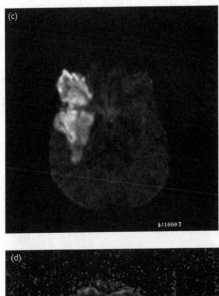

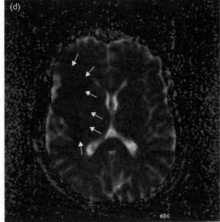

Fig. 5.1 (c) Restriction of diffusion with hyperintensity on DWI and
(d) hypointensity on ADC corresponding to an acute infarct (*white arrows*).

Figure 5.1 (c) and (d) show restriction of diffusion with hyperintensity on DWI
and hypointensity on ADC corresponding to an acute infarct (*white arrows*).

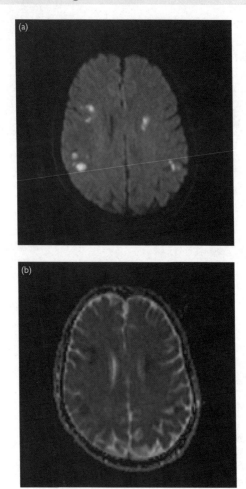

Fig. 5.2 Acute embolic infarcts in patient with atrial fibrillation: (a) DWI axial and (b) ADC map.

Figure 5.2 (a) shows multiple small hyperintense areas on DWI consistent with restriction of diffusion. Figure 5.2 (b) shows matching low signal on the ADC map. Mainly cortical in distribution. Typical appearances for acute embolic infarcts. Subsequent echocardiogram revealed left atrial thrombus.

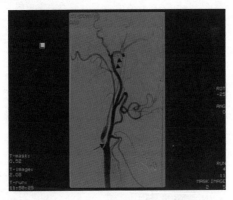

Fig. 5.3 Critical stenosis of internal carotid artery (catheter angiogram).

Figure 5.3 shows tight stenosis at the origin of the ICA with a narrow jet of flow through the stenotic segment (arrow). The calibre of the distal ICA is narrowed due to reduced flow and a degree of vessel collapse (arrowheads).

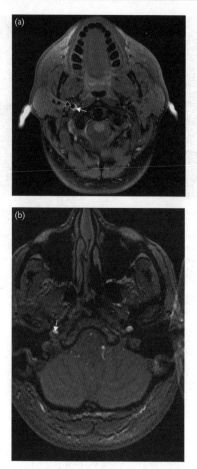

Fig. 5.4 Carotid artery dissection: (a) fat-saturated T_1 axial and (b) axial source image from three-dimensional time-of-flight MRA.

Figure 5.4 (a) shows an expanded right ICA at the skull base with an eccentrically placed lumen, denoted by the flow void (*black arrow*), and a crescent of hyperintensity (methaemoglobin) indicating intramural haematoma (*small white arrows*). Typical appearances of a dissection. In Fig. 5.4 (b) note that the MRA (at a higher level) only demonstrates flow in the eccentric true lumen dissection (*white arrow*).

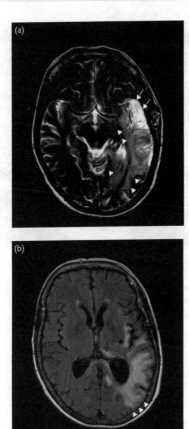

Fig. 5.5 Cerebral vasculitis: (a) axial T$_2$-weighted and (b) axial FLAIR MRI. Extensive area of signal abnormality involving the left temporal, inferior parietal, and occipital lobes with involvement of both grey and white matter.

Figure 5.5 (a) shows a more established area of damage in the lateral and anterior aspects of the left temporal lobe (*white arrows*), while Fig. 5.5 (b) shows more acute involvement in the left inferior parietal lobule/posterior temporal lobe (*white arrowheads*). In (a) there is extensive involvement of the white matter (*white arrowheads*) and in (b) involvement of the left insular cortex (*black arrow*), posterior nuclei of the left thalamus (*open black arrow*), and left occipital lobe. The distribution does not conform to a vascular territory and the disease process has relatively little associated mass effect.

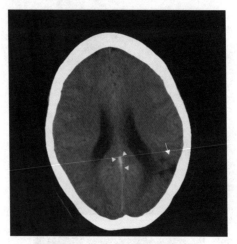

Fig. 5.6 Straight sinus thrombosis (non-enhanced CT).

Figure 5.6 shows a hyperdense and expanded straight sinus (*white arrowheads*). Note the mature venous infarct in the left inferior parietal lobe (*white arrow*).

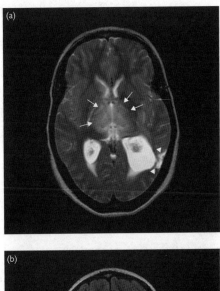

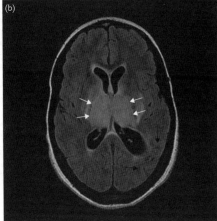

Fig. 5.7 Straight sinus thrombosis: (a) axial T$_2$ and (b) FLAIR.

Figure 5.7 shows abnormal hyperintensity within both thalami and posterior aspects of the lentiform nuclei (*white arrows*). Note the mature damage in the left inferior parietal lobe due to a previous venous infarct (*white arrowheads* T$_2$; *black arrows FLAIR*).

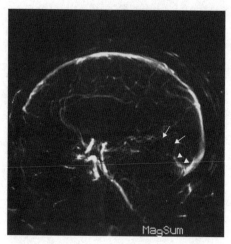

Fig. 5.8 Straight sinus thrombosis (phase contrast MRV).

Figure 5.8 shows absent flow-related signal in the straight sinus in keeping with thrombosis and occlusion (*arrows*). The flow within the distal portion of the straight sinus is preserved (*arrowheads*).

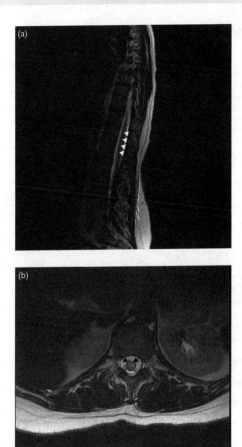

Fig. 5.9 Lower spinal cord infarct: (a) sagittal T$_2$-weighted and (b) axial T$_2$-weighted MRI.

Figure 5.9 shows subtle hyperintensity and expansion is demonstrated in the terminal spinal cord (*closed white arrowheads*). (b) Axial imaging reveals a signal abnormality involving the anterior two-thirds of the cross-sectional profile of the spinal cord (*black arrows*), typical of an anterior spinal artery territory infarct.

Dementia: introduction

Dementia is defined as a syndrome of progressive impairment in two or more areas of cognition sufficient to interfere with work, social function, or relationships. The areas of cognition included in the definition are:

- memory;
- language;
- abstract thinking;
- praxis;
- visuospatial or perceptual skills;
- executive function;
- personality;
- social behaviour.

Epidemiology

At 60 years of age 1% of the population is affected; 40% of those > 85 years. High levels of education may be protective.

Aetiology

Common

Over 65 years

- Alzheimer's disease (AD) (50%).
- Dementia with Lewy bodies (DLB) (20%).
- Frontotemporal dementia (FTD) (10%).
- Vascular dementia (15%).

Under 65 years

- AD (34%).
- Vascular dementia (18%).
- FTD (12%).
- Alcohol-related dementia (10%).
- DLB (7%).
- Other dementias (20%).

Rarer causes

- Corticobasal degeneration (see 📖 'Corticobasal degeneration (CBD)', p. 269).
- CJD.
- CADASIL (cerebral autosomal dominant arteriopathy with subcortical infarcts and leucoencephalopathy).

Treatable causes

- Depressive pseudodementia.
- Normal pressure hydrocephalus.
- B_{12} deficiency.
- Hypothyroidism.
- Syphilis.
- HIV.
- Benign tumours, e.g. subfrontal meningioma.
- Subdural haematoma.
- Obstructive sleep apnoea (OSA) related pseudodementia.

Clinical features

History

- History from patient and relative, carer, or friend.
- Enquire about:
  - Memory problems: forgets names of friends and family; where car parked; recent events; getting lost in familiar environments.
  - Activities of daily living: continue with normal occupation; perform domestic tasks; personal care; operate gadgets (e.g. mobile phone; camera; DVD recorder) as before; make sensible decisions; undertake administrative tasks (e.g. dealing with bills and banks; driving the car).
  - Personality and mental state: change in character; depression; apathy (e.g. stops reading newspapers); changes in personal relationships; impulsive, compulsive, disinhibited, or obsessional behaviour; hallucinations or delusions.
- History of cerebro- and cardiovascular disease.
- Alcohol intake.
- HIV risk?
- Medications.
- Family history, e.g. AD risk ↑ ×4 if one first-degree relative affected, ×8 if two affected.

Examination

- Look for 'head-turning sign'—patients looks to spouse when asked a question.
- Gait: *marche à petits pas* and lower-half parkinsonism (cerebrovascular disease); gait apraxia (NPH); gait ignition failure—difficulty in starting to walk (frontal lobe).
- Focal neurological signs: hemiparesis, visual field defect, primitive reflexes (pout, grasp, rooting).
- Cognitive examination (see Chapter 1, 'Bedside cognitive testing, including language', pp. 24–8).
  - Attention and concentration:
    - count backwards from 20 to 1;
    - months of the year backwards.
  - Language:
    - naming objects;
    - repeating sentence;
    - writing sentence;
    - reading;
    - understanding commands.
  - Memory:
    - orientation;
    - recall (immediate and after 5 minutes);
    - episodic memory (memory for events personally experienced, e.g. birthdays, holidays, funny/sad events);
    - semantic memory (general knowledge about the world, e.g. London capital of England).
- Praxis skills:
  - mime how to comb your hair, use a toothbrush; observe dressing and undressing.

- Executive function (testing ability to plan, organize, abstract reasoning, mental flexibility):
  - verbal fluency test;
  - interpretation of proverbs;
  - cognitive estimates;
  - Luria hand test.

Investigations

First-line

- FBC, ESR.
- Routine chemistry.
- TFT.
- B_{12}.
- VDRL, TPHA.
- CXR.
- MRI (volumetric).
- Neuropsychometric assessment.

Second-line

- CSF examination.
  - beta amyloid 1–42 ↓ 50% in AD; less ↓ in FTD, DLB, and vascular dementia.
  - CSF tau ↑ 2–3x in AD. Also ↑ in FTD, vascular dementia. Specificity 90%, sensitivity 81%.
  - Phosphorylated tau ↑ 2–3x in AD. May be more specific than CSF tau.
- HIV.
- Genetic testing.
- EEG.
- Volumetric MRI.
- SPECT.
- Brain biopsy.

Further reading

Rossor M, Fox NC, Mummery CJ, Schott JM, Warren JD (2010). The diagnosis of young-onset dementia. *Lancet Neurol.*, 9, 793–806.

Alzheimer's disease (AD)

Epidemiology
- Incidence: 1.2 per 1000 person-years among 65–69-year-olds, ↑ to 53.5 in those > 90 years.
- Prevalence 4.4% in those > 65 years.
- Affects F > M.
- Most common > 65 years.

Pathology
Generalized cortical atrophy, especially temporal lobes. Deposits of amyloid A4 protein in cortex with neuritic plaques. Neurofibrillary tangles contain tau and ubiquitin proteins. In cases of amyloid angiopathy, amyloid is found in vessel walls.

Genetics
Familial cases tend to present at a younger age. Familial autosomal dominant cases associated with mutations in three genes:
- APP gene (amyloid precursor protein) on chr 21;
- presenilin 1 and 2;
- apolipoprotein E ϵ4—heterozygotes ↑ risk ×2 of developing AD, homozygotes ↑ risk ×6.

Clinical features
Progressive impairment in at least two cognitive domains that interfere with activities of daily living.
- Memory impairment: episodic (personal experiences) and semantic (store of conceptual and factual knowledge) are affected. Complaints about forgetting day-to-day events, learning new information. Recent past > distant past.
- Visuospatial impairment, e.g. getting lost when driving.
- Constructional and dressing apraxia.
- Language impairment (e.g. word-finding difficulties): alexia, agraphia, acalculia.
- Biparietal variant with deficits in praxis, visuospatial, and visuoperceptual skills. Memory and language only mildly affected early in disease.
- Posterior cortical atrophy variant: visual agnosia, visual disorientation, optic apraxia, simultagnosia, apraxia.
- Presentation with progressive non-fluent aphasia with other deficits appearing later.
- Mini-Mental State Examination (MMSE)—insensitive but practical.
- Physical signs:
  - mild akinetic rigid syndrome;
  - myoclonus.
  - seizures.

Investigations
- MRI to exclude treatable causes (e.g. hydrocephalus).
- Hippocampal volume measurements show correlation with histology. Can be used to monitor disease progression:
  - bilateral hippocampal/entorhinal cortex volume loss disproportionate to atrophy;
  - volume loss with posteroanterior gradient.
- Small vessel white matter hyperintensities on T_2W are common.
- EEG: mild slowing in moderate disease. Non-specific.
- CSF examination (see 📖 'Dementia: introduction', Investigations, p. 200).
- SPECT: bilateral temporal/parietal perfusion/metabolism defects.

Management
- Multidisciplinary team with nurse, counsellor, psychiatrist.
- Essential to consider carer wellbeing.
- Mild cognitive impairment: 10–15% risk of progression to AD. No data on treatment with acetylcholinesterase inhibitors (AChIs).
- AChI and memantine (NMDA receptor antagonist) may improve cognition at least for 6 months. Patients may derive benefit for 2–3 years. If no benefit from one drug, switch. Stop if MMSE < 12. (See Table 5.2 for drugs.)

Table 5.2 Dementia drugs

Drug	Type	Starting dose	Maintenance dose	Side effects
Donepezil	AChI	5 mg od	↑ 10 mg od after 4–6 weeks	Give with meals N&V, diarrhoea, anorexia
Rivastigmine	AChI	1.5 mg bd	↑ 1.5 mg every 2–4 weeks to 3–6 mg bd	N&V, diarrhoea
		4.6 mg/24 hr patch	9.5 mg/24 hr patch	Rash; rotate sites
Galantamine	AChI	4 mg bd	↑ by 4 mg every 2–4 weeks to 12 mg bd	Give with meals N&V, diarrhoea, anorexia
Memantine	NMDA antagonist	5 mg od	↑ by 5 mg every week to 10 mg bd.	Headache, sleepiness, constipation, dizziness

AChI, acetylcholinesterase inhibitor; N&V, nausea and vomiting.

- Psychotic symptoms—consider (initial doses):
  - quetiapine, 12.5–25 mg od;
  - olanzapine, 2.5 mg od;
  - risperidone, 0.25–0.5 mg daily.
- Depression common: consider SSRI (e.g. citalopram 10–40 mg daily).
- Restlessness and agitation: risperidone 0.25 mg or oxazepam 10 mg od–tds.
- Insomnia: temazepam 10–20 mg or zopiclone 3.75–7.5 mg nocte.
- Delirium: exclude medical causes (see 🕮 Chapter 3, 'Delirium', pp. 90–2); haloperidol 0.5 mg od.

Further reading

1. Hort J, O'Brien JT, Gainotti G, et al. (2010). EFNS guideline for the diagnosis and management of Alzheimer's disease. *Eur. J. Neurol.*, **17**, 1236–48.

Frontotemporal dementia (FTD)

Heterogenous group of disorders with variable clinical phenotypes and neuropathology.

Epidemiology
- Second most common cause of early-onset dementia.
- Incidence 9.4–22/100 000.
- Usual onset 45–65 years.
- M = F.

Pathology
Hallmark is selective atrophy of frontal and temporal cortex with neuronal loss, gliosis, and spongiosis.

Two major pathological subtypes:
- FTD with tau-positive inclusions (FTD-tau).
- FTD with ubiquitin positive and TDP 43 positive but tau negative (FTD-TDP).

Genetics
30–50% autosomal dominant inheritance. 50% due to mutations in microtubule-associated protein tau (MAPT) and progranulin (GRN). In familial FTD with MND recent identification of repeat expansion in chromosome 9 orf72 gene.

Clinical features
Behavioural variant FTD (bvFTD)
- Change in personality, social and personal behaviour.
- Apathetic, emotionally blunted.
- Overactive, disinhibited.
- Stereotypic movements, e.g. hand rubbing.
- Perseverative.
- Loss of insight.
- Memory intact.

Progressive non-fluent aphasia (PNFA)
- Pure language deficit.
- Non-fluent effortful speech.
- Loss of prosody.
- Repetition impaired.
- Impairment of well-rehearsed series, e.g. days of the week.
- Anomia.
- Writing affected.
- Comprehension intact.

Note: Alzheimer's patients may develop a similar language disorder in association with abnormalities in other domains.

Semantic dementia (SD)
- Loss of meaning of words.
- Inability to recognize objects and faces.
- Speech is fluent and effortless, but lacks content.
- Semantic paraphasias, e.g. dog for cat.
- Anomia.
- Impaired comprehension.

Note: May be confused with Alzheimer's disease, but memory for day-to-day events and autobiographical details is intact.

Frontotemporal dementia with MND
MND may occur early or late in a subset of patients with FTD. Usually upper limbs and tongue. Rapid progression. Mean survival 3 years.

Investigations
- MRI:
  - bvFTD—atrophy of frontal and paralimbic areas (anterior cingulate, medial frontal, orbitofrontal cortices, hippocampus).
  - SD—asymmetrical atrophy of anterior and inferior lobes, usually left > right.
  - PNFA—inferior frontal lobe and anterior insula, left > right.
- CSF: biomarkers currently unhelpful.

Management
- No drug therapy available.
- Sexual disinhibition may occur. Treat with androgen antagonist (e.g. cimetidine 400 mg od or bd, spironolactone 50 mg od or bd).

Further reading
Seelar H, Rohrer JD, Pijnenburg YA, Fox NC, van Swieten JC (2011). Clinical, genetic and pathological heterogeneity of frontotemporal dementia: a review. *J. Neurol. Neurosurg. Psychiatry*, **82**, 476–86.
Warren JD, Rohrer JD, Rossor MN (2013). Frontotemporal dementia. *BMJ*, **347**, 28–35.

Other dementias

Dementia with Lewy bodies (DLB) and Parkinson's disease dementia (PDD) (occurs in 40% of PD patients). Arbitrarly, PDD if dementia starts one year after parkinsonism.

Epidemiology
Usually sporadic. Most commonly elderly patients.

Pathology
Generalized atrophy, depigmentation of substantia nigra. Lewy body inclusions in cortical neurons. 40% have amyloid deposits.

Clinical features
• Levodopa responsive parkinsonism (less severe in DLB than PDD).
• Cortical symptoms—aphasia, apraxia.
• Fluctuating mental state, e.g. daytime drowsiness.
• Visual hallucinations (animals or humans) and illusions.
• Very sensitive to neuroleptic drugs.
• REM sleep behaviour disorder.
• Autonomic disorder—orthostatic hypotension, bladder disturbance, constipation, impotence.

Investigations
MRI: generalized atrophy. Absence of significant temporal atrophy in a demented patient suggests DLB.

Management
For psychotic symptoms: rivastigmine 1.5–6 mg bd.

Vascular dementia

Epidemiology
Usually > 40 years. Risk factors include hypertension, smoking, vascular disease.

Pathology
Multiple infarcts in cortical and subcortical areas or fibrous and hyaline degeneration of small arteries leading to white matter infarction.

Clinical features
• Recurrent stepwise deterioration.
• Pyramidal signs.
• Pseudobulbar palsy.
• When mainly subcortical disease, slowly progressive syndrome with dysarthria, (lower-half) parkinsonism, gait disorder (*marche à petits pas*) = subcortaical arteriosclerotic dementia.

Investigations
MRI: areas of typical infarction. In subcortical dementia widespread leucoaraiosis, mainly anterior and periventricular.

CADASIL[1]

Clinical features

- Stroke-like episodes.
- Cognitive impairment in variable cognitive domains.
- Strongly associated with migraine.

Investigations

- MRI: extensive white matter T_2W signal change involving the temporal lobes, especially anteriorly, and the subinsular region.
- Genetics: Notch 3 mutation on chromosome 19.

Reference

1 Chabriat H, Joutel A, Dichgans M, Tournier-Lasserve E, Bousser MG (2009). CADASIL. *Lancet Neurol.*, **8**, 643–53.

Creutzfeldt–Jakob disease (CJD)

CJD is a human transmissible spongiform encephalopathy. The prion protein (PrP) gene contains a polymorphic locus at codon 129 encoding methionine or valine. Important in determining susceptibility to sporadic and acquired forms.

- Sporadic CJD, 85–90% cases.
- Familial forms, 10–15% cases:
  - familial CJD;
  - Gerstmann–Sträussler–Scheinker;
  - fatal familial insomnia.
- Iatrogenic CJD (human pituitary derivatives, dura mater and corneal grafts), 1%.
- Variant CJD.

Sporadic CJD

Incidence and epidemiology

One per million per year. In UK 60 cases per annum. Mean age of onset 65 years (range 15–94 years). Peak age group, 7th decade. No sex difference; no definite environmental risk factors identified; similar incidence worldwide. 75% methionine homozygous (MM) at codon 129, 15% heterozygous (MV), 10% valine homozygous (VV).

Pathology

Random misfolding in the prion protein (PrP) or somatic mutation in encoding gene causes the disease. Key pathological features in the brain: spongiform changes, neuronal loss, astrocytosis. PrP deposition demonstrated by immunocytochemistry.

Clinical features

- Rapidly progressive dementia.
- Cerebellar ataxia.
- Myoclonus.
- Pyramidal and extrapyramidal signs.
- Amyotrophy (rare).
- Cortical blindness (rare).

Differential diagnosis

- Alzheimer's disease.
- Cerebral vasculopathy—inflammatory, lymphoma.
- Chronic encephalitis—Hashimoto's encephalitis, SSPE.
- Paraneoplastic encephalitis.

Investigations

- MRI: putamen and caudate hyperintensity on FLAIR and DWI (see Fig. 5.10(a)).
- EEG: periodic triphasic complexes (60%). May be normal early in disease.
- CSF: normal WCC, protein, moderate elevation. ↑ brain-specific protein 14-3-3 (95% sensitivity, but specificity only 28%). (Note: also ↑ if WCC ↑, recent seizures, traumatic brain injury, stroke, AD, encephalitis, paraneoplastic syndromes.)
  - CSF tau 86% sensitivity, 67% specificity.
  - Blood-stained CSF leads to false-positive results.

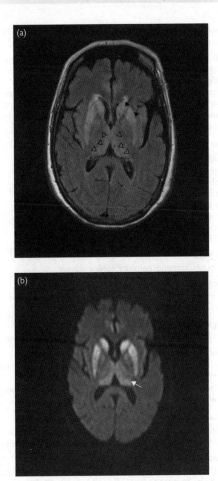

Fig. 5.10 Sporadic Creutzfeldt–Jakob disease (sCJD). (a) FLAIR axial and (b) diffusion-weighted (DWI) MRI.

- Prion genetics even if inherited form not suspected from family history.
- PrP gene codon 129 polymorphism status.

Figure 5.10 shows bilateral symmetric hyperintensity involving the striatal nuclei (*black arrows*) with less prominent involvement of the pulvinar and medial nuclei of the thalami bilaterally (*open black arrowheads*). (b) Note the more conspicuous signal change and increased sensitivity on DWI. In contrast, variant CJD (vCJD) typically demonstrates marked hyperintensity in the pulvinar and medial nuclei of the thalami bilaterally as the most prominent feature—the 'hockey-stick' sign (*white arrow*).

Diagnosing sporadic CJD

Diagnostic criteria

I. Rapidly progressive dementia (if > 2 years diagnosis doubtful).
II. Group of symptoms including:
  - myoclonus;
  - visual or cerebellar symptoms;
  - pyramidal or extrapyramidal features;
  - akinetic mutism.
III. Typical EEG.

Definite diagnosis

Neuropathology/immunochemistry confirmed.

Probable diagnosis

Criterion I plus at least two from criterion II plus criterion III, or 'possible diagnosis' plus positive for protein 14-3-3.

Possible diagnosis

Criterion I plus at least two from criterion II and duration < 2 years.

Management

Supportive. Myoclonus treated with clonazepam, valproate, or piracetam. Results of PRION-1 study: quinacrine (300 mg) an observational study of 107 cases (mixture of sporadic, iatrogenic, variant, and inherited) did not affect clinical outcome.

Variant Creutzfeldt–Jakob disease (vCJD)

vCJD is the human form of bovine spongiform encephalopathy (BSE). Dietary transmission by ingestion of cow products most likely source.

Incidence and epidemiology

In UK 176 (definite/probable) cases (December 2011). Size of future epidemic unknown. Younger patients affected: typically 14–50 years, although older patients reported. All homozygous MM at codon 129.

Pathology

Florid amyloid plaques in cerebrum and cerebellum; spongiform change in caudate and putamen; accumulation of abnormal PrP demonstrated by immunocytochemistry. Widespread accumulation of abnormal PrP in lymphoid tissue (tonsils and spleen).

Clinical features (early)
- Psychiatric symptoms:
  - depression;
  - withdrawal;
  - aggression and irritability;
  - anxiety, fear;
  - hallucinations and delusions.
- Sensory symptoms (thalamic):
  - limb pain;
  - paraesthesiae and dysaesthesiae;
  - numbness;
  - cold or burning sensations.

Later features
- Ataxia.
- Movement disorders—myoclonus, choreiform movements, dystonia.
- Cognitive impairment.
  Progression is slower than for sCJD—mean duration 14 months.

Differential diagnosis
- Wilson's disease (copper, caeruloplasmin levels, 24 hour urinary copper, slit-lamp exam for Kayser–Fleischer rings).
- Alzheimer's disease.
- Cerebral vasculitis.
- Vitamin B_{12} deficiency.
- Infective encephalitis.
- Paraneoplastic syndrome.

Investigations
- MRI: bilateral, symmetrical high signal in the posterior thalamus ('pulvinar sign') (see Fig. 5.10(b)).
- EEG: normal or non-specifically abnormal. Triphasic complexes not seen.
- CSF: normal WCC; protein mild–moderate elevation. 14-3-3 ↑ in 50%. Less sensitive than for sCJD.
- PrP gene codon 129 status.
- Tonsil biopsy may be considered but is not routine. A positive tonsillar biopsy does *not* make a diagnosis of 'definite vCJD'.
- Brain biopsy only if there is a possibility of a treatable disorder that cannot be diagnosed by other methods (e.g. vasculitis).

Management
- Supportive and palliative.
- vCJD is not transmissible by ordinary contact or body fluids but invasive procedures require specific precautions.

Further reading

Knight R, Will R (2004). Prion diseases. *J. Neurol. Neurosurg. Psychiatry*, **75**, 136–42.
Puoti G, Bizzi A, Forloni G, Safar JG, Tagliavini F, Gambetti P (2012). Sporadic human prion diseases: molecular insights and diagnosis. *Lancet Neurol.*, **11**, 618–28.

Epilepsy: introduction

Defined as the tendency to have recurrent seizures. Epilepsy is a manifestation of underlying brain disease. Single seizures or those occurring during acute illness should not be classified as epilepsy.

Incidence

50 per 100 000 per year; 1 in 200 have active epilepsy (in UK, 350 000). Higher incidence in developing countries.

Aetiology

In UK, community surveys show:
- cerebrovascular disease, 15%;
- cerebral tumour, 6%;
- alcohol-related, 6%;
- post-traumatic, 2%;
- genetic disorders, 1%.

Other causes include hippocampal sclerosis, and cortical and vascular malformations. In the tropics, neurocysticercosis is a common cause.

Classification

Basic classification is between generalized (50%) and focal (50%), subdivided into aetiological categories.
- Idiopathic (genetic predisposition with normal development, examination, and EEG).
- Symptomatic (structural abnormality).
- Cryptogenic (structural abnormality supposed but not proven).

Classification of epilepsy (modified abbreviated classification of the International League Against Epilepsy)

Generalized epilepsies and syndromes
- Idiopathic with age-related onset:
  - childhood absence epilepsy;
  - juvenile myoclonic epilepsy (JME);
  - epilepsy with generalized tonic–clonic (T/C) seizures on wakening.
- Symptomatic and cryptogenic:
  - West's syndrome;
  - Lennox–Gastaut syndrome;
  - epilepsy with myoclonic absences.
- Symptomatic
  - myoclonic encephalopathy.

Focal epilepsies and syndromes
- Idiopathic with age-related onset:
  - benign childhood epilepsy with centrotemporal spikes;
  - reading epilepsy.

- Symptomatic:
  - epilepsy with simple partial, complex partial, or secondarily generalized seizures arising from any part of the cortex;
  - epilepsia partialis continua (EPC);
  - syndromes characterized by specific activation.

Undetermined epilepsies and syndromes (focal or generalized)
Epilepsy with continuous spike and wave activity in sleep.

Clinical features

Seizures are paroxysmal stereotypic events. Diagnosis is clinical; eyewitness accounts are crucial. Usually followed by a period of drowsiness. See 📖 Chapter 4, 'Loss of consciousness', pp. 136–7.

Triggers include:
- alcohol;
- fatigue;
- sleep deprivation;
- infections;
- hypoglycaemia;
- stress;
- strobe lighting (photosensitive epilepsy);
- reading, hot water (rare).

Childhood absences
- Rare after age 10 years.
- F > M.
- Brief loss of awareness many times a day. Triggered by hyperventilation.
- Remits in adulthood.
- EEG characteristic—3 Hz spike and wave, no photosensitivity.

Juvenile myoclonic epilepsy (JME)
- Onset before age 30 years.
- Myoclonic jerks in the morning.
- Typical absences.
- Generalized tonic–clonic seizures.
- EEG typical with generalized spike and wave ± photosensitivity.
- Remission rare.

Complex partial seizures
- Associated with underlying structural abnormality, e.g. hippocampal sclerosis, DNET.
- Automatisms (lip-smacking, chewing, swallowing, stereotypical hand movements).
- Déjà vu and jamais vu.
- Olfactory auras (unpleasant).
- Unusual behaviour or emotionality.

Investigations
- Blood investigations:
  - FBC, ESR;
  - renal, liver function, calcium, glucose;

- ECG (rare: ↑ QT interval presenting as morning generalized T/C seizures) (see 📖 Chapter 6, 'Neurological symptoms: cardiac disease', pp. 396–9).
- MRI with specific views of hippocampi if complex partial seizures. Abnormal in 30% of generalized epilepsies and 70% of focal epilepsies. See 📖 Chapter 9.
- EEG (see 📖 Chapter 8, 'EEG and epilepsy', pp. 534–7). Useful in classification of epilepsy but not in the diagnosis of patients who present with loss of consciousness.

Management of epilepsy

General advice

- Tell the patient that it is their duty to inform the DVLA. See
  ℰ <http://www.gov.uk/current-medical-guidelines-dvla-guidance-
  for-professionals>.
- The DVLA defines epilepsy as 2 or more seizures in a 5 year period.
  Group 1 (private car or motorcycle):
  (a) Patients with epilepsy must not drive for 12 months after the last
  seizure.
  (b) A person who has suffered an attack whilst asleep must also
  refrain from driving for at least one year from date of attack. If they
  have had an attack whilst asleep more than three years previously
  and have had no attacks whilst awake since that original attack they
  may be licensed even though attacks asleep continue. If an attack
  whilst awake occurs, one year off driving.
  (c) First seizure: 6 months off driving unless > 20% chance of
  recurrence (abnormal imaging and/or EEG) in which case 12 months.
- Group 2 (lorries, buses, and coaches): see DVLA regulations as higher
  standards required.
- Avoid unsafe activities, e.g. swimming alone, mountain climbing.
- Take showers rather than baths.
- Place guards against open fire places and radiators.

Starting treatment

Single seizures

No treatment unless there is a high risk of recurrence, e.g. abnormal EEG as
in JME or an abnormal MRI. If precipitating factors (e.g. alcohol) identified,
avoidance may prevent recurrence.

After a single unprovoked seizure, risk of recurrence without treatment
is 18–23% with no cause and normal EEG, and 65% if associated with a
neurological abnormality + abnormal EEG.

Prophylaxis

No indication for starting treatment in patients with head injuries, craniotomy, or brain tumours unless seizures occur. In these situations, if patients
on dexamethasone consider using a non-enzyme-inducing drug such as levetiracetam or lamotrigine to avoid drug interaction.

Drug treatment

Aim of treatment is to render patient seizure-free with minimal side effects.
Other factors include sudden unexpected death in epilepsy (SUDEP)—1/200/
year in refractory epilepsy. See Table 5.3 for first- and second-line drugs.

- Factors to be taken into account:
  - age;
  - sex;
  - type of epilepsy;
  - other drugs, e.g. contraceptive pill;
  - other medical conditions, e.g. liver or renal dysfunction.
- Treatment is initiated at low dose gradually titrating to an effective level
  to avoid side effects ('start low, go slow'). See Table 5.4.

Table 5.3 First- and second-line drugs for different types of epilepsy

Type of epilepsy	First-line	Adjunctive AEDS	Notes
Generalized tonic–clonic	Valproate, lamotrigine, carbamazepine, oxcarbazepine	Clobazam, lamotrigine, levetiracetam, valproate, topiramate	Lamotrigine may exacerbate myoclonic seizures. Carbamazepine, oxcarbazepine may exacerbate myoclonic or absence seizures
Focal with or without 2° generalization	Lamotrigine, carbamazepine, levetiracetam, oxcarbazepine, valproate	Carbamazepine, clobazam, gabapentin, lamotrigine, levetiracetam, oxcarbazepine, valproate	Other drugs: tiagabine, zonisamide, lacosamide, pregabalin, phenytoin
Myoclonic seizures	Levetiracetam, valproate, topiramate	Levetiracetam, valproate, topiramate	Other drugs: clobazam, clonazepam, piracetam, zonisamide
JME	Lamotrigine, levetiracetam, valproate, topiramate	Lamotrigine, levetiracetam, valproate, topiramate	Other drugs: clobazam, clonazepam, zonisamide

- If seizures continue, increase dose to maximum tolerated. If seizures still continue, withdraw first drug and try another first-line drug.
- If unsuccessful, adjunctive treatment with a second-line drug should be considered.

Drug monitoring
- Measuring drug levels is indicated in the following situations:
  - suspected poor or erratic compliance;
  - symptoms of toxicity, e.g. nausea, ataxia, confusion, diplopia.
- Valproate levels are only of use for monitoring compliance. Blood levels do not correlate with therapeutic levels as valproate is highly fat-soluble.
- Carbamazepine and valproate are accepted as first-line recommendations for partial (with or without 2° generalization) and generalized seizures, respectively.
- Lamotrigine is used for both types of seizures in women of child-bearing age.

Table 5.4 Antiepileptic drugs: dosages, and side-effects

AED	Dose	Side-effects
Carbamazepine (SR form)*	Start 100 mg/day. ↑ at 2-week intervals 100–200 mg until control achieved. Usually 400–1600 mg/day	Rash, neutropenia, conduction defects, SIADH, numerous drug interactions. May make myoclonus worse. Liver enzyme inducing. Note COC
Sodium valproate	Start 200 mg bd. ↑ at 2-weekly intervals. Max 2.5 g/day. CR form available for od use	Rash, tremor, weight gain, hair loss, pancreatitis, menstrual changes (PCOS), ↓ platelets. ↑ NH_3, encephalopathy, hepatotoxicity, teratogenicity. ↓ IQ in offspring
Lamotrigine*	Start 25 mg/day as monotherapy; ↑ 50 mg 2–weekly. If adjunct to valproate, start 25 mg alternate days for 2 weeks, ↑ 25 mg 2-weekly. Maximum dose, 400 mg/day	Rash, especially with valproate. Multisystem allergic disorder, liver failure, aplastic anaemia
Topiramate	Start 25 mg/day; ↑ 25 mg 2-weekly. Maximum dose 400 g/day	Weight loss, memory problems, renal calculi, paraesthesiae
Levetiracetam	Start 250 mg/day, ↑ 2-weekly. Maximum dose 3 g/day	Weakness, irritability, mood swings. Rare: ↑ seizures
Phenytoin	Start 100 mg/day, then monitor levels to ↑ dose 2-weekly. Note: First-order kinetics—small dose increase → large changes in levels	Gum hypertrophy, acne, hirsutism, coarse facies, osteomalacia, ataxia

* Do FBC, U&E, LFT before starting drug.

- Other add-on therapies available:
  - gabapentin;
  - tiagabine;
  - pregabalin;
  - zonisamide
  - lacosamide.
- Phenytoin and phenobarbital are effective but little used because of long-term side effects. Only indication is in status epilepticus as they can be given IV.
- Clobazam useful adjunct in the short term, especially when cluster seizures occur, e.g. perimenstrually. Dose, 10–20 mg bd.
- Currently controversy regarding osteopenia/osteoporosis and AEDs, especially enzyme inducers. Consider bone scan and vitamin D levels in those with multiple risk factors (age, post-menopause, previous fractures, poor diet, steroids).

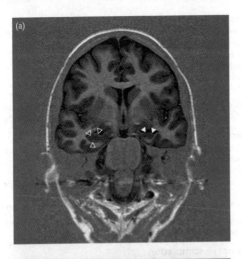

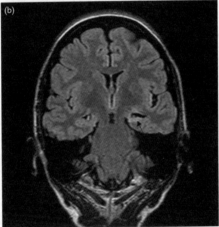

Fig. 5.11 Hippocampal sclerosis: (a) thin-section gradient echo T$_1$-weighted volume; (b) thin-section coronal FLAIR MRI.

Prognosis with drug treatment

By 12 months 60–70% will be seizure-free. After 2 years, withdrawal of drugs can be considered. Predictive factors for relapse:

- syndromic epilepsy, e.g. JME;
- underlying structural pathology;
- severe prolonged epilepsy before remission;
- ↑ age.

Factors that may affect the decision to stop include driving. Patients are advised to stop driving during drug withdrawal and for 6 months thereafter.

Surgery

Should be considered, and patients referred to a specialist centre, in cases with:

- surgically resectable lesion, e.g. DNET;
- temporal lobe seizures where there is evidence of mesial temporal sclerosis (see Fig. 5.11 which shows typical reduction in volume (*white arrowheads*) and hyperintensity (*black arrow*) of the left hippocampus).

In such patients seizure-free rates are 80%, with 3–4% permanent neurological deficit and 1% mortality rates.

Vagus nerve stimulation

An option with no serious side-effects in those with refractory epilepsy, and unsuitable for surgery.

Further reading

Brodie MJ, Kwan P (2012). Newer drugs for focal epilepsy in adults. *BMJ*, **344**, 49–54.

Delgado Nunes V. et al. (2012). Diagnosis and management of the epilepsies in adults and children: summary of updated NICE guidance. *BMJ*, **344**, 47–49.

NICE Clinical Guideline 137 (Jan 2012). The epilepsies: the diagnosis and management of the epilepsies in adults and children in primary and secondary care.

Smith D, Chadwick D (2001). The management of epilepsy. *J. Neurol. Neurosurg. Psychiatry*, **70**, 15–21.

Smith PE (2008). Bare essentials: epilepsy. *Pract. Neurol.*, **8**, 195–202.

Women and epilepsy

Contraception

- Carbamazepine, oxcarbazepine, phenytoin, phenobarbital, primidone, and topiramate (enzyme-inducing drugs) ↓ blood levels of oestrogen and progestogen.
- Sodium valproate, gabapentin, tiagabine, levetiracetam, zonisamide, lacosamide and pregabalin do not affect levels. Recent controversy regarding lamotrigine levels ↓ by COC.
- Recommend COC with at least 50 micrograms oestrogen if on enzyme-inducing drugs. Breakthrough bleeding implies inadequate dose.
- Progestogen-only pill (POP) similarly affected. Recommend change of contraception or use depot injection (Depo-Provera® 150 mg/12 weeks).

Fertility

- Women with epilepsy have lower fertility rates due to multiple factors, e.g. sexual dysfunction in those with temporal lobe epilepsy (TLE).
- Valproate is associated with polycystic ovarian syndrome.

Pregnancy

- Pre-conception counselling essential.
- 90% chance of a normal child and 95% chance of not having a major malformation.
- Start folic acid supplements 5 mg/day to ↓ risks of neural tube defects (NTDs), especially with valproate and carbamazepine.
- Risks and benefits of stopping drug, at least for first trimester, need discussion.
- Lowest possible dose should be used, e.g. risk of spina bifida with valproate significantly reduced if dose < 1000 mg/day. Consider using controlled release preparation to ↓ peak levels.
- Teratogenicity:
  - Incidence of fetal abnormality in general population 2–3%. Risk ↑ to 4–6% with single AED. ↑ with multiple drug therapy.
  - UK Epilepsy and Pregnancy Register: absolute rate of *major* congenital malformations—carbamazepine 2.6%, lamotrigine 3.2%, valproate 6.2%.
  - Valproate has dose-dependent adverse effect of children's neurodevelopment. No such effect shown with carbamazepine. Carbamazepine seems best drug in pregnancy if there is choice (e.g. not recommeded for JME). Contributes to risk of posterior cleft palate.
  - Patients on valproate and carbamazepine should have a series of high-definition USSs to detect anencephaly (11 weeks), NTD (16–18 weeks), congenital cardiac defects (18–20 weeks).
  - Alpha-fetoprotein levels at 18 weeks for NTD.

Epilepsy during pregnancy
- 20% ↑ fits, 50% unchanged, 25% ↓ seizures.
- Carbamazepine, valproate, phenytoin levels ↓ but free drug levels ↑. If well controlled, no changes necessary. Measure levels (free levels if possible) at presentation, so that if fits occur dose changes can be made. Any dose increases may need reversal after delivery.
- Lamotrigine clearance ↑. Dose ↑ necessary.
- First fit during pregnancy needs investigation:
  - eclampsia;
  - higher incidence of structural lesions, e.g. meningioma, AVM;
  - SAH;
  - arterial and venous thromboses.

During labour
Risk of seizure 3% due to lack of compliance, fatigue, dehydration, lack of sleep. Lorazepam can be used.

Vitamin K
Enzyme-inducing drugs (carbamazepine, phenytoin, phenobarbital) affect clotting synthesis. Require vitamin K, 20 mg/day starting 1 month before delivery. Neonate given 1 mg IM at delivery.

Breastfeeding
Only phenobarbital and primidone found in breast milk at high enough concentrations to cause drowsiness.

Further reading
Jackson M (2006). Epilepsy in women. *Pract. Neurol.*, **6**, 166–79.

Seizures versus dissociative non-epileptic attack disorder (NEAD) or pseudoseizures

A major cause of misdiagnosis of epilepsy. However, some patients may have both types of attack. 50% of status cases may be NEAD.

Clinical features of NEAD

- Usually female (ratio 8:1).
- History of childhood physical and/or sexual abuse.
- Triggered by stress.
- Not responsive to multiple drug trials.
- Frequent admissions to hospital.
- Other non-diagnosed physical symptoms.

Differential diagnosis

See Table 5.5.

Investigations

In cases of doubt, videotelemetry helps in diagnosis.

Management

- Establish diagnosis with certainty.
- Explain that the attack is an unconscious response to some form of stress.
- Relaxation techniques, cognitive behaviour therapy.
- Consider withdrawal of AED.

Table 5.5 Charateristics of NEAD compared with those of epileptic seizures

Characteristic	NEAD	Epileptic seizures
Triggered by anger, panic, suggestion	Common	Rare
Onset	Gradual	Sudden
Duration	Prolonged, hours	Minutes
Breathing	Continuous	Apnoeic
Colour	Normal	Cyanosed
Retained consciousness	Yes, elevate arm above face and drop. Patient usually avoids falling on to face. Vibrating tuning fork inserted gently into nostril will wake most patients	Rare
Unusual movements	Pelvic thrusting, back arching, erratic movements. Fighting if held down	Unusual
Eyes	Resistance to forced eye opening	No resistance
Occur in company	Common	Unusual
Tongue biting	Rare	Common
Self-injury	Rare	Common
Incontinence	Rare	Common
Post-ictal confusion	Rare	Common
Prolactin levels before and 20 minutes after	No rise	Elevation but may be normal after prolonged status
Post-ictal EEG	Normal	Slowing

Headache: migraine—introduction and clinical features

Epidemiology

- Common. Prevalence in women 18%; men 6%.
- Mean age of onset 19 years.
- 46% have a family history. Risk of a child developing migraine 70% if both parents are affected, 45% when one parent affected.
- A rare dominantly inherited condition, familial hemiplegic migraine, due to a mutation on chromosome 19 that codes for a subunit of the voltage-gated calcium channel.
- Cerebral autosomal dominant arteriopathy with subcortical infarcts and leucoencephalopathy (CADASIL) may present with hemiplegic migraine and progress to an ischaemic encephalopathy.

Pathophysiology

Migraine is a neurovascular disorder in a genetically predisposed individual. Predisposition is an instability within the trigeminovascular network originating in the brainstem, in particular the dorsal midbrain and dorsolateral pons. Diffuse projections from the locus caeruleus to the cerebral cortex result in impaired cerebral cortical blood flow causing the spreading depression associated with migranous auras.

Clinical features

- Migraine is an episodic headache usually associated with nausea (± vomiting) and photophobia.
- May be preceded by focal neurological symptoms. The aura may not necessarily be followed by headache (previously known as migraine equivalents).
- 30% may have other coexisting headaches, e.g. tension and analgesic overuse headaches.

Headache features

- Unilateral in two-thirds of patients and bilateral in one-third.
- Pain felt behind or along the inner angle of the eye or frontotemporal regions.
- Radiates back to the occiput or the neck.
- Site of headache may be either ipsilateral or contralateral to the focal neurological disturbance.
- Occasional patients may complain of limb pain ipsilateral to the side of the headache.
- Character of the headache is dull at onset and later throbbing (increasing with each pulse). Other patients may only describe a constant headache or even a slight muzzy headache.
- Made worse with movement.

Aura features

- Visual auras include visual hallucinations, scotomas, and fortification spectra (zigzag lines resembling a fortified wall when viewed from above) or teichopsia. Usually white, and shimmer or jitter and move

across the visual field leaving behind an area of impaired vision—scintillating scotomas.
- Other visual phenomena include flashes of light (photopsia).
  Note: Occipital lobe epilepsy causes hallucinations that are circular or of geometric shapes and multicoloured.
- Sensory auras are usually positive, i.e. paraesthesiae rather than numbness, and spread over minutes or hours (5%).
- Other auras: hemiparesis (marching over minutes or hours), dysphasia, olfactory and gustatory hallucinations, and distortion of body parts such as sensation of tongue swelling.

Migraine triggers
- Dehydration (need to have intake of 1.5 L/day).
- Stress and relaxation after stress.
- Sleep: either lack of or unaccustomed excess (lying in).
- Trauma (especially in children).
- Sensory stimulation: glare, flickering lights, smells (e.g. certain perfumes).
- Food and eating habits: missing a meal (hypoglycaemia). Foods including red wine, cheese, chocolate.
- Food additives: monosodium glutamate.
- Caffeine.
- Exercise.
- Excess heat and dehydration.
- Drugs: vasodilators such as glyceryl trinitrate.
- Changes in barometric pressure such as those preceding a thunderstorm.

Migraine variants

Vertebrobasilar migraine
Brainstem symptoms: diplopia, vertigo, incoordination, ataxia, and dysarthria occur in posterior circulation migraine attacks. May also be fainting or loss of consciousness due to involvement of the midbrain reticular formation. In severe cases a stuporous or comatose state may last for a week (migraine stupor). Most cases are associated with other vertebrobasilar symptoms.

Ophthalmoplegic migraine
Extra-ocular paresis—the CN III is most often affected. Paresis may last for days or weeks. Exclude a compressive lesion such as a posterior communicating artery aneurysm.

Retinal migraine
Unusual variant results from constriction of retinal arterioles impairing vision in one eye and is associated with headache behind the same eye. Compressive lesions and a TIA must be excluded.

Benign recurrent vertigo
Increasingly recognized. Migraineurs have abnormalities of the vestibular system. Attacks of vertigo and unsteadiness (may be accompanied by tinnitus, deafness, and headache). Management: anti-migraine therapy, e.g. beta-blockers.

Migraine: differential diagnosis, investigations, and IHS criteria

Differential diagnosis
- Headache occurs in 15% of patients with TIA, 25% with acute ischaemic stroke, 50% with acute intracerebral haemorrhage.
- Other causes of headache with focal neurological disturbance:
  - temporal arteritis;
  - dissection of the carotid and vertebral arteries;
  - meningoencephalitis may resemble an acute migraine attack.
    Note: A lymphocytic pleocytosis may be found in the CSF during a migraine attack.

Investigations

Imaging studies detect a significant abnormality in < 0.5% patients with migraine and a normal neurological examination. Therefore not usually indicated. MRI scans in migraine patients, with and without auras, may reveal small non-specific white matter lesions in 30% of individuals under the age of 40 years. The IHS critera for migraine are shown in Box 5.1.

Box 5.1 Abbreviated International Headache Society (IHS) criteria for migraine

Migraine without aura

a) Headache lasting 4 hours to 3 days.
b) Nausea/vomiting and/or light and noise sensitivity.
c) Two of the following:
  • unilateral pain;
  • moderate or severe intensity pain;
  • aggravation by simple physical activity;
  • pulsating pain.

Migraine with aura

At least three of the following:
• reversible focal brainstem or cortical dysfunction;
• aura develops over > 4 minutes or two auras in succession;
• each aura < 60 minutes;
• headache < 60 minutes following aura.

Suggested criteria for chronic or transformed migraine

a) Daily or almost daily (> 15 days/month) head pain > 1 month.
b) Average headache duration > 4 hours/day (untreated).
c) At least one of the following:
  • a previous history of IHS migraine;
  • history of increasing headache frequency with decreasing severity of migrainous features over at least 3 months;
  • currrent superimposed attacks of headache that meet all the IHS criteria except duration.

Management of acute migraine: the stepped care regimen

Simple analgesia with antiemetics

If nausea and vomiting are not a major symptom, as gastric motility is impaired during a migraine attack.

- Aspirin 900–1200 mg (dissolved) + metoclopramide 10mg or domperidone 10–20 mg.
- Alternative drugs include paracetamol 1000 mg and NSAIDS, e.g. ibuprofen (400–800 mg), naproxen (500–1000 mg), diclofenac (25–50 mg).
- Warn patients of risk of analgesic overuse headache, especially codeine-containing drugs, which results in chronic daily headache.

Triptans

- All drugs in this class (sumatriptan, zolmitriptan, naratriptan, rizatriptan, eletriptan, almotriptan, frovatriptan) have a high efficacy with up to 70% having a response within 2 hours and 40% being pain-free at 2 hours (see Table 5.6).
- Zolmitriptan and rizatriptan available as wafers—do not have necessarily faster action of action.
- Sumatriptan available as nasal spray and injection.
- Drugs work best when taken early, but not during the prodrome or the aura phase.
- Headache recurrence within 12–24 hours occurs in 30%.
- Usual advice is to take a further dose of triptan if headache recurs after 2 hours.
- Some evidence for synergistic benefit using combination of 5-HT agonist + NSAID.
- If no response after three attacks, try another triptan. If three oral triptans fail, try nasal spray or SC sumatriptan.
- Warn patients that overuse may result in chronic daily headache.
- Contraindications: coronary artery disease, cerebrovascular disease, uncontrolled hypertension, peripheral vascular disease, significant hepatic impairment, and pregnancy.
- Side effects: chest discomfort or heaviness; jaw, shoulder, and neck tightness; paraesthesiae; fatigue and dizziness.
- Drug interactions: avoid MAOIs. Propranolol ↑ serum concentration of rizatriptan. Therefore use 5 mg dose. Possible serotonin syndrome when used with SSRIs (tremor, palpitations, flushing, hypertension, agitation).

Table 5.6 Triptan characteristics

More rapid onset	Lower recurrence rate, lower side effects
Sumatriptan 50–100 mg	Naratriptan 2.5 mg
Rizatriptan 5–10 mg	Frovatriptan 2.5 mg
Zolmitriptan 2.5 mg	
Eletriptan 40–80 mg	
Almotriptan 12.5 mg	

Ergotamine preparations

- Still a role for considering ergotamine tartrate in, for example, those patients intolerant to 5-HT agonists. 1–2 mg alone or in combination with caffeine may be given orally at onset or used in those patients who have premonitory symptoms such as cravings, yawning, or fatigue.
- May also be administered by inhaler or suppository.
- Overdosage results in nausea, rebound headache, and peripheral vasoconstriction. The recommended maximum dose per week is 10 mg.
- Dihydroergotamine (DHE) used intravenously in patients with intractable migraine at doses of 0.3–1.0 mg 8-hourly up to total dose of 10 mg (specialist headache units).

Management of migraine

Prophylaxis

- Headache diary useful to monitor frequency and patterns, e.g. relationship to periods, weekends, analgesic and triptan overuse.
- Prophylaxis ineffective if medication overuse.
- Avoid triggers—dietary in only 10%.
- Consider prophylaxis if ≥ 2 attacks per month or one prolonged attack affecting lifestyle.
- Prophylactic drugs (see Table 5.7):
  - beta-blockers;
  - amitriptyline especially if migraine associated with tension headache;
  - sodium valproate;
  - topiramate;
  - pizotifen.

Newer treatment options

- Greater occipital nerve blocks and stimulators: anecdotal reports suggest benefit.
- Botulinum toxin A:
  - episodic migraine: no evidence for benefit compared with placebo.
  - chronic migraine: PREEMPT1 and PREEMPT2 studies—↓ headache days and headache episodes. May also be useful in patients with medication overuse.

Note: Epidemiological link between migraine with aura and patent foramen ovale (PFO). Migraine Intervention with STARFlex Technology (MIST-1) study showed no evidence of benefit of closure.

Table 5.7 Prophylaxis of migraine headache

Drug	Contraindication	Dose (mg)	Side effects	Comments
Beta-blockers	Asthma, peripheral vascular disease, pregnancy			
Non-selective				
Propranolol		20–320	Postural hypotension, fatigue, cold limbs, vivid dreams	Long-acting preparation available
Timolol		10–20		
Nadolol		80–160		
Selective				
Metoprolol		200		Slow release
Atenolol		100		
5-HT² antagonists				
Pizotifen	Pregnancy	0.5–3	Weight gain	Single nocturnal dose
Cypro-heptadine		4–8	Weight gain	Single nocturnal dose
Methysergide	Peripheral vascular and coronary disease, peptic ulcer, pregnancy	1–6	Epigastric pain, cramps, mood changes; rarely, retroperitoneal and pleural fibrosis	Cease treatment for 1 month every 6 months to prevent fibrotic effects. Specialist headache clinic supervision
Amitriptyline	Pregnancy, cardiac conduction defects coronary disease, peptic ulcer, pregnancy	10–150	Dry mouth, drowsiness	Useful if tension headache as well. Combine with beta-blocker
Antiepileptic drugs				
Sodium valproate	Pregnancy, liver disease	500–1500	Weight gain, alopecia, liver dysfunction, tremor, pancreatitis, polycystic ovaries	Chrono preparation. Not licensed for migraine in UK
Topiramate	Pregnancy	25–100	Weight loss, memory and concentration, acute glaucoma	
Gabapentin	Pregnancy		Fatigue, dizziness, diplopia, ataxia	Not licensed for migraine in UK

Note: Flunarizine is an effective prophylactic drug but is not licensed in UK.

Migraine and women

Menstrual migraine

- Hormonal trigger is baseline exposure to high levels of oestrogen followed by a fall in levels.
- Release of uterine prostaglandins occurring around menstruation is an additional mechanism.
- 60% of women report an increase in migraine frequency around menstruation.
- 14% have exclusively menstruation-related migraine.

Management of menstruation-related migraine

Non-hormonal prophylaxis

- NSAIDs:
  - mefenamic acid 500 mg 3–4 times daily or naproxen 500 mg bd 1–2 days before headache and for duration of period (–2 to +3 days of menstruation).
- Ergotamine 1 mg od or bd during vulnerable period.
- Naratriptan 1 mg bd or frovatriptan 2.5 mg bd for 3–5 days.

Hormonal prophylaxis

- Topical oestrogen:
  - transdermal oestrogen (Estradot®), 100 micrograms 3 days before period;
  - estradiol gel 1.5 mg in 2.5 mg gel 3 days before menstruation for 7 days.
- Combined oral contraceptive pill (COC) in patients with irregular periods. If attacks occur in pill-free period, tricycling (three consecutive packets followed by pill-free interval).
- Depot progesterone: inhibition of ovulation so that menstruation ceases. Oral POP not helpful because hypothalamic–pituitary axis not suppressed.
- Other hormonal strategies in conjunction with gynaecologist or endocrinologist: danazol, bromocriptine, tamoxifen.

Migraine, contraception, and stroke

- Migraine can worsen, improve, or remain unchanged when patients are prescribed the COC.
- Migraine may start *de novo* on starting the COC. It is not essential to stop the pill at the first migraine since this may improve over a number of cycles.
- Stop pill in the following situations:
  - new persisting headache;
  - new-onset migraine aura;
  - dramatic increase in headache frequency and intensity;
  - development of unusual and especially prolonged auras.
- Risk of stroke in young women < 45 years of age rises from 5–10 per 100 000 to 17–19 per 100 000 in migraineurs.
- Risk is higher in those with aura than in those without.

- COC is also associated with a small increased risk of stroke. Crucial to assess the other stroke risk factors—smoking, hypertension, hypercholesterolaemia, diabetes, obesity. Risks of stroke need to be weighed against the risks of pregnancy and the psychosocial consequences of unwanted pregnancies.

Guidelines for the use of COC in women with migraine
- Identify risk factors for stroke:
  - ischaemic heart disease or cardiac disease with embolic potential;
  - smoking;
  - diabetes mellitus;
  - hypertension;
  - age > 35 years;
  - obesity (BMI > 30);
  - family history of arterial disease;
  - systemic disease associated with stroke, e.g. sickle cell.
- Identify migraine type, i.e. with or without aura.
- Assess risk of stroke:
  - COC relatively safe: migraine without aura and no other risk factors.
  - Use COC with caution: migraine without aura with one vascular risk factor.
  - COC relatively or absolutely contraindicated: migraine with aura; migraine without aura + 2 or more risk factors.

Migraine, the menopause, and HRT
- At menopause, migraine improves in 65%, worsens in 10%, and is unchanged in 25%.
- Migraine worsens in most who undergo a surgical menopause.
- No evidence that women > 45 years of age with migraine are at increased risk of stroke compared with non-migraineurs.
- Indications and contraindications to the use of HRT similar to women without migraine.
- HRT when necessary for menopausal symptoms may improve or worsen migraine.
- Consider the following strategies:
  - ↓ oestrogen dose;
  - change type of oestrogen (conjugated to synthetic ethinyl oestradiol or pure oestrone);
  - change to a continuous regimen if migraine during withdrawal phase;
  - try oestrogen patch—more steady state level;
  - reduce progesterone dose;
  - change progesterone type;
  - try local progesterone application;
  - withdraw progesterone (with periodic endometrial biopsy and vaginal ultrasound);
  - if osteoporosis main concern, try selective oestrogen receptor modulator (SERMS), e.g. raloxifene instead of oestrogen-containing HRT.

Migraine and pregnancy

- 80% of migraineurs ↓ attacks—especially migraine without aura and those with menstruation-related migraine.
- Migraine patients without aura may experience auras for the first time in pregnancy.
- If first presentation of migraine with aura during pregnancy or if change in usual migraine symptoms, exclude other disorders:
  - cerebral venous thrombosis;
  - AVM;
  - imminent eclampsia.

Management of migraine in pregnancy
Non-drug advice
- To avoid pregnancy-related nausea and vomiting resulting in hypoglycaemia and dehydration:
  - eat frequent small carbohydrate snacks;
  - adequate fluid intake.
- Adequate rest.
- Acupuncture, relaxation techniques.

Drugs
- Minimize drug exposure especially during first trimester.
- If possible, stop prophylactic drugs.
- Acute treatment:
  - Paracetamol: safe in all trimesters and during lactation.
  - Aspirin: probably safe but caution near term due to ↑ risk of post-partum haemorrhage, neonatal bleeding, and premature closure of ductus arteriosus. Avoid during lactation—risk of Reye's syndrome and bleeding in infant.
  - NSAIDs: insufficient data to support use.
  - Codeine: not recommended but occasional use probably safe.
  - Metoclopramide, prochlorperazine, domperidone, chlorpromazine probably safe. Metoclopramide excreted in breast milk; therefore avoid in lactation.
  - Triptans—not recommended;
  - Ergotamine preparations—contraindicated in pregnancy and lactation.
- Prophylaxis during pregnancy:
  - Beta-blockers associated with intrauterine growth retardation—therefore avoid. If necessary use lowest possible dose.
  - Amitriptyline: conflicting data regarding limb deformities and muscle spasms, irritability, and convulsions in neonates. Use if necessary in second trimester only.
  - Pizotifen: limited data available.
  - Sodium valproate: contraindicated due to high risk of fetal deformities.
  - Topiramate: inadequate data.

Further reading

Goadsby P, Sprenger T (2010). Current practice and future directions in the prevention and acute management of migraine. *Lancet Neurol.*, **9**, 285–98.

Primary short-lasting headaches

See Table 5.8 for a description of the primary short-lasting headaches.

Paroxysmal hemicrania

- Rare.
- Important differential diagnosis for cluster headache.
- Shorter duration and higher frequency are clues.
- Patients prefer to sit quietly—behaviour that is rare in cluster headache.
- Secondary causes described include:
  - frontal lobe tumours;
  - idiopathic intracranial hypertension;
  - collagen vascular disease.
- Attacks are triggered by head movement.
- Indometacin is promptly effective.
  - Treatment should start with 25 mg tds. If there is a partial or no response after 10 days, the dose should be increased to 50 mg tds. If necessary, the dose could be increased to 75 mg tds. Side-effects: GI disturbances. Misoprostol and proton pump inhibitors should be used.

Short-lasting unilateral neuralgiform headache with conjunctival injection and tearing (SUNCT)

- Rare.
- Differential diagnosis for trigeminal neuralgia (TGN). SUNCT affects V1, while TGN usually affects V2 and V3.
- Duration of pain 5–250 seconds in SUNCT, < 1 second in TGN.
- Autonomic features are present in SUNCT and rarely in TGN.
- SUNCT is unresponsive to most treatments although lamotrigine is worth trying; TGN usually responds to carbamazepine.
- Both are triggered by cutaneous stimuli.

MRI is necessary to exclude secondary causes such as posterior fossa tumours.

Table 5.8 Primary short-lasting headaches including autonomic cephalgias

Feature	Cluster headache	Paroxysmal hemicrania	SUNCT*	ISH*	Trigeminal neuralgia	Hypnic headache
Sex (M:F)	5:1	1:2	2:1	F>M	F>M	5:3
Pain type	Boring	Boring	Stabbing	Stabbing	Stabbing	Throbbing
Severity of pain	Very severe	Very severe	Severe	Severe	Very severe	Moderate
Location of pain	Orbital	Orbital	Orbital	Any	V2/V3>V1	Generalized
Duration of pain	15–180 min	2–45 min	15–120 s	<30 s	<1 s	15–30 min
Frequency	1–8/day	1–40/day	1/day–30/hour	Any	Any	1–3/night
Autonomic features	+	+	+	–	–	–
Triggers	Alcohol, sleep	Mechanical	Cutaneous	None	Cutaneous	Glyceryl trinitrate
Indomethacin-responsive?	No	Yes	Yes	Yes	No	Yes

*SUNCT, Short-lasting unilateral neuralgiform headache with conjunctival injection and tearing; ISH, idiopathic stabbing headache.

Cluster headache

Epidemiology

Prevalence, 0.1%. Male:female ratio 5:1. Most common age of onset third and fourth decades.

Clinical features

- Episodic cluster: periods lasting 7 days to 1 year separated by pain-free remissions lasting 1 month.
- Chronic cluster: attacks lasting for more than 1 year without remission or remission lasting less than 4 weeks.

Headache features

- Excruciatingly severe unilateral orbital, supraorbital, temporal pain lasting 15 minutes–3 hours but usually 45–90 minutes.
- Abrupt onset and cessation.
- Frequency may range from one every other day to eight per day.
- Associated autonomic features—lacrimation, nasal congestion, rhinorrhoea, facial/forehead sweating, miosis, ptosis, eyelid oedema, conjunctival injection.
- Restlessness or agitation during headache.
- Other features include a striking circannual and circadian periodicity.
- Some also have typical migrainous auras.
- Triggers: alcohol, GTN, exercise.

Differential diagnosis

- Secondary causes such as tumours need exclusion by MRI.
- Features helpful in differentiating CH from migraine include:
  - relatively short headache duration;
  - rapid onset and cessation;
  - periodicity (daily and annually);
  - alcohol precipitates attack within 1 hour rather than several hours as in migraine.
- Paroxysmal hemicrania is similar but more common in females, with briefer and more frequent attacks. Exquisitely responsive to indomethacin.

Management

Acute attacks

- Subcutaneous sumatriptan 6 mg has a rapid effect and a high response rate. This may be used twice daily. Alternatives include sumatriptan 20 mg intranasally, zolmitriptan 5 mg orally.
- 100% oxygen, 7–12 L/min should be used for 20 minutes via a non-rebreathing mask with all apertures sealed up.
- 20–60 mg topical lidocaine 4–6% solution instilled intranasally may be a useful adjunct.

Preventive treatments

Short-term prevention

Short-term regimens are useful for patients with short bouts of CH for a few weeks or help in establishing longer-term preventive measures.

• Prednisolone 60 mg/day for 5 days and tailing off by 10 mg every 3 days.
• Methysergide is useful in patients with clusters lasting a few weeks. Start at 1 mg od, increasing the dose by 1 mg every 3 days to a tds regimen until 5 mg in total. Thereafter the dose can be increased every 5 days by 1 mg to a maximum of 4 mg tds. Prolonged treatment is associated with retroperitoneal, cardiac, and pleural fibrosis. Therefore, a drug holiday for 1 month is recommended every 6 months.
• Ergotamine 1–2 mg PO can be taken 1 hour prior to an attack or at bedtime if they occur predictably. Concomitant use of sumatriptan is contraindicated.

Long-term prevention

Indicated for long bouts of episodic and chronic cluster headaches.

• Verapamil: after a baseline ECG, start at 80 mg bd increasing after 10–14 days to 80 mg tds. Thereafter the dose is increased by 80 mg every 10–14 days, with an ECG prior to each increment, to a maximum dose of 320 mg tds.
• Lithium: after renal and liver function tests, starting dose is 300 mg bd with regular monitoring to achieve a level in the upper therapeutic range. NSAID, diuretic, and carbamazepine use are contraindicated.
• Anecdotal reports of benefit for occipital nerve block, occipital nerve stimulators, and deep brain stimulation (DBS).

Further reading

Cohen AS, Matharu MS, Goadsby PJ (2007). Trigeminal autonomic cephalgias: current and future treatments. *Headache*, **47**, 969–80.

Francis GJ, Becker WJ, Pringsheim TM (2010). Acute and preventive pharmacologic treatment of cluster headache. *Neurology*, **75**, 463–73.

Matharu MS, Goadsby PJ (2002). Trigeminal autonomic cephalgias. *J. Neurol. Neurosurg. Psychiatry*, **72** (Suppl. 2), ii19–26.

Trigeminal neuralgia

Defined as 'sudden, usually unilateral, severe, brief, stabbing pain in the distribution of one or more of the branches of the trigeminal nerve'.

Epidemiology

Usual onset after the age of 40. More common in women.

Clinical features

- Neurological examination, including facial sensation, normal.
- Second and third divisions are most often affected.
- Attacks last < 1 second. Refractory period after an attack. Frequent attacks in a short period may leave a lingering pain.
- Triggers include cutaneous sensory stimuli caused by touch, shaving, eating, talking, and cold draughts.
- Attacks during sleep are rare.
- Secondary weight loss, dehydration, and depression may occur.
- Secondary causes include:
  - Schwannoma of the TG nerve;
  - meningioma compressing the Gasserian ganglion;
  - malignant infiltration of the skull base;
  - in young patients, especially if bilateral, may be due to MS.
  A significant proportion of idiopathic cases are due to arterial or venous compression of the posterior nerve root.

Differential diagnosis

- Temporomandibular joint (TMJ) dysfunction.
- Dental condition, e.g. abscess, cracked tooth.
- Atypical migraine.
- Atypical facial pain.
- Pterygopalatine neuralgia.
- Trigeminal autonomic cephalgias, e.g. cluster headache, SUNCT.

Table 5.9 Drug treatments for trigeminal neuralgia

Drug	Dose (mg)	Side effects
Carbamazepine	300–1000	Drowsiness, ataxia, hyponatraemia, drug interactions
Oxcarbazepine	300–1200	Drowsiness, ataxia, hyponatraemia
Baclofen	30–90	Sedation, drowsiness
Phenytoin	200–300	Sedation, ataxia
Gabapentin*	300–3600	Sedation
Lamotrigine*	100–400	Sedation, rash

*Unlicensed

Table 5.10 Surgical options in the treatment of trigeminal neuralgia

Procedure	Comments
Peripheral branch alcohol injection	Safe; mild sensory loss
Cryotherapy	High recurrence rate: mean, 10 months
Radiofrequency thermocoagulation	Safe; risk of anaesthesia dolorosa Recurrence rate 60% at 5 years
Glycerol injection to Meckel's cave	Safe Recurrence rate 65% at 5 years
Microvascular decompression via posterior fossa approach	Mortality up to 0.4% Complications: CSF rhinorrhoea, cerebellar venous infarction Recurrence rate 25% at 5 years
Gamma knife surgery directed at the TG nerve stereotactically	Long-term effects unknown; 6 months for effect Low recurrence rate

Investigations

MRI of the brain indicated to exclude the secondary causes. In patients < 50 years, 5% may have an abnormality such as trigeminal Schwannoma, Meckel's cave meningioma, or a demyelinating pontine plaque.

Management

Drug treatment

- To avoid side-effects, start at low dose and increase gradually (see Table 5.9).
- Occasionally, combinations of drugs may be necessary to avoid using high doses, e.g. baclofen and carbamazepine.
- In crises consider IV phenytoin (as fosphenytoin 250 mg).

Surgical treatment

In cases refractory to medical therapy or those in whom there are intolerable side effects, surgical options (Table 5.10) should be considered.

Further reading

Cruccu G, Gronseth G, Alksne J, et al. (2008). AAN–EFNS guidelines on trigeminal neuralgia. *Eur. J. Neurol.*, **15**, 1013–28.

Idiopathic intracranial hypertension (IIH)

IIH is a syndrome of ↑ intracranial pressure without hydrocephalus or mass lesion. Normal CSF constituents. Previously referred to as benign intracranial hypertension (BIH) or pseudotumour cerebri.

Epidemiology

- Incidence is 1–3/100 000/year.
- Marked female preponderance.
- Age range: 15–44 years.
- Major risk factors:
  - female;
  - obesity;
  - recent weight gain;
  - hypertension;
  - menstrual irregularity.
- In any atypical patient (e.g. a man or slim female) look for secondary cause—venous thrombosis.

Pathophysiology

Unknown. Possible mechanisms include:
- obstruction to CSF outflow at the level of the arachnoid villi or in the draining veins;
- excess CSF production;
- increased cerebral oedema.

Clinical presentation

Usual symptoms reflect ↑ ICP or papilloedema.
- Daily headache (throbbing) associated with nausea and vomiting.
- Visual symptoms: visual obscurations (loss of vision) lasting a few seconds, visual blurring, and/or visual field loss.
- No localizing neurological signs except uni- or bilateral sixth nerve palsies causing diplopia.
- Cases are reported with third and fourth nerve palsies, internuclear ophthalmoplegia, and skew deviation. There are very atypical and other causes such as venous sinus thrombosis need to be excluded.
- Papilloedema may occasionally be unilateral.
- Papilloedema may be absent in patients with optic atrophy.
- Central visual loss occurring early should raise concern about some other cause of optic disc oedema such as optic neuritis or anterior ischaemic optic neuropathy.
- Central visual loss may occur in IIH if severe disc oedema is associated with retinal oedema, haemorrhages, exudates, or choroidal folds in the papillomacular bundle or the macula.

Differential diagnosis of papilloedema

- Myelinated nerve fibres.
- Crowded optic disc (hypermetropes) with bunching of vessels in a small disc—looks like papilloedema.
- Tilted optic disc. May be associated with visual field defects.
- Optic nerve head drusen. Associated with visual field loss and occasionally with haemorrhage at the optic disc. With drusen, the optic cup is often absent. Drusen may be buried and therefore not visible. On CT, calcification may be seen and ophthalmic ultrasound may be diagnostic.
- Other causes of optic disc swelling apart from papilloedema (which implies ↑ ICP):
  - optic neuritis;
  - ischaemia;
  - neoplastic infiltration.

Diagnosis of papilloedema may be difficult!
- Clues that an apparently swollen disc is not due to papilloedema:
  - blind spot is not enlarged;
  - spontaneous venous pulsation may be present or venous pulsation will appear on minimal orbital pressure;
  - absence of an optic cup in a mild to moderately swollen disc;
  - abnormal vessels at the disc.
- If in doubt, an ophthalmological opinion may be useful.
- Fluorescein angiography is the gold standard. Retinal photos useful for future reference.

Conditions that may produce intracranial hypertension and mimic IIH

Medical disorders
- Addison's disease.
- Hypoparathyroidism.
- Chronic obstructive pulmonary disease.
- Right heart failure with pulmonary hypertension.
- Sleep apnoea.
- Renal failure.
- Severe iron deficiency.

Medications
- Tetracyclines.
- Vitamin A and related compounds.
- Anabolic steroids.
- Withdrawal of corticosteroids.
- Growth hormone administration.
- Nalidixic acid.
- Lithium.
- Norplant levonorgestrel implant system.

Obstruction of venous drainage
- Cerebral venous thrombosis.
- Jugular vein thrombosis.

Imaging studies
- MRI and MR/CT venography should be performed to exclude hydrocephalus, mass lesions, meningeal infiltration, and venous thrombosis. Isodense tumours and subdural collections may be missed by CT. If MRI is unavailable or unsuitable because of the patient's size, CT with contrast should be performed.
- Radiographic signs of raised intracranial pressure in IIH include flattening of the posterior globe (80%) and an empty sella (70%). Slit-like ventricles are *not* a sign of IIH.

Lumbar puncture
- The LP is done with the patient in the lateral decubitus position and the legs extended.
- May be difficult to perform LPs on this group of patients. LPs can be done under X-ray guidance. Radiologists perform the procedure with the patient prone rather than supine—not satisfactory since there are no data to compare the opening pressures in these two positions.
- Normal CSF pressure is < 200 mmH$_2$O. The pressure increases with weight.
- To diagnose IIH, pressure > 250 mmH$_2$O. Levels between 200 and 250 mmH$_2$O are non-diagnostic and need to be repeated. Occasionally, a transducer monitor via a lumbar drain may be needed to clarify the diagnosis.

Management
No evidence of visual loss
Conservative management with:
- Weight loss.
- Diuretics: there are no trials comparing diuretics.
  - Acetazolamide is drug of choice as it reduces the rate of CSF production by the choroid plexus. Starting dose is 125 mg bd increasing to 250 mg tds. If tolerated, the dose can be increased to 250 mg qds. Side effects include paraesthesiae, altered taste, and depression.
  - Furosemide (20–40 mg) is an alternative.
  - Topiramate anecdotal only.
- Headache can be treated with amitriptyline and anti-migraine medication.
- Close follow-up is required with assessment of visual acuity, visual fields (automated or Goldmann), initially at one month and then 3-monthly. Subsequent follow-up depends on the clinical course.

Evidence of visual loss

Surgical intervention needs to be considered. Options are:

- Lumboperitoneal shunting. Side effects include infection, shunt obstruction, low-pressure headache.
- Optic nerve sheath fenestration. Highly specialized procedure. Complications include infection, local haemorrhage.

There are no comparative data on these two procedures.

Repeated LP

- May be unpleasant for the patient.
- Can result in low-pressure headache, which complicates the clinical picture.
- Helpful in some patients with severe headache and also in the management of IIH in pregnancy where drugs are relatively contraindicated.

Further reading

Fraser C, Plant G (2011). The syndrome of pseudotumour cerebri and idiopathic intracranial hypertension. *Curr. Opin. Neurol.*, **24**, 12–17.

Parkinsonism and Parkinson's disease: introduction

Causes of parkinsonism
- Idiopathic Parkinson's disease (PD).
- Parkinsonian-plus syndromes:
  - PSP;
  - MSA;
  - corticobasal degeneration (CBD).
- Secondary parkinsonism:
  - vascular;
  - drug-induced;
  - post-encephalitic;
  - hydrocephalus.
- Degenerative disorders:
  - Alzheimer's disease;
  - Parkinson—dementia—MND complex.
- Genetic disorders:
  - Wilson's disease (consider in all cases < 50 years);
  - Huntington's disease (akinetic rigid (Westphal) variant);
  - Dopa-responsive dystonia.

Epidemiology of PD
- Incidence: 18/100 000.
- Prevalence: 150/100 000.
- In UK, 100 000 cases at any one time.
- M:F ratio: 1.35:1.

Aetiology of PD
- ↑ risk of PD:
  - pesticides;
  - rural residence, farming;
  - MPTP (1-methyl-4-phenyl-1,2,3,6-tetrahydropyridine).
- ↓ risk has been associated with cigarette smoking and caffeine.

Pathophysiology of PD
- Hallmarks of PD are the presence of Lewy bodies + neuronal cell death in the pars compacta of the substantia nigra.
- PD does not develop until striatal dopamine (DA) levels drop to 20% and substantia nigra (SN) cell loss exceeds 50%.
- Functional anatomy involved in PD includes:
  - primary motor cortex;
  - supplementary motor area;
  - striatum (putamen and caudate);
  - globus pallidus;
  - substantia nigra;
  - subthalamic nucleus (STN);
  - thalamus.
- SN acts like an accelerator on the basal ganglia and damage results in slowing.
- STN is a brake and therefore damage causes excessive movement.

Clinical features of parkinsonism and PD

Diagnosis of a parkinsonian syndrome

Bradykinesia: slowness of initiation of voluntary movement with progressive reduction in speed and amplitude with repetition, e.g. thumb and index finger. Plus at least one of the following:

- Rigid ↑ tone.
- Rest tremor:
  - may be the first symptom in 75% of cases of PD;
  - 20% of patients never develop tremor;
  - some patients may also have a postural element to the tremor—this is delayed in onset ('re-emergent') and comes on a short period after the posture is adopted.
- Postural instability not caused by primary visual, vestibular, cerebellar, or proprioceptive dysfunction.

Features supportive of PD: ≥ 3 for definite PD

- Unilateral onset.
- Rest tremor.
- Progressive.
- Persistent asymmetry affecting the side of onset most.
- Good response to levodopa.
- Severe levodopa-induced chorea.
- levodopa response for > 25 years.
- Clinical course > 10 years.

Exclusion criteria for PD

- History of repeated strokes with stepwise progression of parkinsonian features (vascular PD).
- History of repeated head injury.
- History of definite encephalitis.
- Oculogyric crises.
- Neuroleptic treatment at onset of symptoms.
- Sustained remission.
- Strictly unilateral features after 3 years.
- Supranuclear gaze palsy (PSP).
- Cerebellar signs (MSA).
- Early severe autonomic involvement (MSA).
- Early severe dementia (DCLB).
- Babinski's sign (but note striatal toe may mimic).
- Negative response to levodopa (if malabsorption excluded).
- MPTP exposure.

Other features of PD

- Anosmia. 80% of PD patients have ↓ sense of smell. If normal, consider PSP, CBD, or MSA.
- Dystonia:
  - unusual in early disease—consider MSA;
  - more common after levodopa therapy.
- Bladder and bowel symptoms:
  - mild urinary symptoms—frequency, urgency, but rarely incontinence may occur due to detrusor hyperreflexia;
  - in MSA these occur earlier and are more severe;
  - constipation is common.
- Postural hypotension: mild but may be exacerbated by L-dopa and dopamine agonists.
- Speech disorder:
  - hypophonia (monotonous and low volume);
  - tendency to repeat the first syllable (palilalia).
- Sleep disorders:
  - restless legs syndrome;
  - REM sleep behaviour disorder where patients act out their dreams.
- Dementia—in the late stage 20% of patients may have dementia:
  - with memory impairment;
  - with fluctuating confusion;
  - with visual hallucinations;
  - dopaminergic medication may compound the problem.

Differential diagnosis of PD and investigation

Differential diagnosis
- Essential tremor (ET) versus PD:
  - ET 10 times more prevalent than PD.
  - ET is a postural ± action tremor. A severe postural tremor may be present at rest but is not 'pill rolling'.
  - Patients with ET may also have vocal tremor, head tremor ('no–no' or 'yes–yes').
  - In PD there may be jaw tremor, leg rest tremor.

  For further differential diagnoses, see Table 5.11.

Table 5.11 Features of other parkinsonian syndromes

Diagnosis	Clinical features	Response to levodopa
Multiple system atrophy (striatonigral degeneration, sporadic olivopontocerebellar atrophy, and Shy–Drager syndrome)	Early dysautonomia (orthostatic hypotension, impotence, bladder dysfunction) Cerebellar dysfunction Pyramidal signs Stimulus-sensitive myoclonus Extreme forward flexion of neck (antecollis) Mottled cold hands Inspiratory stridor Dysarthria	Good response in 20% and sustained in 13% Dyskinesias or motor fluctuations may occur Cranial dystonia prominent Early wheelchair requirement due to early loss of postural reflexes and ataxia
Progressive supranuclear palsy	Supranuclear vertical gaze palsy Apraxia of eyelid opening Axial rigidity > limb rigidity Early falls Speech and swallowing disturbance Neck extension	Poor
Corticobasal degeneration	Apraxia, cortical sensory changes, alien limb behaviour, pronounced asymmetric rigidity, limb dystonia, stimulus-sensitive myoclonus	None
Vascular parkinsonism	'Lower half' parkinsonism with prominent gait problems; minimal upper limb dysfunction; pseudobulbar palsy, pyramidal signs	Minimal
Dementia with Lewy bodies	Early dementia; rigidity > bradykinesia or tremor; hallucinations; fluctuating cognitive status; exquisite sensitivity to neuroleptics	Motor features respond well Psychiatric side effects

Table 5.12 MRI findings in parkinsonian syndromes

Syndrome	Finding
IPD	Nigral patchy signal loss
MSA	Putamen: ↓ lateral putamen signal on T_2-weighted images due to iron deposition; ↑ signal lateral putamen due to gliosis Pons: 'hot cross bun' sign due to lateral and longitudinal fibres becoming evident on T_2-weighted images (see Fig. 5.12)
PSP	Midbrain atrophy and third ventricular dilatation: 'humming bird sign'
CBD	Asymmetrical atrophy

Investigations

- No diagnostic test for PD. Diagnosis is made on clinical grounds.
- ^{123}I-FP-CIT SPECT scan (DaTscan). Ligand binds to the dopamine re-uptake transporter protein in the presynaptic terminals. ↓ indicates loss of striatonigral neurons. Useful in differentiating ET from PD, but not PD from MSA and PSP.
- Exclude Wilson's disease if onset < 50 years:
  - serum copper, caeruloplasmin;
  - 24 hour urinary copper;
  - slit-lamp examination for Kayser–Fleischer rings.
- MSA patients may have degeneration of Onuf's nucleus—detected as polyphasic potentials with ↑ latency on urethral or sphincter EMG.
  - False positives occur in patients who have had prostatic surgery and in occasional patients with PSP.
  - Sphincter EMG has a sensitivity of 74% and a specificity of 89%.
- Autonomic function tests, if MSA differential. Similarly, a cognitive assessment—dementia is unusual in MSA.
- MRI (see Table 5.12).

Further reading

Jankovic J (2008). Parkinson's disease: clinical features and diagnosis. *Neurol. Neurosurg. Psychiatry*, **79**, 368–76.

Tolosa E, Wennin G, Poewe W (2006). Diagnosis of Parkinson's disease. *Lancet Neurol.*, **5**, 75–86.

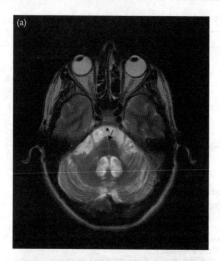

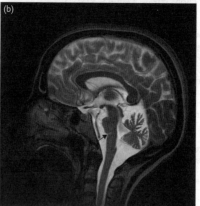

Fig. 5.12 Multisystem atrophy: cerebellar type (MSA-C): (a) axial and (b) sagittal T₂W MRI.

Figure 5.12 shows profound volume loss in the cerebellar hemispheres, vermis, middle cerebellar peduncles, and brainstem which is typical with predilection for the pons and olivary nuceli. (a) Note the prominence of intrapontine CSF clefts (*black arrow*) described as the 'hot cross bun' sign. (b) Sagittal MRI demonstrates pontine volume loss with flattening of the anterior surface and widening of the pontomedullary angle (*black arrow*).

Drug-induced parkinsonism

- Depletion of presynaptic dopamine stores:
  - reserpine;
  - tetrabenazine.
- Dopaminergic blockers:
  - neuroleptic drugs—phenothiazines (chlorpromazine), butyrophenones (haloperidol), thioxanthenes (flupentixol), and substituted benzamides (sulpiride);
  - prochlorperazine prescribed for labyrinthine symptoms and nausea;
  - metoclopramide for GI symptoms;
  - cinnarizine, atypical calcium-channel blocker prescribed for vestibular disorders;
  - combinations of antidepressant and neuroleptics, e.g. Motival®, which contains fluphenazine and nortriptyline, and Parstelin®, which contains trifluoperazine and tranylcypromine.

Clinical features

- Tremor and asymmetry as in PD.
- Patients may have a mixed movement disorder with untreated parkinsonism coexisting with:
  - orofacial dyskinesia;
  - stereotypies;
  - akathisia.
- Parkinsonism may resolve within days of drug being stopped, but may take years especially if depot preparations have been used.
- Elderly patients may be left with residual signs.

Medical management of PD

A multidisciplinary team is essential:
- PD nurse;
- physiotherapist;
- occupational therapist;
- social worker.

Levodopa

Levodopa therapy remains the gold standard of treatment.
- Starting dose is Madopar® (co-beneldopa) or Sinemet 62.5® (co-careldopa) with meals tds.
- Side effects: nausea, vomiting, anorexia. Often resolve spontaneously.
- Consider domperidone 10–30 mg tds.
- Modified release preparations (Madopar® CR and Sinemet® CR) have no beneficial effect in the prevention of motor complications.
- Bioavailablity of these CR preparations is 70% of that of the immediate release preparations.
- CR preparations are especially useful for nocturnal hypokinesia and rigidity.
- Dispersible levodopa preparation useful adjunct in kick-starting immediately on wakening or in the case of sudden 'offs' or during episodes of non-responsiveness.
- Motor complications develop in 50% of all PD patients after 6 years of levodopa therapy.
- Monotherapy with DA drugs is not associated with these complications; hence the rationale for delaying the use of levodopa therapies in younger patients if possible.

Long-term complications of levodopa therapy
- Involuntary movements or dyskinesias:
  - peak-dose choreathetoid dyskinesia;
  - diphasic dyskinesia;
  - dystonia (painful cramp).
- Response fluctuations:
  - end-of-dose deterioration (wearing off);
  - unpredictable on/off switching.
- Psychiatric:
  - confusion;
  - visual hallucinations;
  - delusions;
  - illusions.

Dopamine agonists (DAs)

- DA drugs (Table 5.13) act directly on post-synaptic dopamine receptors without the need for conversion to dopamine.
- DAs have a role as an alternative to levodopa as monotherapy, particularly in younger patients, to delay the use of levodopa and its long-term motor complications.
- In patients already on levodopa who have developed motor complications, DAs can be used with a consequent lowering of levodopa dosage.

Adverse effects

- All DAs: nausea, vomiting, postural hypotension, confusion, hallucinations, somnolence.
- Warn patients about side effects of impulsive behaviour, gambling, and hypersexuality. Enquire about these specifically at follow-up.
- Domperidone 10–20 mg tds is useful for GI side-effects and postural hypotension (peripheral effects).
- Ergot-derived DAs: ankle oedema, erythromelalgia, Raynaud's, retroperitoneal fibrosis, pleural effusions, cardiac valvular disease. Now rarely prescribed because of cardiac side effects.
- Pramipexole may be useful for depressive symptoms.

Table 5.13 Dopamine agonists

Drug	Dosage
Ergot-derived	
Pergolide (rarely used)	3–5 mg/day
Cabergoline* (rarely used)	2–6 mg/day
Non-ergot-derived	
Ropinirole	Starting dose 250 micrograms tds. Weekly increments of 250 micrograms tds, to 1 mg tds. Max. dose 8 mg tds.
Pramipexole	Starting dose 88 micrograms (base) tds ↑ to 1.1 mg tds
	Prolonged preparation available
Rotigotine (patch)	2 mg/24 hour patch ↑ max 8 mg/24 hour

*Long half-life; once-daily dose.

Apomorphine

Apomorphine, a potent D1 and D2 agonist, has poor oral bioavailability. Given by SC injection or continuous infusion.

Indications

- SC injection of apomorphine may be used in assessing the dopaminergic response, pattern, and distribution of dyskinesias in patients on long-term levodopa therapy.
- Intermittent injections are used as rescue for severe 'off' periods in patients already on maximal levodopa and DA therapy. Helpful in painful 'off'-period dystonias as well as 'off'-period sphincter and swallowing difficulty.
- Continuous infusion: consider in all patients with refractory motor fluctuations that cannot be managed on oral therapy and require > 6 apomorphine SC injections.
- Temporary apomorphine therapy should be considered in PD patients undergoing surgery who may be nil by mouth.

Apomorphine challenge test to assess effect

- Start domperidone 30 mg tds 36 hours prior to test.
- No oral anti-parkinsonian drugs for 4–6 hours before challenge.
- Normal breakfast.
- Assess baseline motor function using Unified Parkinson's Disease Rating Scale (UPDRS).
- Measure time to rise from a chair and walk 12 metres.
- Administer apomorphine 1.5 mg SC and observe motor response for 30 minutes.
- Yawning may precede motor response.
- If no significant response, administer 3 mg.
- Increase dose every 30 minutes up to 7–10 mg.
- Positive response is if there is an improvement in UPDRS score of 15–20% or 25% increase in walking time.

Other therapies

Anticholinergic agents

- Limited role and should only be prescribed in young patients with severe tremor and dystonia.
- Trihexyphenidyl (benzhexol) (2–5 mg tds) and orphenadrine (50 mg tds) are the most commonly used.
- Side effects a major drawback especially in elderly patients—confusion, cognitive impairment, nausea, dry mouth, precipitation of closed-angle glaucoma, and urinary retention.

Amantadine

- Previously used in early PD to delay the use of levodopa; with the advent of DA drugs there is little use for this indication.
- New role in the management of drug-related dyskinesias due to glutamate antagonistic properties.
- Dose 100–300 mg/day.
- Side effects: confusion, hallucinations, ankle oedema, livedo reticularis, insomnia (second dose at midday).

Monoamine oxidase B (MAO-B) inhibitors

Selegiline

- Mild symptomatic effect.
- Used as adjunct therapy to levodopa.
- Dose 5 mg bd.
- Side effects: confusion, hallucinations, insomnia (second dose at mid-day).
- New melt preparation given at a lower dose of 1.25–2.5 mg/day.

Rasagiline

- Mild symptomatic benefit.
- Dose 1 mg/day.
- Side effects: dry mouth, hallucinations.

COMT inhibitors

- ↑ the amount of levodopa reaching CNS. ↑ 'on time' and useful for end-of-dose deteriorations.
- Entacapone (200 mg) prescribed with each dose of levodopa. Stalevo® = combination of levodopa (50/75/100/125/150/200 mg doses + carbidopa + entacapone 200 mg, dose range 400–1200 mg/day).
- Side effects: diarrhoea, excess dopaminergic effects, dyskinesias managed by ↓ levodopa.

Duodopa® (co-careldopa gel)

- Infusions via a jejunal tube. Indicated for patients with advanced levodopa-responsive PD with severe motor fluctuations and dyskinesias. Expensive: £25 000–30 000 per year. May be a consideration in those unsuitable for DBS.

Further reading

Grosset DG, MacPhee GJ, Nairn M, et al. (2010). Diagnosis and pharmacological management of Parkinson's Disease: summary of SIGN guidelines. *BMJ*, **340**, 206–9.

Olanow CW, Stern MB, Sethi K (2009). The scientific and clinical basis for the treatment of Parkinson's Disease. *Neurology*, **72** (Suppl. 4), S1–136.

Seppi K, Weintraub D, Coelho M, et al. (2011). Movement Disorder Society Evidence-based Medicine Review Update: Treatments for the motor symptoms of Parkinson's Disease. *Mov. Disord.*, **26** (Suppl. 3), S42–80.

Surgical treatment of PD

Surgical procedures (lesioning and deep brain stimulation) have been developed as a result of a better understanding of the pathophysiology of PD (Table 5.14).

Table 5.14 Functional neurosurgery in PD

Outcome	Posteroventral pallidotomy	Thalamotomy (VIM nucleus)	Bilateral stimulation		
			Thalamic (VIM nucleus)	STN	Pallidal
Dyskinesias	++*	0	0	++	++
Tremor	+*	+*	+++	+	+
'Off' periods	+++	?	0	+++	+++
ADL	++	?	0	+++	+++
Medication	Increased	Unchanged	Unchanged	Reduced(++)	Reduced(+)
Morbidity (%)	5	5	5	?	?
Mortality (%)	2	?	0	?	?

*Contralateral.

Key: +/++/+++ = increasing benefit. 0 = no benefit.

- Major risk with lesion surgery is permanent neurological deficit. However, one-off procedure and no risks of hardware infection. DBS is reversible and titratable.
- A 10-year retrospective meta-analysis of 10 339 patients documented 6573 device-related complications: intracranial haemorrhage 2%; battery failure 2.1%; erosion 14%; lead fracture 14.7%; explantation 15%; infection 16%. Batteries need replacement every 3–5 years.
- STN-DBS greater risk of neuropsychiatric complications than GPi–DBS.
- Only levodopa-responsive motor symptoms benefit from surgery but with less dyskinesia, e.g. 'on' freezing and postural instability do not improve with STN/GPi surgery. Gait freezing and postural instability may be helped by pedunculopontine nucleus (PPN) stimulation. Only drug-resistant tremor may improve with STN-DBS.
- Thalamic DBS helps tremor but not bradykinesia.
- Following STN-DBS ↓ drug doses. After GPi-DBS, ↓ dyskinesia allows ↑ doses to ↑ 'on' time.

- Patient selection for surgery:
  - best in those whose motor symptoms predominate;
  - non-motor symptoms relatively minor;
  - low risk of developing dementia in next 3–5 years, e.g. visual hallucinations a contraindication to surgery. Medication-induced psychosis not a barrier to consideration of surgery;
  - no major active or previous psychiatric illness as DBS can trigger relapse. DBS associated with small risk of suicide.

Further reading

Thevathasan W, Gregory R (2010). Deep brain stimulation for movement disorders. *Pract. Neurol.*, **10**, 16–26.

Management of other problems in PD

Depression

- Affects the quality of life in 40%.
- Pramipexole may have antidepressant action.
- Tricyclic antidepressants: nortriptyline, desipramine.
- Although SSRIs (e.g. citalopram and sertraline) are useful, there is concern that this class of drugs may cause a deterioration of parkinsonian symptoms.
- Mirtazapine (presynaptic α_2 antagonist).
- In severe cases ECT may be an option.

Psychosis

- Occurs in 10–15%.
- Symptoms: mild illusions, visual hallucinations, and paranoid delusions.
- Underlying pathophysiology is combination of development of cortical Lewy body dementia and drugs.

Management

- Treat any infection (UTI, bed sores, etc.).
- Correct any metabolic derangement, e.g. dehydration.
- Reduce and withdraw anticholinergics, selegiline, amantadine, DA, and, lastly, levodopa.
- If necessary, balance between 'mad and mobile' and 'stiff but sane'.
- Consider addition of a newer generation of antipsychotic drugs, e.g. quetiapine. Low-dose clozapine (6.25–50 mg, mean 25 mg) has been shown to be effective. Agranulocytosis occurs in 1.2% of patients.

Dementia

- Features of Lewy body dementia include visual hallucinations, a fluctuating course with lucid intervals, and an exquisite sensitivity to neuroleptic drugs.
- Benefit with the use of cholinesterase inhibitor drugs used in the treatment of Alzheimer's disease, such as donepezil and rivastigmine.

Sleep disturbance

Common problem due to combination of factors.

- Stiffness and rigidity, making it difficult to turn in bed. Consider CR levodopa preparations or cabergoline.
- Bladder disturbance due to detrusor hyper-reflexia resulting in nocturia. Oxybutynin and tolterodine may help.
- Restless legs: CR levodopa or ropinirole or rotigotine patch or pramipexole at night.
- Rapid eye movement (REM) sleep behaviour disorder (RBD) where purposeful nocturnal motor activity occurs. Clonazepam 0.5–2 mg is effective.

Excess salivation due to an inability to swallow

- Can be treated with anticholinergic drugs but will have significant side effects.
- Hyoscine patches behind the ear.
- Instillation of atropine drops 0.5% on the tongue two or three times a day.
- Botulinum toxin injection or deep X-ray therapy (DXT) into the parotid glands if unresponsive and problematical.

'Freezing'

Especially in doorways: visual patterned cues across doorway help. Use of 'laser cane' to step over beam.

Falls and postural instability

- Occur late in the course of the disease and are unresponsive to medication.
- Multidisciplinary assessment with a physiotherapist and OT to acquire walking aids and make appropriate adaptations.

Further reading

Chaudhuri KR, Schapira AH (2009). Non-motor symptoms of Parkinson's disease: dopaminergic pathophysiology and treatment. *Lancet Neurol.*, **8**, 464–74.

Seppi K, Weintraub D, Coelho M, et al. (2011). Movement Disorder Society Evidence-based Medicine Review Update: Treatments for the motor symptoms of Parkinson's Disease. *Mov. Disord.*, **26** (Suppl. 3), S42–80.

Multiple system atrophy (MSA)

Within the spectrum of MSA:
- striatonigral degeneration;
- olivopontocerebellar atrophy;
- autonomic failure.
  Overlap occurs with disease progression.

Epidemiology
- Presentation usually in the sixth decade.
- Life expectancy is around 6 years from onset.
- There are no familial cases reported.

Pathophysiology
- Targeted areas are the striatum, substantia nigra, brainstem nuclei, dentate nuclei of the cerebellum, anteriomedial columns of the spinal cord, and Onuf's spinal nucleus, which innervates urethral and anal sphincters.
- Argyrophilic neuronal and glial cytoplasmic inclusions are positive for α-synuclein.

Clinical features
- Parkinsonian form (MSA-P) presents with an akinetic rigid syndrome. Tremor is less frequent than in PD.
- Olivopontocerebellar variant (MSA–C) presents with ataxia.
- Autonomic involvement with impotence in men, anorgasmia in women, orthostatic hypotension not due to drugs, urinary urgency, and incontinence early in the disease may be a pointer to MSA.
- Bulbar involvement can lead to laryngeal stridor and sleep apnoea.
- Pyramidal involvement not severe: brisk reflexes, extensor plantar responses that in a patient with PD could be due to vascular disease or cervical spondylosis.
- Other clinical signs:
  - dusky blue hands due to autonomic involvement;
  - marked antecollis;
  - painful dystonias;
  - low-amplitude myoclonic jerks of the outstretched fingers (polyminimyoclonus);
  - cognitive problems rare.

Investigations
- Autonomic function tests may confirm the clinical findings.
- Sphincter EMG may show denervation of the external anal sphincter.

MRI
- MSA-P:
  - atrophy of stratum/putamen > caudate;
  - putaminal hypointensity (posterolateral margin) + thin rim of hyperintense signal;
  - ↓ width of pars compacta.
- MSA-C (see Fig. 5.12):
  - pontine atrophy;
  - atrophy of middle cerebellar peduncles, cerebellum + inferior olives;
  - T_2W hyperintensity ('hot cross bun' sign).

Management
- 50% of MSA cases are levodopa-responsive.
- If no response or significant side effects, try amantadine (100 mg bd).
- Orthostatic hypotension:
  - reduce dopaminergic drugs;
  - TED stockings;
  - head-up tilt at night;
  - high salt intake;
  - fludrocortisone (0.1–0.2 mg at night)—side effect, supine hypertension.
  - midodrine 2.5 mg, ↑ to 10 mg tds.
- Bladder urgency: oxybutynin 2.5 mg bd, maximum 5 mg tds.
- Nocturia: intranasal desmopressin 20–40 micrograms at night. Side effect hyponatraemia.

Further reading
Stefanova N, Bücke P, Duerr S, Wenning GK (2009). Multiple system atrophy: an update. *Lancet Neurol.*, **8**, 1172–8.

Progressive supranuclear palsy (PSP)

Also called Steele–Richardson–Olszewski syndrome.

Incidence

Usual onset in sixth and seventh decades. Median survival is 7 years from onset.

Pathophysiology

- Tau-positive neurofibrillary tangles found in the pallidum, substantia nigra, periaqueductal grey matter, and superior colliculi.
- Frontal cortical involvement.

Clinical features

- Presentation with a symmetrical akinetic rigid syndrome with the axial trunk and neck muscles being more affected than the limbs.
- Tremor is uncommon.
- Backward falls early in the course of disease.
- Supranuclear gaze palsy affecting downgaze more than upgaze is the most distinctive feature, with symptoms of difficulty scanning the printed page and walking downstairs.
- Other features:
  - surprised look due to frontalis overactivity;
  - growling dysarthria with palilalia;
  - dysphagia;
  - apraxia of eyelid opening.
- Impairment of frontal lobe executive function with frontal lobe dementia later in the disease with personality change and emotional lability.
- Bladder symptoms unusual and occur late.

Investigations

MRI:
- Midbrain atrophy ('Mickey Mouse ears') due to enlargement of third ventricle + interpeduncular fossa + ↓ AP diameter of midbrain + depression of superior midbrain on sagittal images ('humming bird' sign).
- T_2W hyperintense signal periaqueductal grey matter + globus pallidus.
- Frontotemporal atrophy.

Management

- Response to levodopa is usually poor.
- Amantadine should be tried.
- PEG tube feeding necessary in severe dysphagia.
- Pneumonia is most common cause of death.

Further reading

Warren NM, Burn DJ (2007). Progressive supranuclear palsy. *Pract. Neurol.*, **7**, 16–23.
Williams DR, Lees AJ (2009). Progressive supranuclear palsy: clinicopathological concepts and diagnostic challenges. *Lancet Neurol.*, **8**, 270–9.

Corticobasal degeneration (CBD)

Incidence
Presents in sixth and seventh decades.

Pathophysiology
- Degeneration of posterior frontal, inferior parietal, and superior temporal cortices, thalami, substantia nigra, and cerebellar dentate nuclei.
- Tau deposition in swollen achromatic neurons.

Clinical features
- Striking asymmetry at onset and throughout the disease course, usually involving one limb.
- Combination of akinetic rigidity and cortical features. The latter are:
  - apraxia;
  - cortical sensory loss (simultagnosia and dysgraphaesthesia);
  - 'alien limb phenomenon'—hand may interfere with activities of the other arm or grasp doors and handles.
- Other features:
  - stimulus-sensitive myoclonus;
  - painful limb dystonia;
  - bulbar problems with dysphagia and dysarthria.

Investigations
MRI shows asymmetric cortical atrophy in clinically affected areas.

Management
- Poor response to levodopa.
- Clonazepam, piracetam, and sodium valproate may be used for troublesome myoclonus.
- PEG tube feeding may be necessary in severe dysphagia.

Further reading
Mahapatra R, Edwards MJ, Schott JM, Bhatia KP (2004). Corticobasal degeneration. *Lancet Neurol.*, 3, 736–43.

Peripheral nerve disorders: introduction and clinical approach

Response to physical or metabolic trauma by peripheral nerves is limited to four pathological mechanisms.

1. **Wallerian degeneration** when a nerve is transected with axonal and myelin degeneration of the distal segments. Distal portion will remain electrically excitable for up to 10 days. Denervation potentials are seen in muscles 10–14 days after injury.
2. **Axonal degeneration or axonopathy**: distal axonal loss ('dying back') due to toxins and metabolic disorders such as diabetes. Most common pathological reaction. Presents as a symmetrical length-dependent neuropathy. Axonal regeneration proceeds at the rate of 2–3 mm/day.
3. **Neuronopathy** with nuclear degeneration of the motor anterior horn cells in the spinal cord or the sensory neurons within the dorsal root ganglia (ganglionopathy). Occurs as a result of degenerative processes in motor neuron disease or as a paraneoplastic or autoimmune phenomenon in sensory neuronopathies.
4. **Segmental demyelination** results from direct damage to either the myelin sheath (e.g. GBS) or the Schwann cell (e.g. GBS or CIDP). Repeated episodes of demyelination and remyelination result in a proliferation of Schwann cells—onion bulbs.

Clinical approach

History

- Motor symptoms: difficulty opening jars; tripping due to weakness of ankle dorsiflexion. Proximal weakness (differential diagnosis: myopathies) and/or onset in upper limbs occurs as radiculopathy, radiculoneuropathy (e.g. CIDP), and vasculitis.
- Sensory symptoms: positive sensory symptoms, e.g. pins and needles, burning, tight band-like sensation. Indicative of an acquired rather than an inherited neuropathy.
  - Hypoaesthesia—reduced sensitivity or numbness.
  - Paraesthesiae—abnormal sensations which may be spontaneous or evoked, but are not unduly painful or unpleasant.
  - Dysaesthesiae—unpleasant paraesthesiae.
  - Hyperaesthesia—increased sensitivity to a stimulus.
  - Allodynia—painful sensation resulting from a non-painful stimulus such as light stroking.
  - Hyperalgesia—greater than normal response to a painful stimulus.
  - Hyperpathia—delayed painful after-sensation to a stimulus.
  - Neuropathic pain—burning, gnawing, sharp shooting, or jabbing pains intermittently.

Clinical examination
- Foot deformities such as pes cavus, pes planus, clawing of the toes, or scoliosis may indicate a hereditary neuropathy.
- Nerve thickening (ulnar at the elbow, superficial radial at the wrist, or the common peroneal around the fibular head) may indicate leprosy, CIDP, Refsum's disease, amyloidosis, CMT (I and III), or HNPP.
- Clinical signs that are useful pointers to large fibre involvement (joint position and vibration sense):
  - pseudoathetosis (involuntary movement of the fingers when the hands are held outstretched and the eyes are shut);
  - positive Romberg's sign (increased swaying and unsteadiness with the eyes closed compared with when the eyes are open).
- Small-fibre neuropathies (damage to the unmyelinated and small myelinated fibres). Pain and temperature sensation are impaired, but reflexes may be normal since the afferent fibres of the tendon stretch reflexes lie within the large myelinated fibres.
- In the length-dependent sensory neuropathies, involvement of the anterior intercostal and thoracic nerves will result in a midline area of sensory loss, which could be interpreted as a sensory level falsely implicating spinal cord pathology.
- Autonomic dysfunction:
  - symptoms of orthostatic lightheadedness, impotence, bladder and bowel dysfunction;
  - examination includes pupillary responses to light and accommodation;
  - BP erect and supine (after 3 minutes).
- Clues to a demyelinating neuropathy:
  - postural tremor of the outstretched hands;
  - weakness out of proportion to the degree of wasting;
  - generalized areflexia;
  - thickened nerves.

Diagnosis of peripheral nerve disorders

To reach a diagnosis the following questions need to be answered after the history and examination.
- What is the temporal evolution of the disorder?
  - Acute (days up to 4 weeks), e.g. GBS, vasculitis.
  - Subacute (4–8 weeks).
  - Chronic (> 8 weeks), e.g. CIDP.
- Which parts or combinations of the peripheral nervous system are involved?
  - Motor: distal or proximal, focal, or symmetrical/asymmetrical.
  - Sensory: small fibres (pain and temperature) or large fibres (joint position and vibration).
- Autonomic involvement?
- Cranial nerve involvement?
- Clues to genetic neuropathy? Clues include family history, onset in childhood (motor milestones delayed).

Acute neuropathy

See ☐ Chapter 3, 'Acute neuromuscular weakness', pp. 56–8.

Chronic neuropathy

The following patterns may be recognized in most cases and will help formulate a differential diagnosis (see also Fig. 5.13).

Pattern 1 Symmetrical proximal and distal weakness with sensory loss. Consider CIDP, vasculitis.

Pattern 2 Symmetrical distal weakness with sensory loss. Consider metabolic disorders (e.g. diabetes), drugs and toxins, hereditary neuropathies (e.g. CMT I and II, amyloidosis).

Pattern 3 Asymmetric distal weakness with sensory loss.
- Multiple nerve involvement. Consider vasculitis, hereditary neuropathy with liability to pressure palsies (HNPP), infections (e.g. Lyme disease, leprosy), HIV, infiltration with lymphoma or carcinoma, sarcoidosis. Note: mononeuritis multiplex may eventually develop into a confluent sensory and motor neuropathy.
- Single nerve or root. Consider compressive lesions and radiculopathy.

Pattern 4 Asymmetric distal or proximal weakness without sensory loss. Consider motor neuron disease, multifocal motor neuropathy with conduction block (MMN-CB), neuralgic amyotrophy.

Pattern 5 Asymmetric proximal and distal weakness with sensory loss. Consider polyradiculopathy or plexopathy due to diabetes, malignant infiltration, neuralgic amyotrophy, HNPP.

Pattern 6 Symmetric sensory neuropathy without weakness (mainly small fibre involvement with pain and temperature dysfunction). Consider diabetes, HIV, amyloidosis, Fabry's disease, idiopathic.

Pattern 7 Symmetric sensory loss without weakness (large and small fibre dysfunction). Consider diabetes, drugs, toxins.

Pattern 8 Marked proprioceptive sensory loss. Consider ganglionopathy due to paraneoplastic disorders, Sjögren's syndrome, B$_6$ and *cis*-platinum toxicity, HIV.

Pattern 9 Neuropathy with autonomic involvement. Consider diabetes, amyloid (familial or acquired), porphyria, GBS.

Pattern 10 Neuropathy with cranial nerve involvement (most often the facial nerve). Consider Lyme disease, HIV, CIDP, sarcoidosis, malignant infiltration, Gelsolin familial amyloid neuropathy (Finnish), Tangier disease.

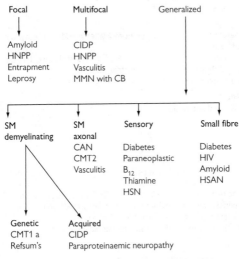

Fig. 5.13 Algorithm for the diagnosis of peripheral neuropathy: CAN, chronic axonal neuropathy; CIDP, chronic inflammatory demyelinating neuropathy; CMT, Charcot–Marie–Tooth disease; HIV, human immunodeficiency virus; HNPP, hereditary neuropathy with liability to pressure palsies; HSAN, hereditary sensory and autonomic neuropathy; HSN, hereditary sensory neuropathy; MMN with CB, multifocal motor neuropathy with conduction block; SM, sensorimotor.

Investigations in peripheral nerve disorders

Nerve conduction tests (NCT)

Necessary in most cases (see 📖 Chapter 8) to:
- distinguish demyelinating neuropathy (20%) from axonal neuropathy (80%);
- identify features distinguishing hereditary from acquired neuropathy (e.g. uniform slowing of motor conduction velocities in hereditary neuropathy);
- detect clinically asymptomatic abnormalities;
- distinguish symmetrical length-dependent neuropathy from asymmetric patchy neuropathy which suggests a vasculitic or inflammatory aetiology.

Blood tests

First-line
- Haematology: FBC, ESR, B_{12} (+ homocysteine and/or methylmalonic acid), folate.
- Biochemistry: renal and liver function, Ca, fasting glucose, HbA_1c immunoglobulins, and protein electrophoresis.
- Immunology: ANA, dsDNA, ENA (anti-ro and la).

Second-line
- Antineuronal antibodies.
- ACE.
- Lyme.
- HIV.

Third-line
- Vasculitic neuropathy: hepatitis B, C, cryoglobulins, complement C3, C4, c-ANCA, p-ANCA.
- Genetic tests: chr 17 (duplication for CMT 1a, deletion for HNPP), P0, connexin 32, familial amyloid polyneuropathy (FAP) mutations.
- Specific antibody tests: GQ1b (Miller Fisher syndrome), GM1 (MMN with CB), anti-MAG (IgM paraproteinaemic neuropathy).

Radiology

- CXR (sarcoidosis, malignancy).
- MRI brachial, lumbosacral plexus with gadolinium (CIDP, infiltration).

CSF examination

Should be considered in any progressive undiagnosed neuropathy.
- ↑ CSF protein, pleocytosis, oligoclonal bands indicate demyelination or inflammatory process.
- Cytology examination for malignant cells.

Nerve biopsy

- Sural, superficial peroneal, superficial radial, or dorsal ulnar nerve biopsy should be considered in the following situations:
  - vasculitis (nerve and muscle biopsy may ↑ yield);
  - CIDP if NCT and CSF not supportive;
  - amyloid neuropathy;
  - possible hereditary neuropathy with no FH and genetic tests negative;
  - complex neurological syndromes with PN involvement.
- Diagnostic yield is low in chronic axonal neuropathy.
- Nerve selected depends on clinical and NCT involvement. If normal NCT, yield is poor.

Complications
- Infection.
- Persistent pain and numbness.

Diabetic neuropathies

Epidemiology

Most common cause of neuropathy worldwide. 8% have neuropathy at diagnosis; 50% after 25 years.

Diagnosis of diabetes mellitus (DM)

- Type 1: beta cell destruction (autoimmune).
- Type 2: relative insulin deficiency.

Criteria for diagnosis of DM

- Symptoms of DM (polyuria, polydipsia, weight loss) + random plasma glucose > 11.1 mmol/L *or*
- Fasting plasma glucose > 7.8 mmol/L *or*
- 2 hour plasma glucose after GTT (75 g glucose load) > 11.1 mmol/L.
- $HbA_1c \geq 6.5\%$ (may vary in different ethnic groups).

Classification of diabetic neuropathies

Diabetic polyneuropathy

Clinical features

- Distal symmetrical sensory > motor neuropathy starting in the toes and progressing to knees when fingers and hands become affected ('glove and stocking'). Complaints of numbness, tingling, and symptoms of a painful small fibre neuropathy (burning, stabbing).
- Weakness restricted to small muscles of feet.
- Absent ankle and/or knee jerks.
- Associated autonomic function abnormality correlates with severity of neuropathy:
  - postural hypotension;
  - loss of sinus arrhythmia;
  - impotence;
  - gastroparesis;
  - nocturnal diarrhoea.
- Retinopathy.
- Nephropathy with proteinuria.

NCT

Length-dependent changes, mixed axonal and demyelinative changes with small amplitudes and slowing.

Nerve biopsy

Indicated if prominent autonomic dysfunction early for amyloid; marked or rapid progression with motor signs to exclude CIDP and vasculitis.

Management

- Foot care: regular assessment for callus and ulcer formation. Podiatric referral.
- Ophthalmological and renal assessment.
- Strict control of hyperglycaemia.
- Neuropathic pain control (gabapentin, pregabalin, carbamazepine, duloxetine, amitriptyline, lamotrigine).

Diabetic cachectic neuropathy (or acute painful neuropathy of DM)
- Usually in elderly men with poor diabetic control and profound weight loss.
- Symptoms of small fibre neuropathy: burning, allodynia, hyperaesthesia.
- Spontaneous recovery with good diabetic control.

Insulin neuritis
Onset with insulin treatment. Acute painful neuropathy that improves with good diabetic control.

Diabetic lumbosacral radiculo-plexus-neuropathy (Bruns–Garland syndrome)
Usually seen in males, > 50 years with type 2 DM.

Clinical features
- Abrupt-onset severe pain in back, hips, anterior thighs. Followed by progressive proximal weakness and wasting, but may involve distal muscles.
- Usually unilateral but occasionally bilateral.
- Associated with weight loss.

Differential diagnosis
Vasculitis, malignant infiltration.

Investigations
- NCT: changes of distal sensory diabetic neuropathy.
- EMG: denervation changes in paraspinal, proximal, and distal muscles.
- Consider MRI (with contrast) of lumbosacral spine and plexus for infiltration.
- CSF for malignant cells.
- Nerve biopsy (of intermediate cutaneous nerve of thigh) not usually indicated. Shows microvasculitis.

Management
Strict diabetic control; pain management. Role of steroids and IV Ig unclear. Most recover spontaneously.

Diabetic truncal radiculoneuropathy
Abrupt onset with burning radicular pain over thoracic spine, ribs, chest, or abdomen. Weakness of abdominal or respiratory muscles. Spontaneous recovery.

Cranial neuropathies
Third and sixth nerves affected. Third nerve palsy associated with orbital pain in 50%. Pupil spared. MRA needed to exclude a posterior communicating artery aneurysm. Recovery in 3 months.

Mononeuropathies
Increased susceptibility to compression injuries: carpal tunnel syndrome, ulnar and common peroneal nerves. If associated with wasting, local decompression should be considered. Results not as good as in non-diabetics.

Further reading
Little AA, Edwards JL, Feldman EL (2007). Diabetic neuropathies. *Pract. Neurol.*, **7**, 82–92.

Chronic inflammatory demyelinating polyneuropathy (CIDP)

CIDP, which can be considered a chronic form of GBS, is important to recognize as a cause of chronic neuropathy because it is treatable. Incidence 0.15/100 000. Prevalence: 1.24–1.9/100 000. Mean age of onset, 47 years.

Clinical presentation

- Most patients will have weakness and some sensory symptoms. Distribution usually symmetrical distal and proximal.
- Clues to diagnosis:
  - upper limb onset;
  - postural tremor;
  - pseudoathetosis;
  - weakness out of proportion to wasting;
  - large fibre sensory loss;
  - generalized areflexia, thickened nerves.
- 10% purely motor; 10% purely sensory (ataxic).
- Cranial nerve involvement rare: third and seventh.
- Autonomic and respiratory complications unusual.

Clinical course

Monophasic progression > 8 weeks, relapsing–remitting, chronic progressive.

Clinical variants

- Focal or multifocal monomelic (single limb) presentation.
- Sensory ataxic variant. May resemble ganglionopathy due to a paraneoplastic disorder or Sjögren's syndrome.
- Diabetes and CIDP. Diagnosis must be considered in any diabetic patient with predominant motor or ataxic neuropathy. May be difficult to confirm due to axonal changes on NCT due to diabetes. ↑ protein levels in the CSF occur in diabetic patients.
- Hereditary neuropathy and CIDP. Cases are reported of HMSN Ia with superimposed inflammatory CIDP responding to treatment. Clues include significant positive sensory symptoms and/or a rapid deterioration in motor signs.
- CNS involvement in CIDP. Combination of CNS involvement on clinical presentation, such as an internuclear ophthalmoplegia, with demyelinating lesions on MRI scans. Relapses may occur as a result of the central or peripheral pathology.

Investigations

Nerve conduction studies

- MCV slowing (variable not uniform).
- DML prolonged.
- F wave prolonged.
- Conduction block away from usual sites.
- Temporal dispersion.
- Denervation on EMG indicates axonal loss.

See 📖 Chapter 8, 'Technical summary of nerve conduction studies (NCS)', pp. 542–3.

CSF
- Cell count < 10 cells.
- Protein > 1 g (80%).
- Oligoclonal bands may be positive.

Indications for biopsy
Discrepancy between clinical findings and NCT: 48% demyelination, 21% axonal; 21% mixed; 18% normal.

Differential diagnosis
- Hereditary: CMT Ia, Ib, X-linked; HNPP; Refsum's disease.
- Toxic: amiodarone, perhexiline.
- Paraproteinaemic: myeloma, POEMS, Waldenström's macroglobulinaemia.
- Amyloid neuropathy.

Management
See Table 5.15.

Treatment
See Fig. 5.14.

Table 5.15 CIDP: management options

	Corticosteroids	IV Ig	Plasma exchange
Response rate (%)	65–95	70	80
Response speed	Slow	Rapid	Rapid
Relapses	No	Yes	Yes
Cost	Cheap	Expensive	Moderate
Complications	Long-term: weight gain, ↑BP, DM, osteoporosis	Blood product	Invasive, sepsis, cardiovascular complications

Second-line (no RCT data)
- Azathioprine, 2.5 mg/kg/day, as immunosuppressant and/or steroid-sparing agent.
- Cyclophosphamide, oral 1–2 mg/kg/day or IV 1–3 mg (pulsed).
- Ciclosporin: starting 3–7 mg/kg/day, maintenance 2–3 mg/kg/day.

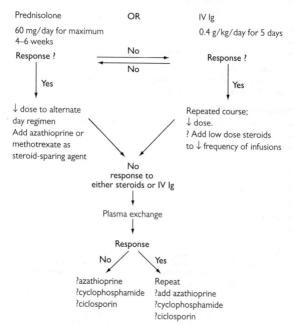

Fig. 5.14 Treatment flow chart for CIDP.

CIDP in association with monoclonal gammopathy

The findings of IgG, IgA, and IgM paraproteins of unknown significance (MGUS) in association with CIDP is common.

- Patients with IgG and IgA + clinical + neurophysiological findings consistent with CIDP should be treated as such.
- All patients with a monoclonal protein must be evaluated for a myeloproliferative disorder with:
  - urinary protein electrophoresis;
  - skeletal survey;
  - bone marrow examination.
- levels of paraprotein should be regularly monitored as risk of developing a myeloproliferative disorder.

Patients with IgM monoclonal proteins reacting to myelin-associated glyco-protein (MAG) have a distinctive syndrome:

- Usually over the age of 50 years.
- Slowly progressive, distal, symmetrical, sensory > motor features.
- Sensory ataxia.
- Postural tremor.
- Disproportionate prolongation of the DML compared with proximal CV.
- Nerve biopsy shows decompaction and widening of myelin lamellae by protein deposition.
- Treatment response to steroids and IV Ig is poor. Small case series suggest that rituximab (monoclonal antibody against CD20) may stabilize the disease or in some cases show improvement.

Further reading

Joint Task Force of the EFNS and the PNS (2010). European Federation of the Neurological Societies/Peripheral Nerve Society Guideline on Management of Chronic Inflammatory Demyelinating Polyradiculoneuropathy: report of a joint task force. *J. Peripher. Nerv. Syst.*, **15**, 1–9.
Nobile-Orazio E, Gallia F, Tuccillo F, Terenghi F (2010). Chronic inflammatory demyelinating poly-neuropathy and multifocal motor neuropathy: treatment update. *Curr. Opin. Neurol.*, **23**, 519–23.

Multifocal motor neuropathy with conduction block (MMN-CB)

MMN-CB is an acquired chronic demyelinating neuropathy which can be considered as part of the spectrum of CIDP. Mimics MND.

Epidemiology

100 times less common than MND. M:F ratio 3:1. Mean age of onset 41 years.

Pathophysiology

Immune-mediated supported by association with GM1 antibody and treatment response.

Clinical features

- Progressive asymmetric distal weakness of upper > lower limbs.
- Cramps and twitching in affected limb.
- No sensory symptoms or signs.
- Weakness > atrophy in early stages.
- In affected limb, fasciculations, myokymia, and reduced reflexes.
- Cranial nerve involvement (bulbar) rare.

Differential diagnosis

- Motor neuron disease (spinal muscular atrophy variant).
- CIDP.
- Lead poisoning.
- Hexosaminidase A deficiency.

Investigations

- High titres of GM1 antibody in 80%.
- CSF normal.
- NCT: sensory studies normal; small CMAPS; conduction block (CB) outside usual entrapment sites. Reduced MCV in segments with CB. Localized denervation.

Treatment

- IV Ig 0.4 g/kg/day effective. Regular infusions necessary.
- In some patients steroids may cause deterioration.
- Oral or IV cyclophosphamide can be tried in resistant cases.

Further reading

Vlam L, van der Pol WL, Cats EA, et al. (2011). Multifocal motor neuropathy: diagnosis, pathogenesis and treatment strategies. *Nat. Rev. Neurol.*, **8**, 48–58.

Vasculitic neuropathy

Epidemiology

Rare. Encountered in patients with systemic vasculitides or connective tissue disorders. Vasculitis may be restricted to peripheral nerves only. 6–12/million/year.

Aetiology

- Systemic necrotizing vasculitis
  - Polyarteritis nodosa
  - ANCA-associated (Churg–Strauss syndrome, Wegener's granulomatosis, microscopic polyangiitis).
- Vasculitis associated with connective tissue disorders
  - Rheumatoid arthritis.
  - Sjögren's syndrome.
  - SLE.
- Hypersensitivity vasculitis
  - Drug-induced vasculitis.
  - Malignancy.
- Infections
  - Bacterial: Lyme disease, TB, syphilis.
  - Viral: HIV, herpes zoster, CMV.
- Isolated peripheral nerve vasculitis (IPNV).

Clinical features

- Mononeuritis multiplex progressing stepwise. In ↓ order of frequency:
  - common peroneal;
  - posterior tibial;
  - ulnar;
  - median;
  - radial;
  - femoral;
  - sciatic.
- 25% have a symmetrical sensory motor neuropathy at presentation.
- Dysaesthetic pain, 75%.
- Asymmetric onset clue to vasculitis.
- Localized swelling.

Investigations

- Laboratory tests for underlying vasculitis or inflammatory disorder:
  - FBC, ESR;
  - renal and liver function;
  - urinalysis;
  - ANA, dsDNA, ENA, ANCA, RhF;
  - C3, C4;
  - cryoglobulins;
  - hepatitis B, C;
  - ACE;
  - Lyme disease;
  - HIV.

- CXR.
- NCT:
  - patchy asymmetric neuropathy;
  - clinically asymptomatic lesions.
- Nerve ± muscle biopsy. See 📖 'Investigations in peripheral nerve disorders', pp. 274–5.

Management

- Discuss mangement with local vasculitis experts—usually rheumatologists or nephrologists.
- IPNV, commonly a monophasic illness, may not require cyclophosphamide; steroids only may suffice—depends on severity.
- Variety of protocols for treatment. Note: pulsed cyclophosphamide (IV or PO) as effective as continuous oral but with less side effects and bladder toxicity.

Induction

IV cyclophosphamide 10–15 mg/kg (max 1 g) + IV methylprednisolone 1 g pulses. Every 2 weeks × 6. Oral steroids 20–30 mg continued if systematically unwell, but stop within 3 months if possible.
- Measure WBC at 7, 10, 14 days.
- If WBC < 3 (polymorphs < 2.5), ↓ dose for next pulse.
- If WBC at day 14 < day 10, delay treatment for 1 week.
- ↓ dose of cyclophosphamide if renal impairment.
- H_2 antagonist (e.g. ranitidine 150 mg bd).
- Bladder toxicity minimal with pulsed cyclophosphamide—mesna optional. Advise at least 3 L per day on day of infusion and 24 hours later.
- Co-trimoxazole 480 mg bd 3 × week for *Pneumocystis jiroveci* prophylaxis.

Maintenance

- Pulses 3-weekly × 4, then monthly 6–12 months.
- If in remission at 1 year consider azathioprine or methotrexate.

Further reading

Collins MP, Dyck PJ, Gronseth GS, et al. (2010). Peripheral Nerve Society Guideline on the classification, diagnosis, investigation and immunosuppressive therapy of non-systemic vasculitis neuropathy: executive summary. *J. Peripher. Nerv. Syst.*, **15**, 176–84.

Schaublin GH, Michet CJ, Jr, Dyck PJ, Burns TM (2005). An update on classification and treatment of vasculitic neuropathy. *Lancet Neurol.*, **4**, 853–61.

Carpal tunnel syndrome

Compression of the median nerve in the carpal tunnel at the wrist by adjacent tissue or ↑ interstitial pressure is the most common compression neuropathy.

Epidemiology

- Incidence 120 per 100 000 (women); 60 per 100 000 (men).
- Prevalence 9% of women and 0.6–2% of men.
- Peak age group 45–54 years.

Aetiological factors

- ↓ space in tunnel:
  - rheumatoid arthritis;
  - osteophytes, degenerative changes due to old fractures.
- ↑ susceptibility of nerves to pressure:
  - diabetes mellitus;
  - HNPP.
- Others:
  - pregnancy and lactation;
  - hypo- and rarely hyperthyroidism;
  - acromegaly;
  - primary amyloid and familial amyloidosis;
  - chronic renal failure and dialysis (deposition of β_2-microglobulin);
  - work involving repetitive and strenuous use of wrists and hands.

Clinical features

Frequently bilateral.

Symptoms

- Numbness, paraesthesiae, and pain in palmar aspect of thumb, first and second fingers, and lateral aspect of third finger. Sensory symptoms frequently involve other fingers. Pain and discomfort can extend proximally to the arm and shoulders.
- Typically worse at night, and also when holding a newspaper, telephone, or steering wheel.

Signs

- Sensory impairment first three finger tips.
- Weakness of abductor pollicis brevis (APB).
- Wasting of APB a late sign. Elderly patients may have APB wasting with few symptoms.
- Tinel's sign—tapping distal wrist crease causes paraesthesiae in median nerve distribution. Sensitivity 23–60%; specificity 64–87%.
- Phalen's sign—sustained flexion of wrist at 90° for 60 seconds results in paraesthesiae. Sensitivity 10–90%. Specificity 33–86%.
- Flick sign–patient makes flicking movement of wrist to alleviate symptoms. Sensitivity 93%. Specificity 96%.

Differential diagnosis
- C6 or C7 radiculopathy—usually unilateral associated with neck pain, symptoms on dorsal aspect rather than palmar, not worse at night. Weakness of biceps, brachioradialis (C6) or triceps (C7) with loss of reflex. Median innervated muscles (C8 and T1) not affected.
- Thoracic outlet syndrome (lower trunk of brachial plexus)—wasting of thenar muscles but sensory disturbance in C8 and T1 dermatomes.
- Thalamic infarcts can produce sensory symptoms in the hand that mimic CTS but symptoms are constant and associated with perioral paraesthesiae.

Investigations
- Check T$_4$, glucose, FBC, ESR. Consider serum protein electrophoresis.
- The best diagnostic tests for carpal tunnel syndrome are nerve conduction studies ± needle electromyography (NCS/EMG).
  - The characteristic nerve conduction findings include impaired median sensory and motor conduction velocities across the carpal tunnel region in comparison with either the ulnar fibres from the same hand or other segments of the median nerve (see 📖 Chapter 8, Fig. 8.7, p. 545).
  - Sensory fibres are affected before motor fibres.
  - Needle EMG is used to confirm denervation of the abductor pollicis brevis muscle in severe cases, and normal EMG of median-innervated muscles in the forearm can also help exclude a median motor neuropathy proximal to the carpal tunnel region.
  - Carpal tunnel syndrome can be categorized as mild/early, moderate/intermediate, or severe/advanced on the basis of the NCS/EMG findings.
- Imaging (not routinely used):
  - high resolution ultrasound;
  - MRI.

Management
Depends on severity of symptoms, neurological deficit, occupation, other medical conditions.
- Wrist splints: keep hand in neutral position to ↓ intracarpal pressure. 70% symptom relief in short term.
- Intracarpal injection of corticosteroid. Relapses common.
- Oral medications—only prednisolone 10–25 mg/day for 2 weeks shown to be superior to placebo in providing short-term benefit in one study. Diuretics and NSAIDs ineffective.
- Surgery—open carpal tunnel release or more recently endoscopic carpal tunnel release both effective, with 80–90% of patients improving.

Further reading

Bland J (2007). Clinrefical review: carpal tunnel syndrome. *BMJ*, **335**, 343–6.

Ulnar neuropathy

Neuroanatomy

- Fibres arise from C8 and T1 roots, pass through lower trunk, and medial cord of brachial plexus (see 📖 Chapter 2, 'Innervation of the upper limbs', pp. 36–40).
- Passes through condylar groove behind medial epicondyle of distal humerus followed by passage through the cubital tunnel–roof aponeurotic arch and fibres of flexor carpi ulnaris (FCU), floor–medial elbow ligaments, and muscle fibres of FCU.
- Branches to FCU and flexor digitorum profundus (FDP) 4,5 high in forearm.
- Palmar cutaneous branch arises mid forearm.
- Dorsal cutaneous branch arises 5 cm above wrist.
- At wrist nerve passes through Guyon's canal.
- Divides into superficial (pure sensory) and deep terminal (pure motor supplying all ulnar innervated hand muscles) branches.

Most frequent site of damage is elbow. Distal (hand, wrist) rare.

Clinical features

- Paraesthesiae, numbness of fourth and fifth digits. Initially intermittent, later constant.
- May complain of pain and discomfort around elbow.
- Look for wasting first dorsal interosseous muscle (FDIO), hypothenar eminence, forearm muscles (FCU + FDP).
- Claw hand (*main en griffe*).
- Examine FDIO, abductor digiti minimi (ADM), FDP 4,5. APB (median), FPL (anterior interosseous nerve).
- Frequently, damage at elbow may spare FCU and FDP 4,5 owing to fascicular sparing.
- Examine:
  - palmar cutaneous branch;
  - dorsal cutaneous branch;
  - superficial terminal branch;
  - medial cutaneous branch.
- Sensory loss 2–3 cm above wrist crease = C8/T1 or medial cutaneous nerve of forearm (therefore brachial plexus or mononeuritis multiplex).
- Palpate ulnar nerve at elbow for tenderness, thickening, or prolapsing of nerve on flexion.
- Elicit Tinel's sign at elbow by gentle tapping.

Differential diagnosis:

- (Rare) lacunar infarcts in thalamus or corona radiata.
- Spinal cord—anterior horn cell disease, syringomyelia.
- Roots—C8, T_1 radiculopathy.
- Brachial plexus—TOS, infiltration (look for Horner's syndrome = Pancoast tumour).
- MMN with block, CIDP.
- Vasculitis.
- HNPP.

Aetiology:

- At elbow:
  - External pressure, e.g. leaning on hard surfaces, wheelchair and bedbound patients, sleeping with arm flexed, perioperative due to poor positioning.
  - Repeated flexion/extension causes narrowing of cubital tunnel and chronic entrapment (cubital tunnel syndrome). In extreme flexion, nerve is stretched around epicondyle.
  - Trauma associated with fracture or blunt trauma.
  - Soft tissue injury.
- At wrist:
  - around Guyon's canal—pressure, e.g. cycling, occupational;
  - ganglion.
- Other causes:
  - multifocal motor neuropathy with block;
  - leprosy;
  - soft tissue and nerve tumours;
  - diabetics ↑ vulnerability to pressure.

Investigations

- NCT/EMG useful to ensure that no other nerves are involved to suggest MMN or HNPP or vasculitis:
  - 'inching studies' may help to localize the lesion but are not always reliable;
  - imaging—MRI elbow and increasingly MR neurography; ultrasound.
- Check glucose.

Grading of severity

- Grade 1 (mild) = sensory symptoms ± signs. No wasting or weakness.
- Grade 2 (moderate) = sensory symptoms and signs. Mild wasting + weakness grade 4 or 4+.
- Grade 3 (severe) = constant sensory symptoms + sensory loss. Moderate/severe atrophy + weakness grade 4 or less.

Management of ulnar neuropathies at elbow

- Conservative:
  - avoid pressure, wear elbow support pad (available from sports shop) even at night if tendency to sleep with elbow flexed, and avoid repetitive flexion/extension movements (e.g. weight-lifting);
- Surgical—refer to experienced surgeon preferably one who specializes in peripheral nerve surgery:
  - if bony abnormality at elbow;
  - soft tissue mass;
  - cubital tunnel decompression (may only become apparent during operation);
  - medial epicondylectomy.
- Grades 1 and 2: conservative measures with close follow-up. If worse consider surgery.
- Grade 3: consider surgery early to avoid further weakness. In very severe neuropathy with marked wasting and minimal strength (grade 2 or less) of ulnar innervated muscles may need to consider tendon transfer operations as perhaps too late for decompression.

Further reading

Stewart JD (2010). *Focal peripheral neuropathies* (4th edn). West Vancouver: JBJ Publishing.

Muscle disorders: classification and features

Classification
Major classification between inherited and acquired disorders.

Inherited disorders
- Muscular dystrophy.
- Myotonic dystrophy.
- Congenital myopathies.
- Metabolic myopathies.
- Mitochondrial myopathies.
- Channelopathies.

Acquired disorders
- Inflammatory myopathies.
- Endocrine myopathies.
- Drug-induced myopathies.
- Metabolic myopathies.
- Toxic myopathies.

Clinical features

History
- Symptoms suggestive of proximal myopathy: difficulty rising from sitting position, reaching high shelves.
- Difficulty using aerosols: long flexors in IBM.
- Myalgia or tenderness.
- Exercise-related muscle cramps and pains (glycogen and lipid metabolic myopathies).
- Symptoms of myoglobinuria (dark urine).
- Dysphagia.
- Developmental history: delayed milestones, difficulty playing sports at school.
- Family history.
- Drugs, e.g. statins.

Examination
- Proximal weakness in upper and lower limbs.
- In inclusion body myositis (IBM) finger flexors and quadriceps particularly involved.
- Distal limb muscle involvement is seen in IBM but also in the inherited distal myopathies and the scapuloperoneal syndrome.
- Involvement of extraocular muscles:
  - oculopharyngeal muscular dystrophy (OPMD) in association with bulbar and limb involvement;
  - chronic progressive external ophthalmoplegia (CPEO) in isolation or as part of the Kearns–Sayre mitochondrial syndrome.
- Facial muscles are involved in:
  - myotonic dystrophy;
  - facioscapulohumeral (FSH) dystrophy.

- Severe weakness of the neck extensors leading to a 'dropped head':
  - due to an inflammatory myopathy that may be very localized;
  - also in MG and MND.
- Muscle hypertrophy, confined to the calves, is typically seen in Duchenne (DMD) and Becker (BMD) muscular dystrophies. More general hypertrophy is a feature of myotonia congenita.
- Myotonia (slow relaxation) feature of myotonic dystrophy (MD) and channelopathies.
- Muscle contractures occur in:
  - Emery–Dreifuss muscular dystrophy;
  - fibrosing myositis found in scleromyxoedema.
- Depressed or absent reflexes may suggest an associated neuropathy (unless there is profound muscle wasting of the appropriate muscles). Consider:
  - paraneoplastic;
  - mitochondrial disorders.
- Skin rashes. Characteristic skin rash of dermatomyositis over face and the extensor surfaces of the MP and IP joints (Gottron's sign).

Muscle disorders: investigations

Biochemical studies

- Serum creatine kinase (CK) best indicator of muscle disease. ↑ up to 3× normal may occur following:
    - strenuous exercise;
    - IM injections and EMG studies;
    - viral infections.
- Highest levels of CK in inflammatory myopathies, acute rhabdomyolysis, and early stages of DMD when the patient is still ambulant.
- Serum CK levels are normal in most congenital myopathies, myotonic syndromes, and corticosteroid and thyrotoxic myopathies.
- In asymptomatic individuals ↑ CK level may indicate:
    - predisposition to malignant hyperthermia;
    - McArdle's disease;
    - early inflammatory myopathy;
    - carriers of DMD and BMD gene.
- In chronic denervating disorders such SMA and MND, CK levels ↑ but never greater than 10× normal.
- Myoglobinuria will result in a positive urinary benzadine dip test, which also reveals haematuria and haemoglobinuria.
- Venous lactate ↑ at rest or after exercise in patients with:
    - mitochondrial myopathy;
    - defects of the respiratory chain.
- Lactate production is ↓ or absent in the metabolic myopathies due to defects in:
    - glycogenolysis (myophosphorylase or phosphorylase b kinase deficiency);
    - the glycolytic pathway (phosphofructose kinase and lactate dehydrogenase deficiency).

The forearm exercise test

- Venous blood samples are taken for estimation of lactate and ammonia at rest and at 1, 2, 4, 6, and 10 minutes after a one-minute period of repetitive maximum isometric contractions of the forearm flexor muscles.
- Normally, there is a 2- or 3-fold ↑ in lactate concentration within the first 2 minutes after exercise. ↓ or absent in patients with defects in the glycogenolytic and glycolytic pathways.
- In patients with myoadenate deaminase deficiency ammonia production is reduced or absent.

Neurophysiology studies (NCT EMG)

See 🕮 Chapter 8.

EMG features of a myopathic disorder are:
- Motor unit action potential (MUAP) duration and amplitudes will be ↓.
- ↑ number of polyphasic motor unit potentials.
- With voluntary contraction there is early recruitment of ↑ numbers of short-duration MUAPs with a full interference pattern.

- Spontaneous fibrillation potentials, positive sharp waves, and complex repetitive discharges prominent in inflammatory myopathies, toxic myopathies, e.g. chloroquine myopathy, metabolic myopathy such as hypothyroid myopathy, and some cases of DMD.
- In myotonic disorders pronounced increase in insertional activity with a diagnostic waxing and waning ('dive bomber') of myotonic discharges due to electrical instability of the muscle cell membrane.

Muscle biopsy

- Ideal muscle to biopsy is one that is only moderately affected (MRC grade 4).
- Select muscle that has not been the site of IM injections or EMG studies (may take at least a month for such changes to heal).
- Muscles that are very weak and/or atrophied will show non-specific endstage changes and will be of little diagnostic use.
- Selection of needle versus open biopsy will depend on experience and availability.
- Open biopsy preferred in cases of inflammatory myopathies and where quantitive or molecular analyses required.
- Some of the muscle tissue obtained should be frozen for histological, histochemical, and immunohistochemical investigations. Latter technique will diagnose, using monoclonal antibodies, enzyme deficiencies, storage disorders, and the various dystrophinopathies and sarcoglycanopathies.
- Tissue should also be fixed in glutaraldehyde for electron microscopy, essential in the diagnosis of mitochondrial myopathy and IBM.

Molecular diagnosis

Molecular diagnosis is an increasingly important method of diagnosis but muscle biopsy remains the gold standard, especially in *de novo* cases.

Muscular dystrophies

- X-linked recessive:
  - DMD, mutations in dystrophin gene (found in 70% cases);
  - BMD, mutations in dystrophin gene;
  - Emery–Dreifuss, mutations in EMD gene (encoding emerin).
- Autosomal dominant:
  - Myotonic dystrophy, DM protein kinase gene mutation;
  - FSH, deletions in 4q;
  - OPMD, PABP2 gene;
  - Emery–Dreifuss, mutations in LMNA gene (encoding lamin A and C);
  - Limb girdle dystrophies, mutations in genes coding for myotilin, lamin A/C, caveolin.
- Autosomal recessive:
  - Limb girdle dystrophies, various mutations including calpain 3, sarcoglycans.

Other investigations
- Imaging with MRI useful in detecting atrophy and hypertrophy or defining the extent of a polymyositis and guide to biopsy.
- NMR spectroscopy may be useful in the evaluation of patients with glycolytic and mitochondrial dysfunction.
- ECG, 24 hr tape, echo essential for patients with DMD and BMD, MD, and Emery–Dreifuss.

Further reading
Merrison AFA, Hanna MG (2009). The bare essentials: muscle disease. *Pract. Neurol.*, **9**, 54–65.

Dermatomyositis, polymyositis, and inclusion body myositis

Clinical features of dermatomyositis (DM) and polymyositis (PM)

- DM, presentation subacutely over weeks but may be acute.
- PM, slower presentation over weeks or months.
- In DM the characteristic skin rash may precede muscle disorder:
  - heliotrope (blue–purple) rash with oedema on upper eyelids;
  - erythematous rash over cheeks, upper chest, upper posterior chest ('shawl sign');
  - erythematous scaly eruption over knuckles (Gottron's sign);
  - dilated capillary loops at base of fingernails;
  - lateral and palmar areas of hands become rough and cracked with 'dirty' horizontal lines ('mechanic's hands').
- Extramuscular complications:
  - in both DM and PM, interstitial lung disease in 10% associated with anti-Jo 1 antibodies;
  - myocarditis and conduction abnormalities may occur;
  - in severe disease dysphagia may occur.

Clinical features of inclusion body myositis (IBM)

- Presentation is chronic over months and years.
- Most common acquired inflammatory disorder in those > 50 years.
- Distribution of muscle weakness is clue to diagnosis:
  - weakness and atrophy may be asymmetric;
  - distal and proximal weakness especially finger flexors and ankle dorsiflexors;
  - marked quadriceps weakness presents as falls;
  - mild facial weakness may occur;
  - dysphagia may be present early or late.

Investigations
See Table 5.17.

Management of DM and PM

Corticosteroids

- Early aggressive management associated with better outcome unless very indolent.
  - IV methylprednisolone 500 mg for 5 days, followed by oral prednisolone 1 mg/kg daily.
  - When CK normal and clinical improvement reduce by 5 mg alternate days over 2 months. Thereafter, dose gradually reduced, monitoring CK and clinical state.
  - Note: Consider osteoporosis prophylaxis with baseline bone scan—bisphosphonate with Ca and vitamin D supplements.

Table 5.17 Inflammatory myopathies

Characteristics	Polymyositis	Dermatomyositis	Inclusion body myositis
Age at onset	>18 years	Any age, 2 peaks: 5–15 & 45–60 years	>50 years
Female:male ratio	2:1	2:1	1:3
Familial association	No	No	Rarely
Association with: connective tissue diseases	Yes	Scleroderma, MCTD	No
Systemic autoimmune diseases	Yes	No	No
Malignancy	No	RR 1.3–2.1	No
Viruses	HIV, HTLV-1	No	No
Muscle involvement	Proximal symmetrical	Proximal symmetrical	Distal, proximal, asymmetrical, finger flexors, quadriceps
Atrophy	+	+	++
Serum CK (I)	Up to 50×	Up to 50×	Normal to 10×
EMG	Myopathic	Myopathic	Myopathic + mixed large units; 30% have signs of an axonal neuropathy
Muscle biopsy	Peri- & endomysial infiltrate, inflammatory infiltrate	Perifascicular atrophy. Perivascular & perifascicular, inflammatory infiltrate, microvasculopathy	Endomysial infiltrate, rimmed vacuoles
Cells	CD8 + T cells, macrophages Uniform expression of Class 1 MHC products on all fibres.	B cells, CD4 + T cells, macrophages	CD 8 + T cells, eosinophilic inclusions
EM		Tubulovesicular inclusions in capillary endothelium	Helical filaments, fibrils

RR, relative risk.

- Consider starting immunosuppressant drugs at the same time to reduce steroid dose:
  - azathioprine 2.5 mg/kg/day (check TPMT levels), guided by lymphocyte response;
  - methotrexate (up to 20–25 mg/day), weekly with folic acid;
  - other options: ciclosporin up to 5 mg/kg/day; oral cyclophosphamide 2 mg/kg/day; mycophenolate 2 g daily.

IV immunoglobulin

Effective but expensive; used in resistant cases.

Physiotherapy

- Maintain residual strength.
- Prevention of contractures.
- Supply of orthotics.

OT assessment

Home visit for advice re home access, stairs, grab rails in bathroom, etc.

Monitoring

- Primarily muscle strength and function rather than CK.
- Rising CK may herald relapse, but relapse may occur without CK rise.
- Steroid-induced myopathy a possible concern.

Management of IBM

- Corticosteroids, immunosuppressant drugs, and IV Ig have not been shown to be of significant functional benefit.
- Trial of steroids may be considered if marked inflammatory cells on biopsy or very high CK.

Further reading

Amato AA, Barohn RJ (2009). Evaluation and treatment of inflammatory myopathies. *J. Neurol. Neurosurg. Psychiatry*, **80**, 1060–8.

Channelopathies

Channelopathies in neurology

Migraine
- Familial hemiplegic migraine (FHM):
  - FHM 1: mutations in CACNA1A gene encoding Ca$_v$2.1 P/Q voltage-dependent calcium channel. Same gene causes FHM 1 and also SCA 6 (allelic disorders). See 🕮 Chapter 4, 'Ataxia', pp. 144–7.
  - FHM 111: mutations in voltage-gated sodium channel SCN1A.

Episodic ataxias
- Episodic ataxia type 1: mutations in potassium-channel KCNA1 gene.
- Episodic ataxia type 2: mutations in calcium-channel gene CACN1A.

Muscle channelopathies
See Table 5.16.
- Myotonia = delayed relaxation of skeletal muscle after voluntary contraction. Usually most marked after initial muscle contraction and improves after repeated muscle activity.
- Andersen's syndrome. AD, K$^+$-sensitive periodic paralysis, ↑ QT interval, ventricular arrhythmias, dysmorphic features (hypertelorism, mandibular hypoplasia, low-set ears). Caused by mutations on KCNJ2 gene on chr 17q23.
- Hyperekplexia, AD, hypertonia, exaggerated startle response, brisk brainstem reflexes. Mutations in glycine receptor gene.
- Malignant hyperthermia syndrome. Most common cause of death during anaesthesia (1:7000–50,000). ↑ risk with use of depolarizing muscle agents in combination with inhaled gases.
  - Genetics—heterogenous with the following loci identified:
    — Mutations in ryanodine receptor calcium-release channel (RYR1) leads to Ca^{2+} from sarcoplasmic reticulum. Also SCN4A, CACNL2A, CACNA1S.
  - Clinical features
    — muscle rigidity, spasms, rhabdomyolysis;
    — sympathetic hyperactivity, tachycardia, hyperventilation;
    — fever;
    — cyanosis.
  - Investigations:
    — O$_2$ consumption;
    — PCO_2;
    — K$^+$;
    — ↑ CPK;
    — lactic acidosis.
  - Treatment:
    — dantrolene 2 mg/kg every 5 minutes (max 10 mg/kg);
    — hyperventilation;
    — HCO$_3$;
    — cooling;
    — maintain urine output;
    — avoid Ca, Ca antagonists, beta-blockers.

Table 5.16 Clinical, molecular, and pathophysical features of muscle channelopathies

	HypoPP	HyperKK	Myotonia congenita	Paramyotonia congenita
Mode of inheritance	AD	AD	AR (Becker's)/ AD (Thomsen's)	AD
Gene	CACNA1S-SCN4A	SCN4A	CLCN1 on chr 7q35	SCN4A on chr17q35
Mutations	CACNA1S (60%), SCN4A (10%)	SCN4A (55%)	CLCN1 (95%)	SCN4A
Penetrance	↓ females	> 90%	> 90%	> 90%
Prevalence	1:100 000	1:200 000	1:100 000	
Onset	1st–2nd decades	1st decade	1st–2nd decade	Neonate–infancy
Duration of attacks	Hours–days	Hours	Hours	Cold, associated weakness lasts minutes or days when associated with hyperK PP
Triggers	Rest after exercise, carbohydrate load	Rest after exercise, K+-rich foods	Cold, stress, pregnancy	Cold, exertion, spontaneous
Ictal K+	↓	↑, normal	Normal	Some association with hyperK PP
EMG myotonia	No	Yes	Yes	Yes + ↓ CMAP with cooling
Fixed proximal weakness	Yes	Yes	±	±
Cardiac arrhythmia	No	No	No	No
Response to K+	Improves weakness	Triggers weakness	No effect	Weakness is K+ sensitive
Treatment				
ACZ	Yes	Yes	No	Yes (weakness)
DCP	Yes	Yes	No	Yes (weakness)
Thiazides	No	Yes	No	Yes (weakness)
Mexiletine	No	Yes/no	Yes	Yes (myotonia)

Acz, acetazolamide; DCP, dichlorophenamide; hyperKK, hyperkalaemic periodic paralysis; hypoPP, hypokalaemic periodic paralysis.

Epilepsy
- Generalized epilepsy with febrile seizures plus syndrome (Dravet syndrome):
  - mutations in SCN1B, GABA receptor gene (GABRG2), SCNA2A.
- Autosomal dominant nocturnal frontal lobe epilepsy;
  - mutations in nicotinic acetylcholine receptor CHRNA4 and CHRNB2.

Further reading

Graves TD, Hanna M (2005). Neurological channelopathies. *Postgrad. Med.*, **81**, 20–32.

Meola G, Hanna MG, Fontaine B (2009). Diagnosis and new treatment in muscle channelopathies. *J. Neurol. Neurosurg. Psychiatry*, **80**, 360–5.

Motor neuron disease: introduction and clinical features

Incidence: 2/100 000/year; prevalence 5/100 000. In UK, 1200 new cases per year. Age of onset: median 60 years, but up to 10% present < 40 years.

Aetiology

- 5–10% autosomal dominant inheritance.
- 20% of these have a mutation in gene for Cu, Zn superoxide dismutase (SOD1).
- Clustering in some areas, e.g. Guam (genetic and dietary factors).

Clinical features

Typical MND (amyotrophic lateral sclerosis)

- 70% of cases.
- Asymmetric onset of weakness in upper or lower limb (e.g. foot drop or hand weakness) or dysarthria or dysphagia. Note: dysphagia without dysarthria unusual.
- Variable mixture of upper and lower motor signs, e.g. weak wasted triceps with brisk reflex.
- Widespread fasciculation may only be evident if patient examined carefully. Observe muscles for a few minutes.
- Fasciculating tongue (difficult sign in early stages).
- Neck flexion weakness.
- Corticobulbar signs, e.g. brisk jaw jerk, forced yawning.
- ⇈ plantar responses.
- Abdominal reflexes retained.
- Sensory symptoms occasionally but no signs.
- Median survival 3–4 years.

Progressive bulbar palsy

- 20% cases.
- More common in elderly women.
- Onset with dysarthria and/or dysphagia. Note: dysphagia without dysarthria very unusual.
- Limb involvement later, perhaps years.
- Median survival 2–3 years.

Progressive muscular atrophy (PMA)

- 10% of cases.
- LMN weakness of arms or legs (e.g. 'flail arm variant' or Vulpian–Bernhardt syndrome).
- Most develop bulbar symptoms.
- Median survival 5 years; some 10 years.

Primary lateral sclerosis

- Slowly progressive, symmetrical upper motor neuron syndrome.
- Survival 15–20 years.

ALS–frontal lobe dementia syndrome
- 5% of cases.
- Presentation with frontotemporal dementia.
- Later develop signs of MND.
- 3% of cases (30% of MND patients have frontal cognitive changes).

Other presentations to the neurologist
- Respiratory failure.
- Wasted hand.
- Weight loss.
- Dropped head.

Other causes of motor neuron disorders

Genetic
- Spinal muscular atrophy (proximal and distal onset; autosomal recessive).
- Brown–Vialetto–von Laere syndrome (early-onset bulbar and spinal MND with sensorineural deafness) and Fazio–Londe syndrome (infantile onset, bulbar, autosomal recessive)—due to mutations in SLC52A3 gene with riboflavin deficiency.
- Hexosaminidase deficiency.
- X-linked bulbospinal muscular atrophy (Kennedy's syndrome)—mutation in androgen receptor gene:
  - facial and tongue fasciculations;
  - proximal symmetrical weakness;
  - gynaecomastia;
  - diabetes;
  - sensory neuropathy (on NCS).
- Hereditary spastic paraparesis.

Acquired
- Infections (poliomyelitis, HTLV-1, HIV).
- Prion disease (amyotrophic form of CJD).
- Toxins (lead, mercury).
- Endocrinopathies ($\uparrow$ T_4, hyperparathyroidism, insulinoma).

Mimics of MND
- Spondylotic myeloradiculopathy (cervical and lumbar).
- Multifocal motor neuropathy with conduction block.
- Foramen magnum lesions.
- Syringomyelia.
- Spinal dural fistulae.
- Inclusion body myositis.
- Myasthenia gravis.
- Benign cramp fasciculation syndrome.

Motor neuron disease: investigations and management

Investigations

First-line
- FBC, ESR.
- Biochemistry including Ca^{2+}, glucose, T_4, CPK, immunoglobulins, and protein electrophoresis; VDRL + TPHA.
- Autoantibody screen.
- CXR.
- MRI, e.g. craniocervical junction, lumbar spine.
- EMG and NCT (see 📖 Chapter 8).

Second-line
- CSF examination: protein may be slightly ↑; > 5 cells, markedly elevated protein, oligoclonal bands may suggest another diagnosis (e.g. motor variant of CIDP, meningeal infiltration, HIV, or syphilis).
- ACh receptor antibodies.
- Anti-GM1 antibodies (MMN with CB).
- Anti-neuronal antibodies.
- Lead and mercury levels.
- Hexosaminidase levels (white cell enzymes).
- Muscle biopsy (inclusion body myositis).
- Nerve biopsy (if sensory abnormalities on NCT) for vasculitis.

Management

Involvement of a multidisciplinary team
- Specialist MND nurse.
- Physiotherapist.
- Orthotics (neck brace, ASO).
- OT.
- SALT (communication aids, swallowing assessments).
- Dietician.
- Respiratory team.
- Gastroenterology.
- In the later stages, palliative care.

Drug treatment
- Riluzole, 50 mg bd ↑ life expectancy by 3 months. Important psychologically for patient and family. LFTs need monitoring.

Symptomatic treatment
See Table 5.18.

Nutrition
- Consider PEG or radiologically inserted gastrostomy (RIG). Indications:
  - risk of aspiration;
  - > 10% loss of body weight despite nutritional supplements;
  - dehydration.
- PEG relatively safe if VC > 1 L; if VC < 1 L, RIG safer.

Table 5.18 Symptomatic treatment in MND

Symptom	Treatment
Cramps	Quinine sulfate 200 mg bd; carbamazepine, phenytoin, baclofen
Sialorrhea	Home suction device; atropine eye drops 0.5%, one drop instilled sublingual bd; hyoscine transdermal patches; amitriptyline 10 mg; glycopyrronium bromide liquid
Thick secretions, weak cough	Carbocisteine 250–750 mg tds; assisted cough
Emotional lability	SSRI (citalopram)
Depression	Psychological support; antidepressants

Respiratory support

Respiratory insufficiency may occur insidiously and requires regular assessment.

- Symptoms: orthopnoea, dyspnoea on mild exertion or talking, poor sleep, excessive daytime sleepiness (Epworth sleep score > 9), fatigue, impaired concentration, morning headache.
- Signs: ↑RR, paradoxical diaphragmatic movement, weak cough, tachycardia, confusion.
- Measure FVC sitting or standing and supine. If supine < 25% sitting, significant diaphragmatic weakness is present. FVC ≤ 80% predicted indicative of respiratory insufficiency.
  - Measurement may be difficult in patients with facial weakness or bulbar involvement.
  - Sniff nasal pressure may be more accurate.
    ≤ 40 mmHg = respiratory insufficiency.
- Blood gases (ear lobe) PCO_2 ≥ 6.5 kPa = respiratory failure.
- Nocturnal desaturation on overnight oximetry.
- Non-invasive ventilation (NIV) utilizes nasal or face masks and non-invasive inspiratory positive pressure devices (NIPPY).

Further reading

Andersen PM, Abrahams S, Borasio GD, et al. (2012). EFNS guidelines on the clinical management of amyotrophic lateral sclerosis (ALS): revised report of an EFNS task force. *Eur. J. Neurol.*, **19**, 360–75.

NICE (2010). *Motor neurone disease: non-invasive ventilation.* NICE Clinical Guideline 105.

Multiple sclerosis: introduction and clinical features

Multiple sclerosis (MS) is an inflammatory demyelinating disorder of the CNS defined by episodes disseminated in time and neuroanatomical location.

Epidemiology

- In the UK, 90 000 individuals affected.
- Incidence 7/100 000/year, prevalence 100–150/100 000.
- Female:male ratio 2:1.
- Rare before puberty and after the age of 60 years.
- Peak incidence in thirties and forties.
- Incidence higher with increasing latitude.
- Recent data suggest that, owing to its immunomodulatory effects, low vitamin D levels may be a risk factor for the development of MS as well as affecting disease course.

Pathogenesis

- Two phases—initial inflammatory process (relapsing–remitting phase) followed by a degenerative phase (secondary phase).
- Primary progressive MS—degenerative from onset.
- An association with HLA DR15 and DQ6 suggests genetic susceptibility triggered by an environmental factor (e.g. infection with EBV or HHV6).

Clinical features

Subacute evolution of symptoms over days; symptoms reach a plateau and resolve over days or weeks.

- Transverse myelitis:
  - weakness, sensory symptoms;
  - urinary urgency and retention;
  - flexor spasms;
  - spastic quadri- or paraparesis;
  - sensory level.
- Brainstem:
  - ataxia;
  - diplopia;
  - dysarthria;
  - facial numbness;
  - internuclear ophthalmoplegia;
  - gaze palsy;
  - rubral tremor.
- Cerebellum:
  - ataxia, dysarthria, nystagmus.

- Optic neuritis: visual loss, painful eye movements, RAPD (relative afferent pupillary defect), impaired colour vision (Ishihara colour plates), ↓ acuity, optic atrophy.
- Cerebral hemispheres:(subcortical white matter):
  - poor memory;
  - disinhibition (late);
  - dementia (late).
- Cortical:
  - epilepsy (10%).
- Characteristic symptoms/signs:
  - Lhermitte's phenomenon. Neck flexion causes paraesthesiae or tingling down the spine due to a cervical cord plaque. Other causes: B_{12} deficiency, cervical spondylosis, or tumour.
  - Uhthoff's phenomenon: worsening of symptoms (e.g. vision) when body temperature is raised (e.g. during exercise).
  - Internuclear ophthalmoplegia.
    — Other causes: vascular, Wernicke's encephalopathy, pseudo-INO in MG.

Course of disease

- 85% present with relapsing–remitting disease (RRMS).
- After 10–15 years, 50–60% enter the secondary progressive phase, some with relapses (SPMS).
- 10% have primary progressive disease (PPMS) with gradual accumulation of disability:
  - average age of onset 40 years.
  - males affected > females.

Multiple sclerosis: investigations and diagnosis

Investigations

MRI

See Figs 5.15 and 5.16.

- T_2W high signal changes seen in the corpus callosum, periventricular white matter, brainstem, and cerebellum.
- In patients > 50 years white matter lesions are less specific as they are found in normal individuals and those with cerebrovascular disease and migraine.

Evoked responses

- Visual evoked response (VER): delay is the most sensitive method of demonstrating previous optic neuritis even after clinical recovery.
- Somatosensory evoked potential (SSEP) and brainstem evoked potential (BSEP) less useful.

CSF oligoclonal bands (OCBs)

- Presence of OCBs in the CSF not in the serum are indicative of inflammation confined to the CNS.
- Positive in 95% of clinically definite MS.
- May be present in other disorders, such as paraneoplastic syndromes, vasculitis, autoimmune disorders, infections.

Diagnosis of MS

See Box 5.2 for the revised McDonald criteria for diagnosis of MS.

- MS is a clinical diagnosis with a prerequisite for evidence of lesions disseminated in time and place and the exclusion of mimics.
- It is not possible to diagnose MS after a single monophasic episode even if there are multiple lesions on MRI as there is no dissemination in time. However gadolinium enhancement found in some but not all lesions would indicate dissemination in time.
- After an isolated episode of demyelination an abnormal brain MRI suggests that the likelihood of suffering a further attack, and therefore of making a diagnosis of MS, is 80% compared with 20% if brain MRI is normal.

Box 5.2 Revised McDonald criteria for diagnosis of MS[1]

Two or more episodes; objective clinical evidence of two or more lesions
- No additional tests required.

Two or more episodes; objective clinical evidence of one lesion
- Dissemination in space shown by MRI (see Box 5.3 for Barkhof–Tintoré criteria) or two or more MRI lesions consistent with MS + OCBs in CSF or await further clinical episode at a different site.

One episode; objective clinical evidence or two or more lesions
- Dissemination in time shown by MRI at least 3 months later shows one or more Gd enhancing lesions or two scans are done, the first at least 30 days after onset of episode and the second at least 30 days later with one or more new T_2 lesions on the second scan or second clinical episode.

One episode; objective clinical evidence of one lesion
- Dissemination in space shown by MRI or two or more MRI lesions consistent with MS + OCBs in CSF *and*
- Dissemination in time shown by MRI or second clinical episode

Insidious neurological progression suggestive of MS
- One year of disease progression and two of the following:
  - positive brain MRI (nine T_2 lesions or four or more T_2 lesions with positive VER);
  - MRI spinal cord lesions;
  - OCBs in CSF.

[1]Polman CH, Reingold SC, Edan G, et al. (2005). Diagnostic criteria for MS: 2005 revisions to the McDonald criteria. *Ann Neurol.*, **58**, 840–6.

Box 5.3 Barkhof–Tintoré criteria

Greatest accuracy in predicting clinically definite multiple sclerosis, achieved with ≥ 3 positive features.
- At least one Gd enhancing lesion or nine T_2 hyperintense lesions if no Gd enhancing lesion present.
- At least one or more infratentorial lesions.
- At least one or more juxtacortical lesions.
- At least three or more periventricular lesions.

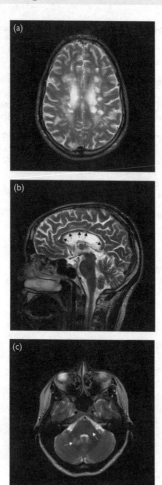

Fig. 5.15 Multiple sclerosis. (a), (c) T$_2$-weighted axial; (b) sagittal T$_2$-weighted MRI. Multiple rounded or ovoid deep cerebral white matter lesions with surrounding areas of ill-defined less pronounced hyperintensity are typical. There is marked involvement of the corpus callosum demostrated axially and sagittally (*black arrows*). Involvement of the posterior fossa is common; in this case, lesions in the middle cerebellar peduncles are particularly suggestive of MS ((c) *white arrows*.) (a), (b) Note that there is loss of white matter volume and thinning of the corpus callosum in keeping with the later stages of disease progression.

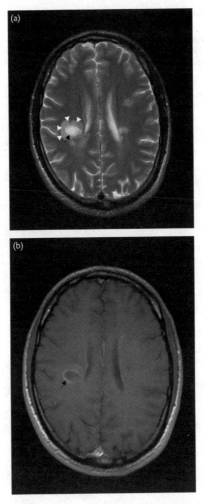

Fig. 5.16 Acute presentation of MS. (a) Axial T$_2$-weighted and (b) axial post-contrast enhanced MRI. Several rounded hyperintense lesions in the deep cerebral white matter. The largest in the right corona radiata ((a) *black arrow*) is surrounded by a halo of slightly less hyperintensity ((a) *white arrowheads*) and demonstrates an incomplete ring of enhancement ((b) *black arrow*).

Differential diagnosis

ADEM
- Usually antecedent infection or immunization.
- Monophasic.
- Fever, headache, meningism.
- Seizures.
- Coma.
- Multifocal neurological deficits.
- Bilateral ON.
- CSF pleocytosis, elevated protein.
- OCB positive in 30% and may disappear.
  - MRI shows larger lesions; involve grey matter; mass effect; uniform enhancement.

Neurosarcoidosis
- Systemic features (lungs, skin, uveitis).
- Meningeal enhancement on MRI with Gd.
- Other investigations: ACE, CXR, gallium or PET scan, lacrimal gland biopsy.

See Fig. 5.17.

Neuromyelitis optica (NMO)
- Optic neuritis and myelitis occur simultaneously or in rapid succession.
- MRI brain normal.
- OCB negative.
- NMO IgG antibody positive.

See 📖 'Neuromyelitis optica', pp. 322–3.

Other mimics
- SLE.
- Behçet's disease.
- Lyme disease.
- Primary CNS vasculitis.
- Leucodystrophies.

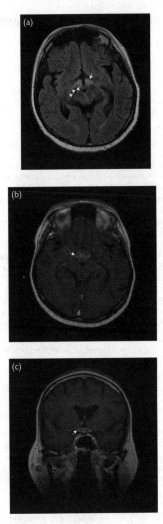

Fig. 5.17 Neurosarcoidosis: (a) FLAIR axial; (b), (c) axial and coronal post-contrast enhanced MRI. There is hyperintensity, expansion, and peripheral enhancement of the optic chiasm and hypothalamus (*white arrows*) with extension of abnormal signal posteriorly along the right optic tract ((a) *white arrowheads*).

Multiple sclerosis: management

Acute relapses

- Corticosteroids hasten recovery.
    - IV methylprednisolone 1 g daily for 3 days or 500 mg daily for 5 days.
    - Oral methyprednisolone 500 mg–2 g daily for 3–5 days.
- Side effects (intravenous): flushing, psychiatric disturbance, insomnia, hyperglycaemia, hypertension. Exclude infection prior to treatment (MSU). Rarely, aseptic bone necrosis reported.

Disease-modifying treatments (DMTs)

- Interferon beta is a natural cytokine with effects on the immune system. Three preparations are available:
    - IFN beta-1b (Betaferon®)—250 micrograms SC on alternate days;
    - IFN beta-1a (Avonex®)—30 micrograms IM once weekly;
    - IFN beta-1a (Rebif®)—22–44 micrograms SC 3× weekly.
- Glatiramer acetate (Copaxone®) is a combination of amino acids—30 micrograms SC daily.
- All drugs ↓ frequency of relapse by a third, i.e. from three to two relapses over 3 years.
- IFN beta reduces progression of disability compared with placebo through prevention of relapses. It is not clear if this is sustained.
- The effect of IFN beta in secondary progressive disease is unclear, but it probably does not have significant impact if no relapses. May be effective in those with superimposed relapsing disease.
- IFN beta shows no effect in primary progressive disease.
- Neutralizing antibodies: ↓ efficacy of IFN beta. Cross-react with all preparations and switching preparations ineffective. Role of routine testing unclear.

In patients with aggressive disease or unresponsive to IFN, there are second- and third-line treatment options.

Second-line therapy:

Fingolimod is a sphingosine-1-phosphate receptor ligand which prevents egree of lymphocytes from lymph nodes into the CNS.

- FREEDOMS and TRANSFORM trials—↓RR by 50%.
- Oral dose 0.5 mg daily.
- Side effects: influenza virus infections, diarrhoea, ↑LFT, macular oedema. Transient bradycardia, ↓AV conduction, heart beat after first dose. All patients need cardiac monitoring before, during, and for 6 hours after first dose or if treatment has been interrupted for one day or more in first two weeks, > 7 days during weeks 3 + 4 or > two weeks after one month of treatment.

Third-line therapy:

- Natalizumab (Tysabri®) 300 mg IV once every 4 weeks. ↓ relapse rate up to 81% at 2 years and up to 64% ↓ disability over 2 years. Risk (low, around 1 in 1000) of progressive multifocal leucoencephalopathy (PML). Expensive (£20,000/year). Best administered in specialized centres with careful monitoring protocols for PML (risk stratification by measuring anti-JCV antibodies in blood now possible).
- Mitoxantrone maybe as effective as natalizumab but side effects include cardiotoxicity and risk of acute leukaemia.

Other treatment options:
- Teriflunomide is a dihydroorotate dehydrogenase inhibitor. Oral dose 14 mg once daily. Effect on relapses, disease progression, and MRI activity comparable to first-line therapies.
- Dimethyl fumarate. Oral preparation 240 mg bd. Relapse rate reduced by 50%. Conflicting data on disease progression. MRI activity reduced by 80–90%.
- Alemtuzumab (Campath 1H®) and rituximab under trial—both unlicensed to date.
- IV Ig reduces relapse rate. Effect on disease progression unclear.
- Plasma exchange for rapidly progressive disease.

Symptomatic treatment

Spasticity
Note: treating spasticity may unmask weakness and ataxia.
- Treat any infections (UTI, pressure sores), constipation, pain.
- Physiotherapy essential.
- Baclofen starting 5 mg/day ↑ to 100 mg daily in three divided doses. Limited by side effects of sedation, muscle weakness.
- Tizanidine starting 2 mg/day ↑ to 8 mg tds. LFTs need monitoring.
- Dantrolene starting 25 mg/day ↑ to 100 mg tds. Monitor LFTs.
- Gabapentin starting at 100 mg ↑ 800 mg tds helps tonic spasms or phasic spasticity.
- Clonazepam useful for night-time spasms and stiffness in combination with daytime baclofen or tizanidine.
- Cannabinoids: oromucosal spray (Sativex®) contains dronabinol and cannabidol available as an add-on treatment for spasticity. Trial results difficult to interpret because of unblinding and difficulty in spasticity assessment scales. Four-week trial reasonable.
- Focal spasticity, e.g. adductor spasm use botulinum toxin. Should be combined with physiotherapy programme.
- In severe lower limb spasticity resistant to therapy, intrathecal baclofen via a pump.

Ataxia and tremor
- Inadequate trials: consider propranolol, clonazepam, carbamazepine, ondansetron.
- In selected patients with localized, especially distal, tremor and minimal disability, role for DBS or thalamotomy.

Bladder dysfunction
Three aspects of neurogenic bladder dysfunction (all three may be present simultaneously):
- detrusor hyper-reflexia characterized by reduced capacity, urgency, frequency, and incontinence;
- detrusor/sphincter dyssynergia associated with urgency, delayed emptying, retention;
- bladder hyporeflexia characterized by incomplete emptying and increased residual urine.

Symptomatic treatment includes the following:
- Even distribution of fluid intake (2 L/day).
- Pelvic floor exercises help urgency and incontinence.

- Measure residual urine volume by catheter or bladder USS. If > 100 mL consider intermittent self-catheterization (ISC). May be limited by disability unless performed by carer.
- Detrusor hyper-reflexia treated with anticholinergics. Check post-micturition residual after starting unless using ISC:
  - oxybutynin 2.5 mg bd–5 mg bd;
  - oxybutynin XL 5 mg od;
  - tolterodine 2–4 mg/day;
  - tolterodine XL 4 mg od;
  - solifenacin 5–10 mg/day.
- Nocturia managed by: ↓ fluid intake in the evening; intranasal desmopressin 10–20 micrograms. Side effect, hyponatraemia.

Fatigue

Fatigue is common and is worsened by heat.

- Exclude other causes, e.g. ↓ Hb, ↑ T_4, depression.
- Fatigue management classes with aerobic training.
- Screen for depression and treat.

Drug treatments—inadequate trials. Consider:

- amantadine 100–200 mg daily;
- modafinil 100–200 mg daily;

Disease-modifying drugs may improve fatigue.

Paroxysmal symptoms

Duration seconds to minutes occurring up to 30 times a day. They include trigeminal neuralgia, Lhermitte's phenomenon, tonic spasms (painful contractions of the limbs), dystonic spasms, and spasms of myelopathic pain. All respond dramatically to low-dose carbamazepine (50–100 mg). Alternative drugs include oxcarbazepine and gabapentin.

Impaired ambulation

- Physiotherapy input essential.
- Recent study suggests fampridine may have a possible benefit. High cost and contraindicated in patients with seizures.

Further reading

Compston A, Coles A (2008). Multiple sclerosis. *Lancet*, **372**, 1502–17.

Rice CM (2014). Disease modification in multiple sclerosis: an update. *Pract. Neurol.*, **14**(1), 6–13.

Sorensen PS (2014). New management algorithms in multiple sclerosis. *Curr. Opin. Neurol.*, **27**(3), 246–59.

Thompson A, Toosey A, Ciccarelli O (2010). Pharmacological management of symptoms in multiple sclerosis: current approaches and future directions. *Lancet Neurol.*, **9**, 1182–99.

Neuromyelitis optica

Inflammatory demyelinating disorder which is distinct from multiple sclerosis.

Epidemiology

- Incidence 0.4/million/year. Prevalence: 4/million.
- Higher incidence in Asian, Afro-Caribbean, and South American populations.
- Female predominance > 3:1. Mean age of onset 40 years.

Pathophysiology

- Identification of the disease-specific antibody NMO-Ig against the aquaporin-4 water channel located in astrocytic foot processes at the blood–brain barrier (BBB) suggests humorally mediated inflammatory disorder.
- Pathology:
  - Extensive necrosis, demyelination, and cavitation involving grey and white matter.
  - Perivascular inflammatory infiltrates and complement deposition on blood vessels implicate these sites of immune-mediated damage.

Clinical features

- Transverse myelitis (TM)—usually extensive longitudinally.
- Optic neuritis (ON)—unilateral or bilateral.
  - TM and ON can occur simultaneously, in rapid sequence, or separated by many years.
  - Consider diagnosis in apparent idiopathic relapsing myelitis or steroid-responsive optic neuritis or if poor recovery.
- Usually relapsing disorder (> 80%). Occasionally monophasic.
- Compared with MS, in NMO:
  - more TM and ON and less recovery;
  - other regions of CNS spared but disease spectrum widening with more experience.
- Hypothalamic involvement with DI, ↓ T_4, galactorrhoea.
- Evidence of other autoimmune disorders, e.g. MG, SLE, pernicious anaemia.

Differential diagnosis

- MS.
- Sarcoidosis.
- CNS vasculitis.
- Behçet's disease.
- Paraneoplastic.
- Leber's optic atrophy and autosomal dominant optic atrophy due to nuclear mitochondrial gene OPA1 mutations.

Investigations
- Blood tests: 40% have positive autoantibodies, including ANA.
- NMO antibody positive: sensitivity 73%, specificity 91%.
- CSF: ↑ lymphocytes and/or neutrophils; ↑ protein; usually (> 80%) no oligoclonal bands.
- MRI: extensive cord lesion ≥ 3 vertebral segments. Patchy enhancement. Brain: 60% have lesions usually atypical for MS around periaqueduct and hypothalamus.

Treatment
No data from large RCTs.
- Relapses treated with IV methylprednisolone 1 g × 3 followed by a steroid taper 1 mg/kg/day over months. Aim for maintenance dose 10–20 mg on alternate days.
- In steroid non-responders or in cases of rapid relapse—plasma exchange.
- Prevention of relapses with azathioprine 2.5 mg/kg. Mycophenolate mofetil an alternative. In resistant cases anecdotal reports suggest rituximab or mitoxantrone may be helpful.

Further reading
Papadopoulos MC, Verkman AS (2013). Aquaporin 4 and neuromyelitis optica. *Lancet Neurol.*, **11**(6), 535–44.

Myasthenia gravis: introduction, clinical features, and investigations

Epidemiology
- Prevalence 50–125/1 000 000.
- Peak incidence:
  - females in the second and third decades;
  - another peak affecting mainly males in the sixth and seventh decades.

Pathophysiology
- $\downarrow$ in the number of nicotinic AChRs at the neuromuscular junction (NMJ).
- Also conformational change, simplification, and $\uparrow$ gap at the NMJ.
- As a result of the decrease in receptors, the endplate potentials (EPPs) $\downarrow$ amplitude and fail to trigger a muscle action potential. Neuromuscular fatigue occurs as increasing numbers of fibres fail to fire with repeated contractions.
- AChR antibodies are pathogenic: present in 85% of generalized and 50% of ocular MG patients. No correlation between the titres of antibody and disease severity.
- Subgroup of patients with seronegative MG have antibodies to the muscle-specific kinase (MuSK) protein (up to 50% of seronegative cases).
- Thymus is abnormal in 75% of patients: hyperplasia (85%) and thymoma (15%).
- Other autoimmune conditions associated with MG: thyroiditis, Graves' disease, rheumatoid arthritis, SLE, pernicious anaemia, Addison's disease, vitiligo, NMO.

Clinical features
- Painless muscle weakness $\uparrow$ with exercise is the clinical hallmark.
- In early stages, weakness may be transient and variable; often misdiagnosed as a functional disorder.
- In 15–20%, only the ocular muscles are involved: ptosis and/or diplopia.
- In 85% the weakness is generalized.
- Presenting features are ocular (70%), limb weakness (10%), generalized muscle weakness (9%), dysphagia (6%), dysarthria and dysphonia (5%), jaw weakness (4%), and neck weakness (1%).
- Rarely, may present as respiratory failure and isolated foot drop.
- Certain muscles are preferentially affected: neck and finger extensors.
- Vital capacity measurement lying and standing essential. Peak flow measurement is unhelpful.
- Reflexes and sensory testing are normal.
- Patients with long-standing disease may be left with fixed muscle weakness.
- MG may be exacerbated by:
  - hyperthyroidism (found in 3%);
  - occult infection;
  - drugs—aminoglycosides (e.g. gentamicin), quinine, penicillamine, anti-arrhythmic drugs, botulinum toxin, anaesthetic agents (e.g. succinylcholine).

Investigations

Serum AChR antibody test
Highly specific for MG.

Repetitive nerve stimulation
Sensitive in 50–60% of cases (see 📖 Chapter 8).

Single-fibre EMG studies
Detect delay or failed neurotransmission in pairs of muscle fibres supplied by a single nerve fibre. Specialized technique positive in 90% but is not specific to MG and may be found in other NMJ disorders.

Tensilon® (edrophonium) test:
Uses a rapid-onset (30 seconds) short-acting (5 minutes) cholinesterase inhibitor drug given IV. If there is unequivocal improvement in a muscle that can be tested objectively, the test is positive.
- Difficult to interpret in borderline cases.
- Potential cardiac side effect of the test (bradycardia)—therefore performed with full resuscitation measures available.
- Two observers should be present.
- Sequence of test is as follows:
  - IV atropine 600 micrograms before edrophonium (optional);
  - test dose 3 mg edrophonium;
  - if no response, 7 mg given.

Post-contrast CT or MRI:
Mediastinum looking for thymoma.

Other tests
Striated muscle antibody occurs in 90% of patients with thymoma compared with 30% in all MG patients. Thyroid function, thyroid antibodies, vitamin B_{12}, and intrinsic and gastric parietal cell antibodies.

Differential diagnoses

Generalized MG
- Lambert–Eaton syndrome.
- Botulism.
- Drug-induced myasthenia (penicillamine).
- Congenital myasthenic syndromes.
- Inflammatory myopathies.
- Motor neuron disease (bulbar onset).

Ocular MG
- Disinsertion syndrome.
- Thyroid ophthalmopathy.
- Mitochondrial disease (progressive external ophthalmoplegia).
- Intracranial mass lesion (cavernous sinus).
- Wernicke's encephalopathy.
- Oculopharyngeal muscular dystrophy (OPMD).

Myasthenia gravis: management

Cholinesterase inhibitors

Pyridostigmine bromide acts within 1 hour with duration of action of 4 hours.

- The 2–4–6 starting regimen can be used:
  - 30 mg twice daily: 2 days;
  - 30 mg five times daily: 4 days;
  - 60 mg/30 mg/60 mg/30 mg/60 mg: 6 days;
  - 60 mg five times daily thereafter.
- The maximum dose is rarely > 300 mg/day.
- Higher doses cause muscle twitching and increased weakness. Overdosage causes a cholinergic crisis with bulbar and respiratory muscle weakness. Patients need to be warned.
- Side effects: caused by effects on muscarinic smooth muscle NMJ—abdominal pain and diarrhoea that responds to propantheline 15–30 mg PRN.

Prednisolone

- Steroids indicated in patients who are not adequately contolled with cholinesterase inhibitors and are unsuitable for thymectomy.
- Prednisolone usually started as an inpatient because of the risk of deterioration which occurs in 50% of MG patients at 7–21 days (steroid dip).
- Initial starting dose of 10 mg on alternate days is ↑ every 2 or 3 days to a dose of 1–1.5 mg/kg on alternate days.
- Improvement begins after 2–4 weeks with maximal benefit at 6–12 months.
- After 3 months, or when remission is evident, the dose is slowly tapered to the minimum required. A small dose may be required on the off day to prevent fluctuation of strength.
- A few patients may be able to do without steroids.
- All patients should be started on osteoporosis prevention with a bisphosphonate. HRT should be considered in post-menopausal women.
- Patients should be advised to carry a steroid card.

Azathioprine

- Azathioprine, with its actions predominantly on T cells, is used:
  - for those in whom corticosteroids are contraindicated;
  - for those with an insufficient response to corticosteroids;
  - as a steroid-sparing agent.
- Combination of steroids and azathioprine acts synergistically.
- TPMT levels need to be measured to predict the risk of haematological side effects.
- Starting dose is 50 mg/day for 1 week increasing by 50 mg/week to a dose of 2.5 mg/kg/day.

- Desirable haematological endpoints are:
  - WBC < 3500/mm^3;
  - lymphocyte count < 1000/mm^3;
  - MCV > 100 fL.
- Blood tests (FBC and LFT) necessary every week for 2 months and then 3-monthly for the duration of treatment.
- Therapeutic benefit may not be apparent for up to 12 months.
- Side effects:
  - 5% have a hypersensitivity reaction with nausea, abdominal pain, fever, rash, or arthralgia, in which case the drug must be stopped;
  - bone marrow suppression;
  - hepatotoxicity.

Other immunosuppressants

- Methotrexate is also used as a steroid-sparing agent (7.5–20 mg once weekly + folate).
- Mycophenolate mofetil 1 g bd.
- In patients intolerant of azathioprine, ciclosporin 2–5 mg/kg/day in two divided doses (total dose 125–250 mg twice daily) may be considered. Side effects include nephrotoxicity and hypertension. Trough drug levels need monitoring.
- Rituximab (anti-CD20 B-cell monoclonal antibody) 375 mg/m^2 IV four times weekly—anecdotal reports of benefit in resistant cases.

Plasma exchange and IV immunoglobulin

- Both may be used for patients in myasthenic crisis with severe bulbar and respiratory compromise.
- Patients may also be pre-treated prior to thymectomy.
- Patients with seronegative MG may also respond. The effects last 4–6 weeks.
- Plasma exchange: five exchanges, 3–4 L per exchange over 2 weeks.
- IV immunoglobulin: 0.4 g/kg/day for 5 days.

Thymectomy

- Procedure should be carried out in units with adequate surgical and postoperative experience of management of MG patients.
- Mortality rate in such institutions is the same as for general anaesthesia.
- Postoperative anticholinesterase medication is given IV at a dose of 75% of the preoperative oral dose.

Indications

- Prevention of local spread of a thymoma. If complete removal cannot be achieved, postoperative radiotherapy is necessary. Some patients with thymoma may become weaker after thymectomy and require further immunosuppressive treatment.
- Therapeutic benefit in MG (generalized and less often in ocular myasthenia): results in complete remission in some patients or a reduction in immunosuppressive medication in others.

- No RCTs in patients under the age of 45 years with AChR antibodies: general consensus on its benefit.
- Surgery should be considered before starting corticosteroids if clinically feasible.
- Controversy in patients > 45 years and those who are AChR antibody negative.
- In children surgery should be deferred until after puberty since the thymus has a role in the development of the immune system.
- Benefits of thymectomy may not be evident until months or years after surgery.

Summary of MG management
See Fig. 5.18.

Ocular MG
- In patients with pure ocular MG who do not completely respond to pyridostigmine, corticosteroids are necessary. Low doses may often be adequate.
- Thymectomy is an option in younger AChR-antibody-positive patients.
- If the extraocular muscle weakness is consistent, prisms may help the diplopia.
- Ptosis props help to hold up the eyelids.
- Where deficits are chronic and static, corrective surgery may be an option.

Women and MG
- 14% of babies born to mothers with MG develop neonatal MG due to the placental transfer of maternal antibodies.
- Weakness may be apparent days after birth and last for days or months. Treatment is not necessary.
- Some patients have antibodies to fetal as well as adult AChRs. This may result in recurrent miscarriage or give rise to fetal deformities such as arthrogryposis multiplex congenita or facial deformities.
- Corticosteroids and azathioprine are both teratogenic. Adequate advice on contraception and pre-pregnancy counselling are necessary.

Further reading
Farrugia ME, Vincent A (2010). *Curr. Opin. Neurol.*, **23**, 489–95.
Jacob S, Viegas S, Lashley D, Hilton-Jones D (2009). Myasthenia gravis and other neuromuscular junction disorders. *Pract. Neurol.*, **9**, 364–71.
Keesey J (2004). Clinical evaluation and management of myasthenia gravis. *Muscle Nerve*, **29**, 484–505.

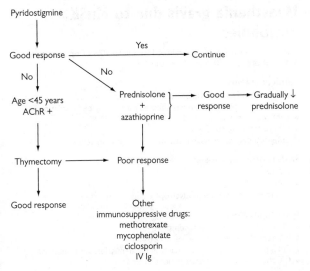

Fig. 5.18 Flowchart for the management of MG.

Myasthenia gravis due to MuSK antibodies

- Accounts for 5–8% of generalized MG. Up to 50% of seronegative MG.
- Age of onset: 2–70 years. M:F ratio 1:3.

Clinical features
- Predominantly affects bulbar, ocular, and facial muscles.
- Neck and respiratory muscles affected rarely. May be in isolation.
- Limb weakness usually mild.
- May deteriorate suddenly.
- Long-standing cases have facial and bulbar muscle atrophy.

Differential diagnosis
- MND.
- IBM.
- Oculopharyngeal musculodystrophy.

Investigations
- MuSK antibody +; ACh receptor ab–.
- Edrophonium test may be weakly positive.
- EMG may show NMJ abnormality in facial muscles. Limbs normal.
- CT chest—no thymic enlargement.

Management
See Fig. 5.18.
- More difficult to treat than seropositive MG.
- Poor response to acetylcholinesterase inhibitors.
- Poor response to immunosupression with corticosteroids and azathioprine.
- Good response to PE.
- Rituximab tried in resistant cases.
- Thymectomy doubtful benefit. Inadequate data.

Further reading
Guptill JT, Sanders DB, Evoli A (2011). Anti-MuSK antibody myasthenia gravis: clinical findings and response to treatment in two large cohorts. *Muscle Nerve*, **44**(1), 36–40.

Paraneoplastic disorders: introduction

- Term applies to all non-metastatic neurological conditions in which no specific aetiology, such as vascular, metabolic, or treatment-related causes, can be identified.
- Important to note that a particular antibody can be found in a number of different syndromes and that one syndrome can be associated with different antibodies.
- Usually a neurological presentation in a patient not known to have cancer.
- Clinical picture is usually with a subacute progressive syndrome, but may rarely be one with slow progression, relapses, and remissions or a benign course.
- Since there is evidence of a biologically effective immune response against the tumour, tumours may initially remain small or only locally invasive.

See Table 5.19 for antibodies and cancer types associated with paraneoplastic disorders.

Table 5.19 Paraneoplastic disorders, associated antibodies, and cancer types

Syndrome	Paraneoplastic antibody	Associated cancer
Lambert–Eaton myasthenic syndrome (LEMS)	VGCC	SCLC
Subacute cerebellar degeneration	Anti-Hu	SCLC
	Anti-PCA-2	SCLC
	Anti-Yo	Ovary, breast
	Anti-Ta/Ma2	Testis
	Anti-Ri	Breast, SLCC
	Anti-Tr = Anti-DNER	Hodgkin's lymphoma
Opsoclonus/myoclonus (children)	Anti-Hu	Neuroblastoma
Opsoclonus/myoclonus (adult)	Anti-Ri	Breast
	Anti-Hu	SCLC
	Anti-Ma	Various
	Anti-Ta/Ma2	Testis
Subacute sensory neuropathy/neuronopathy	Anti-Hu	SCLC
	Anti-amphiphysin	SCLC
	ANNA-3	SCLC
	Anti-CRMP5/CV2	SCLC, thymoma, breast
Limbic encephalitis	Anti-Hu,	SCLC
	Anti-CRMP5/CV2	SCLC, thymoma
	Anti-AMPA	Breast, lung
	Anti-GABAb	SCLC
Limbic encephalitis, + brain stem, + hypothalamic syndrome	Anti-Ta/Ma2	Testis
Encephalitis, + seizures + neuropsychiatric features + autonomic dysfunction + movement disorder	Anti-NMDA receptor	Ovarian teratoma
Encephalomyelitis, +/– rigidity	Anti-Hu	SCLC
	Anti-Ri	Breast, SCLC
	CV2/CRMP5	SCLC, breast
	Anti-glycine	Thymoma
	Anti-Ma	Various
Retinopathy	Anti-Hu	SCLC
	Anti-recoverin	SCLC
Stiff person (anti-GAD) syndrome	Anti-amphiphysin	Breast

Anti-AMPA, alpha-amino-3-hydroxy-5-methylisoxazole-4-propionic acid; anti-DNER, delta/notch-like epidermal growth factor-related receptor; anti-GAD, anti-glutamic acid decarboxylase antibody; anti-PCA-2, anti-Purkinje cell antibody; SCLC, small cell lung cancer; VGCC, voltage-gated calcium channel.

Paraneoplastic syndromes: central nervous system

Limbic encephalitis

- Presents with short-term anterograde with variable retrograde memory disturbance.
- May be associated with denial and confabulation.
- Epileptic seizures (as a partial non-convulsive status).
- Acute confusional state; psychiatric symptoms (such as personality change, hallucinations, depression) may coexist.
- MRI (Fig. 5.19): hyperintensity signal change in mesial temporal lobes.
- CSF: mild pleocytosis and oligoclonal bands.
- Pathologically, there is neuronal loss in the amygdala and hippocampi.
- Differential diagnosis includes:
  - voltage gated K^+ channel complex antibodies (usually LG1-1) (see Chapter 3, 'Acute encephalitis (including limbic encephalitis)', pp. 130–1);
  - tumours;
  - infective meningoencephalitis (HSV);
  - thiamine deficiency;
  - venous thrombosis;
  - vasculitis.

Encephalomyelitis with or without rigidity (spinal interneuronitis)

- Generalized disorder may occur.
- Cognitive change.
- Seizures.
- Brainstem, cerebellar, and myelopathic symptoms and signs.
- Patients present initially with sensory symptoms such as dysaesthesiae followed by the development of stiffness and rigidity.
- Painful stimulus-sensitive spasms.
- Myoclonus.
- Profuse sweating.
- Natural history is progression to death in 3 years.
- Differential diagnosis includes stiff person syndrome with anti-GAD antibody and prion disease.

Cerebellar degeneration

- Rapidly evolving syndrome over days and weeks.
- Affects gait, speech, trunk, and limbs.
- Vertigo, nausea, vomiting, and downbeat nystagmus.
- Differential diagnosis:
  - tumours;
  - demyelination syndromes;
  - infections (viral cerebellitis);
  - drugs.
- MRI: cerebellar atrophy.
- CSF: mild pleocytosis with oligoclonal bands.

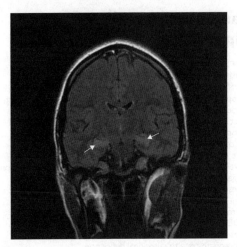

Fig. 5.19 Limbic encephalitis (coronal FLAIR MRI). Symmetric hyperintensity and swelling of the hippocampus bilaterally (*white arrows*). While paraneoplasia is the most common aetiology, potassium channelopathies, status epilepticus, and hypoxic injury are other causes.

Opsoclonus, myoclonus, and ataxia
- 'Dancing eyes, dancing feet syndrome' occurs as a result of damage to the fastigial nucleus of the cerebellum or may arise from dysfunction of omnipause neurons in the pons.
- Opsoclonus is defined as involuntary, chaotic, and repetitive rapid eye movements. In children this is due to either a neuroblastoma or a viral infection.

Rhombencephalitis
- Generalized brainstem syndrome may occur with gaze palsies; respiratory involvement with central sleep apnoea.
- Differential diagnosis:
  - infections such as listeria;
  - inflammatory conditions such as Behçet's disease.

Retinopathy
- Rare.
- Associated with melanoma.
- Symptoms include painless loss of visual acuity, photosensitivity, abnormalities of colour vision (cone symptoms), and night blindness (rod symptoms).
- Electroretinogram is flat even though vision may be relatively preserved.
- Differential diagnosis: vascular and vasculitic disorders such as giant cell arteritis; optic neuritis; drugs and toxins; Leber's optic atrophy.

Paraneoplastic syndromes: peripheral nervous system

Sensory neuropathy/neuronopathy (dorsal root ganglionopathy)

- Typically patients present with an asymmetrical painful sensory neuropathy that gradually evolves to loss of proprioception with pseudoathetosis and a severe sensory ataxia.
- Onset may be in the upper limbs, which is unusual in peripheral neuropathies.
- Rate of progression variable.
- There may be motor involvement.
- Nerve conduction tests may show both axonal and demyelination changes.
- In sensory neuropathy/neuronopathy sensory action potentials are absent with no or minimal motor abnormalities.
- Differential diagnoses:
  - CIDP;
  - vasculitis;
  - neuropathy due to nutritional deficiencies;
  - Sjögren's syndrome;
  - vitamin B_6 excess.

Motor neuron syndromes

- Three groups identified in cancer patients with motor neuron syndromes:
  - some are anti-Hu positive and will go on to develop involvement of other areas of the nervous system;
  - patients, usually women, who present with an upper motor syndrome that resembles primary lateral sclerosis and also have breast cancer;
  - patients who have both amyotrophic lateral sclerosis and cancer coincidentally.
- There may be an association between lymphoma and cancer.
- Differential diagnosis includes multifocal motor neuropathy with conduction block, which is associated with anti-GMI antibodies.

Autonomic neuropathy

- Autonomic failure may be a paraneoplastic manifestation with postural dizziness, abdominal pain, diarrhoea, gastroparesis, pseudo-obstruction, and oesophageal achalasia.
- Differential diagnoses include:
  - Guillain–Barré syndrome;
  - amyloid neuropathy;
  - autonomic variant of multiple system atrophy.

Lambert–Eaton syndrome (LEMS)

- In 60% of cases this is a paraneoplastic disorder usually associated with small cell lung cancer.
- 40% autoimmune (usually female and younger patients).
- Voltage-gated calcium-channel antibody does not discriminate between the two.
- Clinical presentation:
  - proximal weakness around the pelvic girdle with or without weakness around the shoulder girdle;
  - weakness improves with sustained or repeated exercise;
  - reflexes reappear after exercise (post-tetanic accentuation);
  - cranial nerve involvement occurs in 30% (dysphagia, dysarthria, ptosis, and diplopia);
  - autonomic involvement is manifested with symptoms of a dry mouth.
- EMG studies show:
  - reduced amplitude of the CMAP after a single supramaximal stimulus;
  - an increase after exercise (post-exercise facilitation);
  - a decremental response to repetitive stimulation at 3 Hz with an incremental response > 200% at > 30 Hz.
- Single-fibre studies reveal increased jitter.
- Edrophonium test may be positive in LEMS but never to the extent seen in myasthenia gravis.
- Other causes of myopathy also need to be considered.

Paraneoplastic syndromes: investigations and management

Tumour identification
- Careful clinical examination should include looking for:
  - clubbing;
  - skin examination for melanoma;
  - lymphadenopathy at all palpable sites;
  - breast palpation;
  - testicular palpation;
  - PR examination;
  - PV examination (by gynaecologist if necessary).
- Tumour markers:
  - PSA (prostate-specific antigen);
  - CEA (carcinoembryonic antigen) for GI malignancy;
  - CA125 (for ovarian cancer).
- Imaging:
  - CXR;
  - CT or MRI of chest, abdomen, and pelvis;
  - mammography;
  - increasing role for the use of positron emission tomography (PET) in detection of cancers if the above investigations are negative, but note may be negative in adenocarcinomas and testicular tumours.

Management
Treatment of the tumour, if possible, should be the first line of management. Paraneoplastic peripheral syndromes and those due to Hodgkin's disease seem to have the best response.

Immunological therapy
- No controlled data.
- First-line treatment: consider IV methylprednisolone 1 g/day for 3 days.
- IV immunoglobulin 0.4 g/kg/day—anecdotal reports of benefit especially in stiff person syndrome.

Symptomatic treatment
- Opsoclonus: clonazepam, propranolol.
- Myoclonus: clonazepam, valproate, piracetam.
- LEMS: 3,4-diaminopyridine, pyridostigmine.
- Stiff person syndrome: diazepam, clonazepam, baclofen.

Further reading
Antoine JC, Camdessanché JP (2007). Peripheral nervous system involvement in patients with cancer. *Lancet Neurol.*, **6**, 75–86.

Dalmau J, Rosenfeld MR (2008). Paraneoplastic syndromes of the central nervous system. *Lancet Neurol.*, **7**, 327–30.

Titulaer MJ, Soffietti R, Dalmau J, et al. (2011). Screening for tumours in paraneoplastic syndromes: report of an EFNS task force. *Eur. J. Neurol.*, **18**, 19–27.

Vertigo, dizziness, and unsteadiness: introduction

- Common problem.
- Differentiate between labyrinthine symptoms (vertigo and dizziness) and unsteadiness (staggering, off-balance), which may be due to a variety of neurological and general medical disorders, e.g. posterior fossa tumours.
- In the elderly, the clinical picture may result from multiple pathologies.

Vertigo

- Vertigo is an illusion of movement, which is typically rotational but can also be tilting or swaying.
- The underlying mechanism is an asymmetry of neural activity between the right and left vestibular nuclei.
- Vertigo is always temporary even after vestibular nerve section because of neurochemical compensatory changes in the brainstem.
- Other clinical features of vertigo:
  - nausea and vomiting;
  - worse with head movement, and patients prefer lying still.

Acute first episode of vertigo
See 📖 Chapter 4, 'Acute vertigo', pp. 138–41.

Recurrent episodes of spontaneous vertigo
Classified by duration of the vertigo.

Vertigo lasting a few seconds:
- Benign paroxysmal positional vertigo (BPPV). (See 📖 'Benign paroxysmal positional vertigo (BPPV)', pp. 344–7.)

Vertigo lasting minutes or hours
- Ménière's disease:
  - Due to intermittent endolymphatic hypertension.
  - Produces attacks of severe vertigo, nausea, and vomiting with low-frequency hearing loss, tinnitus, and a sense of fullness in the affected ear.
  - Audiogram essential: low-frequency hearing loss.
  - In the early stages the caloric and audiogram tests may be normal, but with repeated episodes progressive hearing loss will be apparent and may fluctuate.
  - Treatment: ↓ sodium intake aiming for a urinary sodium of less than 50 mmol/day. Thiazide diuretics: bendroflumethiazide 2.5 mg. Surgical options as a last resort include endolymphatic sac surgery and intracranial vestibular nerve section. Transtympanic gentamicin labyrinthectomy will stop the disabling vertigo but will not prevent hearing loss.

- Migraine:
  - Vertigo may form part of the aura in vertebrobasilar migraine and is followed by a typical throbbing headache.
  - Increasingly recognized is that some migraineurs only suffer from vertigo and nausea without a significant headache component. Standard migrainous prophylactic drugs such as beta-blockers are helpful.
- Rarely, partial seizures may present with vertigo. Usually history of epileptic seizures.
- A postoperative, post-traumatic, or cholesteatoma-associated perilymph fistula may produce vertigo, especially on straining. This is associated with hearing loss.
- Episodic ataxia (see 'Hereditary ataxias', pp. 350–1).

Dizziness, unsteadiness, or 'off balance': neurological causes

Important to assess and examine carefully for the following possible causes.

Peripheral labyrinthine disorder (PLD)

- Patients with an uncompensated PLD complain of constant 'dizziness'.
- History of a previous acute vestibular neuritis or significant head injury.

Neurological examination:

- Assess the gait looking for unsteadiness especially on turning; tandem gait with eye closure is impaired in vestibular disorders and also in patients with large fibre neuropathy and posterior spinal cord pathology.
- Positive Romberg's test—due to bilateral vestibular failure or loss of ponten sense in feet.
- Unterberger's test (see 🕮 Chapter 4, 'Acute vertigo', pp. 138–41) may indicate vestibular abnormality but will not differentiate between central and peripheral causes.
- The head impulse test (see Fig. 4.1), if positive, implies absent lateral semicircular canal function on the affected side.
- Eye movements assessed for nystagmus, pursuit, and saccades.
- Corneal reflexes should be tested in case of an acoustic neuroma, although other signs will be found.
- Hearing tested at the bedside using Rinne's and Weber's tests.
- The external auditory meati and tympanic membranes must be viewed with an auroscope.
- Hallpike's test (see Fig. 5.20) must always be performed.
- Caloric testing is helpful in confirming lateral canal paresis.
- Patients with bilateral vestibular failure (usually due to gentamicin toxicity) complain of vertigo, oscillopsia, and unsteadiness. Positive Romberg's test. There is a degradation of visual acuity with rapid head movements due to an inability to fixate.

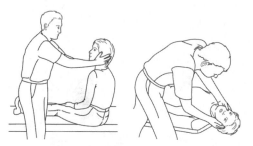

Fig. 5.20 Dix–Hallpike manoeuvre.

Cerebellar disorder

- Broad-based gait or poor tandem gait.
- Eye movements usually reveal broken-up pursuit and hypometric saccades.
- Finger–nose and heel–shin ataxia.
- Aetiology (see 📖 Chapter 4, 'Ataxia', pp. 144–7):
  - tumours;
  - drugs;
  - paraneoplastic;
  - hereditodegenerative (SCA, MSA).

Basal ganglia disorders

- Progressive supranuclear palsy may present with unsteadiness and a tendency to fall backwards.
- Autonomic dysfunction in MSA and PD will result in postural dizziness due to hypotension.

Hemispheric lesions

- Parietal lobe lesions may present with unsteadiness of gait and no other signs.
- Frontal lobe lesions cause gait disorders which are described as unsteadiness.
  - Aetiology: tumours or small vessel disease.

Hydrocephalus

- Normal pressure hydrocephalus (Hakim's triad of gait instability, urinary incontinence, and cognitive impairment).

Spinal cord disorders

- MS.
- B_{12} deficiency.

Peripheral neuropathy

- Large fibre neuropathy affecting proprioceptive fibres will cause unsteadiness and a positive Romberg's sign.
- Associated autonomic neuropathy will cause postural hypotension: diabetes, amyloid, HIV.

Primary orthostatic tremor

- Unsteadiness on standing only. Auscultate calf muscles.

Benign paroxysmal positional vertigo (BPPV)

BPPV is characterized by brief attacks of rotatory vertigo provoked by rapid changes in head position relative to gravity.

Incidence

Most common cause of dizziness, about 20%.

Pathophysiology

- BPPV is a mechanical disorder due to the movement of debris (canalolithiasis) within the endolymph to the most dependent part of the canal during changes of head position.
- Posterior semicircular canal is the most commonly affected, followed by the horizontal and, least often, the anterior semicircular canal.

Clinical features

- Antecedent events include head trauma and viral infections with or without acute labyrinthitis. In some, may occur during the course of a progressive inner ear disease such as Ménière's disease.
- Typical symptoms:
  - vertigo on turning over in bed, lying down, or sitting up from the supine position;
  - vertigo on looking up or bending forward.
- Diagnosis is made by the observation of the typical features of peripheral positional nystagmus (Table 5.20) using Hallpike's manoeuvre (Fig. 5.20).
- Typical features of posterior canal BPPV with a normal CNS examination. No further investigation unless:
  - no response to repositioning manoeuvres;
  - nystagmus is atypical (e.g. downbeating nystagmus);
  - in these circumstances MRI indicated.

Treatment
In cases with a positive Hallpike's test:
- Epley liberatory manoeuvre (Fig. 5.21).
- Semont's manoeuvre (Fig. 5.22); Brandt–Daroff positional exercises.
- These manoeuvres are effective in 80–90% of cases.

The natural history for BPPV is spontaneous resolution with exacerbations, but the condition persists in 30% if untreated.

In patients with a typical history but negative Hallpike's test, manoeuvres for the horizontal and anterior canals should be performed, i.e. variations of the Hallpike test.

Table 5.20 Characteristics of peripheral versus central positional nystagmus

Symptom/sign	Positional nystagmus	
	Peripheral	Central
Latency (time to onset of nystagmus or vertigo)	0–40 s (mean 7.8 s)	No latency
Duration	< 60 s	Symptoms, signs persist
Fatiguability (lessening signs/symptoms with repetition)	Yes	No
Nystagmus	Fixed direction, torsional towards the lowermost ear	Variable
Intensity of symptoms and signs	Severe vertigo with nausea	Mild. Nausea rare. Marked nystagmus
Reproducibilty	Inconsistent	Consistent

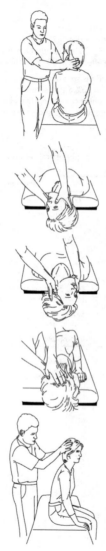

Fig. 5.21 Epley's manoeuvre. Treatment of left posterior canal BPPV.

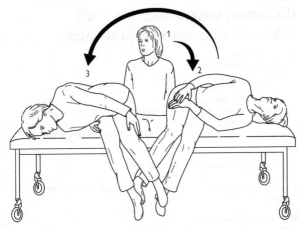

Fig. 5.22 Semont's manoeuvre. Treatment of left posterior canal BPPV.

Instructions for Semont's manoeuvre
1. Sit on edge of the bed.
2. Lie down sideways to position which brings on vertigo.
3. Change sides.
4. Remain until symptoms subside.
5. Sit up for 30 seconds.
6. Lie down on appropriate side for 30 seconds.

Continue this sequence of positioning until symptoms resolve. Repeat exercises 3–4 times a day until two consecutive vertigo-free days.

Dizziness, unsteadiness, or 'off balance': non-neurological causes

Cardiological

- If symptoms suggest presyncope consider:
  - vasovagal attacks;
  - carotid hypersensitivity;
  - postural hypotension;
  - cardiac arrhythmias such as paroxysmal atrial fibrillation and Stokes–Adams attacks.
- Severe aortic stenosis causes presyncope, especially during exertion.

Ophthalmological

- Cataracts and macular degeneration.
- Visual field defects may cause subtle unsteadiness.
- Eye movement disorders such as an internuclear ophthalmoplegia (INO).

Differential diagnoses

- MS.
- Cerebrovascular disease.
- Wernicke's encephalopathy.

Hyperventilation

- May be due to anxiety as a result of any of the above diagnoses and will compound the symptoms of dizziness and unsteadiness.
- Hyperventilation may be a sign of asthma or other lung disorder such as a PE or interstitial lung disease.
  - CXR and lung function tests necessary.
  - Constant sighing may be a clue to chronic hyperventilation.
  - ↓ PCO_2 symptoms include paraesthesiae, cold extremities, light-headedness and dizziness, chest discomfort, and a sense of weakness especially on the left.
  - Reproduce symptoms by asking patient to force hyperventilate for 3 minutes.
  - Hyperventilation is not a diagnosis. Identify underlying cause, which may be anxiety due to, for example, worry about underlying serious disease, psychological distress, or pain.

Other general medical causes

Check FBC, renal, liver, thyroid function, Ca, PO_4, glucose.

Further reading

Barraclough K, Bronstein A (2009). Vertigo. *BMJ*, **339**, 749–52.

Bronstein A, Lempert T (2007). *Dizziness: a practical approach to diagnosis and management*. Cambridge: Cambridge University Press.

Neurogenetic disorders: introduction

- 10% of neurological patients have single-gene mutation disorders.
- Family history essential. May require contacting other hospitals, consultant colleagues, and GPs.
- Examination of other family members helpful.
- Absence of FH may be due to:
  - autosomal recessive or X-linked inheritance;
  - new mutation;
  - non-paternity;
  - reduced penetrance;
  - variable phenotypes;
  - phenomenon of anticipation—milder disease in preceding generations.
- Distinction between diagnostic and predictive (or presymptomatic) testing.
  - Diagnostic test: symptomatic patient. Purpose of test is to determine cause.
  - Predictive test. At-risk but asymptomatic individual tested to determine if the mutant gene is present. Risk of developing the disease depends on penetrance.
- Pretest counselling mandatory.
- Signed consent mandatory.
- Request form requires detailed FH and clinical phenotype.
- Prenatal testing by chorionic villous biopsy available for some disorders. Counselling essential and discussions regarding any interventions, i.e. termination if test is positive.

Hereditary ataxias

Early-onset ataxias (< 20 years)

Autosomal recessive disorders: Friedreich's ataxia

Gene

Trinucleotide (GAA) mutation in Frataxin gene. 96% have an expansion in both alleles. Others have a point mutation in one allele and expansion in the other. Diagnosis excluded if two normal-sized alleles.

Clinical features
- Gait ataxia.
- Pyramidal weakness and signs, extensor plantars.
- Axonal peripheral neuropathy (absent ankle jerks).
- Optic atrophy.
- Abnormal eye movements: nystagmus, broken pursuit, hypometric saccades, macrosaccadic square-wave jerks.
- Deafness.
- Skeletal abnormalities:
  - pes cavus;
  - scoliosis.
- ECG abnormalities: widespread T-wave inversion.
- Diabetes or glucose intolerance.

Differential diagnoses
- Vitamin E deficiency.
- Abetalipoproteinaemia.
- Ataxia telangiectasia (conjunctival telangiectasia, IgA deficiency, frequent infections, risk of malignancy; ATM gene).
- Mitochondrial disorders.
- Cholestanosis (cerebrotendinous xanthomatosis). Tendon xanthomas, ataxia, spasticity, neuropathy, cataracts.
- ARSACS (with demyelinating neuropathy). Autosomal recessive spastic ataxia of Charlevoix-Saguenay. Mutations in SACS gene. Diagnosis by gene testing and optical coherence tomography (OCT)—changes in retinal fibre layer.

Late-onset ataxias (> 20 years)

Usually autosomal dominant (ADCA). All have features of cerebellar ataxia (Table 5.21).

Episodic ataxias

See Table 5.22 for characteristics.

Further reading

Durr A (2010). Autosomal dominant cerebellar ataxias: polyglutamine expansions and beyond. *Lancet Neurol.*, 9, 885–94.

Table 5.21 Characteristics of autosomal dominant cerebellar ataxias (ADCA)

Clinical features	Gene
ADCA type I (complex)	
± Pyramidal signs ± supranuclear ophthalmoplegia ± extrapyramidal signs ± peripheral neuropathy ± dementia	SCA1, SCA2, SCA3, SCA12, SCA17
ADCA type II	
Pigmentary retinopathy ± any other signs for type I (above)	SCA7
ADCA type III	
Pure cerebellar ± mild pyramidal signs. Late onset	SCA6

Table 5.22 Characteristics of episodic ataxias EA1 and EA2

Features	EA1	EA2
Age at onset (years)	3–20	3–30
Duration of attack	Minutes	Hours–days
Interictal myokymia	+	–
Response to acetazolamide	+/–	++
Progressive ataxia	No	Sometimes. Interictal nystagmus
Seizures	Sometimes	No
Gene	K^+ channel, KCNA1	Na^+ channel, CACNA1A

Genetic neuropathies

Classification:

- Neuropathy sole or major part of presentation:
  - Charcot–Marie–Tooth disease (CMT);
  - hereditary neuropathy with liability to pressure palsies (HNPP);
  - hereditary sensory and autonomic neuropathy (HSAN/HSN);
  - distal hereditary motor neuropathies (dHMN);
  - hereditary neuralgic amyotrophy (HNA).
- Neuropathy part of multisystem hereditary disorders:
  - familial amyloid polyneuropathy (FAP);
  - neuropathy associated with metabolic disorders, e.g. adrenoleucodystrophy, Fabry's disease, metachromatic leucodystrophy, Tangier's disease;
  - porphyrias;
  - disorders with defective DNA;
  - neuropathies associated with mitochondrial disorders (MERRF, NARP, MINGIE, SANDO, POLG1);
  - neuropathies associated with other genetic disorders, e.g. hereditary ataxias.

Figures 5.23 and 5.24 show flowcharts for genetic neuropathies.

Charcot–Marie–Tooth disease (CMT)

- Common condition: prevalence 1/2500.
- NCT helps to classify into:
  - Demyelinating: upper limb MCV < 38 m/s with SAPs ↓ or absent. Other clues: homogeneous slowing. Patchy slowing may indicate CMT1 X (GJB1, connexin 32) or acquired demyelinating neuropathy.
  - Axonal: upper limb MCV > 38 m/s.
  - Intermediate: upper limb MCV 25–45 m/s may indicate CMT1 X.

Autosomal dominant demyelinating neuropathy (CMT1)

- CMT1a most common form of CMT1 (70%). Caused by duplication in peripheral myelin protein 22 gene (PMP22) on chromosome 17p11.2. Note up to 10% sporadic. 1% (usually more severe) due to point mutations.
- CMT1b. AD. (10%) Caused by mutations in human myelin protein zero (MP0) on chromosome 1q22–q23.
- CMT1c. Classic CMT. Caused by mutation in LITAF/SIMPLE gene.
- CMT1d caused by mutations in early growth response 2 gene (EGR) on chromosome 10. Rare. Severe phenotype; cranial nerve involvement.
- CMT1f: NEFL gene. Rare. Early onset, tremor, and cerebellar ataxia.
- Dejerine–Sottas disease (and congenital hypomyelinating neuropathies) which present in the first decade and are more severe due to point mutations in PMP22, MPZ, and EGR2.

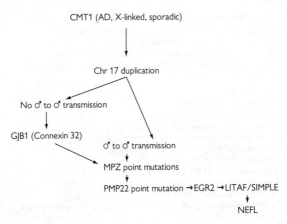

Fig. 5.23 EGR2, early growth response 2; GJB1, gap junction protein beta 1; LITAF, lipopolysaccharide-induced tumour necrosis factor; MPZ, myelin protein zero; NEFL, neurofilament light polypeptide; PMP22, peripheral myelin protein 22; SIMPLE, small integral membrane protein of lysosome.

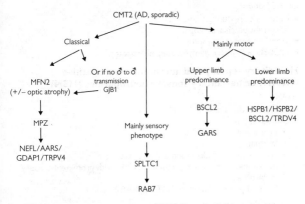

Fig. 5.24 AARS, alanyl-tRNA-synthetase; BSCL2, Berardinelli–Seip congenital lipodystrophy; GARS, glycyl tRNA synthetase; GDAP1, ganglioside-induced differentiation-associated protein 1; GJB1, gap junction protein beta 1; HSPB1, heat shock protein beta-1; HSPB2, heat shock protein beta-2; MF2, mitofusin 2; MPZ, myelin protein zero; NEFL, neurofilament light polypeptide; RAB7, member RAS oncogene family; SPLTC1, serine palmitoyltransferase, long-chain base subunit-1; TRPV4, transient receptor potential vanilloid 4 protein.

Autosomal dominant axonal neuropathy (CMT2)
Fewer genes identified. In sporadic and AD axonal neuropathy:
- mitofusin 2 (20%) (mitochondrial GTPase);
- if no male-to-male transmission or sporadic or index case female: consider GJB1. If negative: MPZ, neurofilament light chain (NEFL), HSP22, and HSP27.

Intermediate cases
- Check chr 17 first. If negative and no male-to-male transmission check GJB1 encoding connexin 32 (CMTX):
  - males more severely affected than females;
  - females may be axonal, males demyelinating;
  - neurophysiology—patchy demyelination,
  - rarely, CNS involved (plantars ↑).
- If negative: MPZ, PMP22, and EGR2 point mutations.
- Autosomal recessive demyelinating neuropathy (CMT4).
- Autosomal recessive axonal neuropathy (AR CMT2).
- 13 genes identified including PMP22, MPZ, and EGR2 which usually cause CMT1.
- Infantile onset, severe.

Hereditary neuropathy with liability to pressure palsies (HNPP)

Autosomal dominant. Gene: PMP22 deletion or nonsense mutations.

Clinical features
- Recurrent pressure palsies.
- Recurrent brachial plexopathy.
- Transient sensory symptoms.
- NCT shows patchy, demyelinating neuropathy.

Hereditary sensory and autonomic neuropathies (HSAN) or hereditary sensory neuropathies (HSN)

HSAN I
- Autosomal dominant.
- Clinical features:
  - prominent sensory loss;
  - lancinating pains;
  - complications of ulceration and amputation;
  - motor involvement—may resemble CMT with prominent sensory involvement;
  - SPTLC1 gene—similar to CMT2 or RAB7.

HSAN II
- Autosomal recessive.
- HSN2 gene identified.
- Clinical features:
  - early onset first two decades;
  - sensory symptoms in limbs and trunk, ulcerations.

HSAN III (Riley–Day syndrome, familial dysautonomia)
- Autosomal recessive.
- Mutations in IKBKAP gene.
- Clinical features.
  - autonomic symptoms predominate;
  - sensory and motor involvement.

HSAN IV
- Autosomal recessive.
- Mutations in NTRK1 gene.
- Clinical features:
  - congenital insensitivity to pain;
  - anhidrosis;
  - recurrent episodes of fever;
  - self-mutilating behaviour;
  - mental retardation;
  - loss of unmyelinated fibres on biopsy.

HSAN V
- Autosomal recessive.
- Mutations in NTRK1 and NGFB genes.
- Clinically similar to HSAN IV but no retardation or anhidrosis.
- Loss of small myelinated fibres on biopsy.

Further reading

Pareyson D, Marchesi C (2009). Diagnosis, natural history and management of Charcot–Marie–Tooth disease. *Lancet Neurol.*, **8**, 654–67.

Reilly M, Murphy SM, Laurá M (2011). Charcot–Marie–Tooth disease. *J. Peripher. Nerv. Syst.*, **16**, 1–14.

Inherited myopathies

Inherited myopathies with limb–girdle weakness

Duchenne's (DMD) and Becker's (BMD) muscular dystrophies (X-linked dystrophy)

- DMD: incidence 3/1000 per live born ♂; prevalence 3/100 000.
- BMD: incidence 0.3/1000; prevalence 0.3/100 000.

Clinical features

- BMD is the milder form with better prognosis.
- Presentation in early childhood with walking difficulty and toe walking.
- Other features:
  - Gower's manoeuvre;
  - calf hypertrophy; contractures.
- Wheelchair dependent around age 10–12 years in DMD.
- Scoliosis compromises respiratory function.
- Cardiomyopathy occurs in both DMD and BMD.

Diagnosis

- CK ↑ > 10 000.
- Mutation in dystrophin gene found in 70%.
- If DNA studies negative, muscle biopsy with dystrophin stains and immunohistochemistry studies necessary for other limb–girdle muscular dystrophies.

Management

- In DMD corticosteroids ↑ muscle strength, ↑ muscle mass, ↓ progression. Mechanism unknown; may be due to ↓ muscle protein degradation rather than immunosupression. Recommended starting dose in ambulatory boys 0.75 mg/kg daily (maximum dose 40 mg). Azathioprine and ciclosporin no benefit.
- Ventilatory support increases quality of life and life expectancy.

Limb–girdle muscular dystrophy syndromes

Clinical features

- Range of phenotypes from non-specific limb–girdle weakness to those resembling the X-linked muscular dystrophies.
- Facial weakness not a feature.
- Variable cardiac and respiratory complications.

Genetics

See Table 5.23.

Diagnosis

Muscle biopsy mandatory to identify abnormal protein by immunohistochemistry in order to focus DNA studies.

Proximal myotonic myopathy (PROMM)

- Autosomal disorder similar to myotonic dystrophy but with limb–girdle rather than distal weakness.
- Muscle pain and stiffness prominent features.
- Gamma GT levels ↑.
- Genetic defect in zinc finger gene on chromosome 3.

Table 5.23 Genetics of limb–girdle muscular dystrophy (LGMD) syndromes

Syndrome	Chromosome	Protein
Autosomal dominant		
LGMD1A	5q	Myotilin
LGMD1B	1q	Lamin A/C
LGMD2C	3p	Caveolin
Autosomal recessive		
LGMD2A	15q	Calpain
LGMD2B	2p13	Dysferlin
LGMD2C	13q	γ-Sarcoglycan

Inherited myopathy with distal weakness

Miyoshi's myopathy (allelic LGMD2b)

- Autosomal recessive.
- Onset in teens with weakness and wasting of gastrocnemius muscle progressing to involve more proximal muscles.
- CK markedly ↑.
- Muscle biopsy shows dystrophic changes.

Welander's myopathy (TIA1 mutation)

- Autosomal dominant.
- Onset between fourth and sixth decades.
- Weakness in the upper limbs (wrist and finger extensors) and wasting of hand muscles followed by foot drop and leg weakness.
- CK normal or slightly ↑.
- DNA diagnosis.
- Muscle biopsy shows myopathic changes with rimmed vacuoles.

Nonaka myopathy (hereditary inclusion body myopathy type 2)

- Autosomal recessive.
- Onset with tibialis anterior weakness and wasting.
- DNA diagnosis GNE gene.

Other inherited myopathies

Facioscapulohumeral (FSH) muscular dystrophy

- Autosomal dominant.
- Prevalence: 1–2/100 000.

Clinical features

- Onset in teens with facial weakness. Weakness of scapular fixators results in upward displacement ('chicken wings').
- Frequent "formes frustes".
- Deltoid is spared but there is weakness of humeral muscles (biceps and triceps).
- Leg weakness is common, affecting hip flexors, quadriceps, and tibialis anterior.
- Asymmetric weakness, usually worse on the right, is the rule.
- Risk of being wheelchair bound is 20%.
- No cardiac complications.

Diagnosis
- CK normal to ↑ several-fold.
- EMG myopathic.
- DNA diagnosis by demonstration of a truncated region at chromosome 4q35.
- Muscle biopsy may show inflammatory changes, confusing the diagnosis.

Emery–Dreifuss muscular dystrophy

See 📖 'Muscle disorders: classification and features', pp. 292–3, and 📖 'Muscle disorders: investigations', pp. 294–6.
- X-linked and autosomal dominant inheritance.

Clinical features
- Progressive scapulohumeral peroneal weakness.
- Thin muscles.
- Contractures of cervical extensors, biceps, and long finger extensors characteristic.
- Cardiac conduction defects with atrial paralysis with absent or small P waves causing sinus bradycardia requiring pacing.

Diagnosis
- Muscle biopsy required for immunocytochemistry to demonstrate absence of lamin A/C and emerin. DNA diagnosis.
- DNA diagnosis: distinguish lamin A/C mutations (EDMD2, all LGMD1B) from emerin mutations (EDMD1). (This is important as EDMD2 patients should have prophylactic ICD, and EDMD1 patients manage with a simple pacer.)

Further reading

Bushby K (2009). Diagnosis and management of the limb girdle muscular dystrophies. *Pract. Neurol.*, **9**, 314–23.

Bushby K, Finkel R, Birnkrant DJ (2010). Diagnosis and management of Duchenne muscular dystrophy. Part 1: Diagnosis, pharmacological and psychosocial management. *Lancet Neurol.*, **9**, 77–93.

Myotonic dystrophy (MD)

MD is a multisystem disorder characterized by myopathy and myotonia. The incidence is 1/8000 live births.

Genetics

- Autosomal dominant disorder with full penetrance but variable expression.
- Gene abnormality is an expansion in the CTG trinucleotide repeats in the dystrophica myotonica protein kinase gene.
- Anticipation, increased clinical severity in succeeding generations, is well recognized.

Clinical features

Phenotype varies from a lethal severe congenital myopathy to late-onset cataracts.

- Neuromuscular:
  - myotonia;
  - distal muscle weakness (hand and foot drop) with progression to proximal muscles;
  - facial weakness;
  - temporalis, masseter, and sternomastoid wasting and weakness.
- CNS:
  - somnolence;
  - cognitive impairment.
- Cardiac:
  - conduction defects with heart block and tachyarrhythmias due to fibrosis in the conduction system and SA node;
  - cardiomyopathy;
  - risk of sudden death and anaesthetic complications.
- Eyes: cataracts.
- Endocrine:
  - diabetes mellitus and impaired GTT;
  - testicular atrophy;
  - repeated miscarriages and menstrual irregularities;
  - frontal hair loss.
- Smooth muscle involvement:
  - oesophageal problems;
  - respiratory infections;
  - recurrent cholecystitis.

Investigations

- Serum CK may be ↑.
- EMG: myopathic and myotonic features.
- DNA testing for triplet expansion > 5–30 in the DM-PK gene.

Management
- Genetic counselling especially as the severe congenital form occurs in the offspring of affected females with > 100 repeats.
- Prenatal diagnosis available.
- Myotonia if symptomatic; mexiletine if ECG QT interval normal.

Further reading
Turner C, Hilton Jones D (2010). The myotonic dystrophies. *J. Neurol. Neurosurg. Psychiatry*, **81**, 358–367.

Inherited movement disorders

Parkinson's disease (PD)

LRRK2

- Autosomal dominant (incomplete penetrance).
- 2% prevalence in sporadic Parkinson's patients.
- Recommended testing in patients > 40 years with first-degree relatives and also high-risk populations (Ashkenazi Jews and North African Arabs).
- No definite clinical hallmarks though abduction–adduction leg tremor and early-onset leg dystonia may be more frequent.
- Good response to levodopa and deep brain stimulation.

PARK 2 (Parkin)

- Autosomal recessive.
- Young-onset PD but onset at 70 years also described.
- 50% cases onset < 50 years.
- Excellent response to levodopa.
- Marked sleep benefit.
- Hyper-reflexia.
- Early dystonia.
- Very slowly progressive.

PARK 1 (alpha synuclein)

- Autosomal recessive.
- Rare.

Huntington's disease

- Autosomal dominant with full penetrance:
  - expansion of CAG trinucleotide repeat > 36 repeats;
  - expansion size inversely related to age of onset;
  - ↑ expansion with each generation—'anticipation';
  - prenatal diagnosis available.

Clinical features

- Onset in fourth and fifth decades.
- Movement disorders:
  - chorea, initially fidgetiness;
  - parkinsonism—juvenile-onset Westphal variant;
  - dystonia.
- Psychiatric features:
  - change in personality.
- Dementia.
- Other features:
  - slowed saccades;
  - head thrust or blinking to generate saccades;
  - progressive weight loss.

Differential diagnosis
- Dentatorubropallidoluysian atrophy (DRPLA).
- ADCA I.
- Hallervorden–Spatz disease (autosomal recessive, caused by mutation in the pantothenate kinase gene (PANK 2)).
- Neuroferritinopathy (autosomal dominant, adult onset neurodegenerative disorder associated with iron accumulation in the basal ganglia).

Dystonia

Primary (Oppenheim's) dystonia
- Prevalence 1/3000. Common in Ashkenazi Jews.
- Autosomal dominant:
  - DYT I gene on chr 9 (coding for torsin A protein);
  - low penetrance (30%);
  - variable expression.

Clinical features
- Childhood onset.
- Initially focal (foot); variable spread to segmental or generalized.
- Craniocervical muscles spared.

Dopa-responsive dystonia (DRD)—Segawa's disease
- Autosomal dominant:
  - mutation in gene for GTP cyclohydrolase 1;
  - AR form due to mutation in tyrosine hydroxylase gene.

Clinical features
- Childhood lower limb onset progressing to generalized dystonia.
- Diurnal variation in symptoms.
- Mild parkinsonism.
- Paraparesis presentation.
- Also cases described similar to cerebral palsy.
- Exquisite response to levodopa.

Management
- Therapeutic trial of levodopa in all cases of dystonia < 30 years: Sinemet 275 tds for 3 months.
- In equivocal cases phenylalanine loading test.

Further reading

Albanese A, Asmus F, Bhatia KP, et al. (2011). EFNS guidelines on diagnosis and treatment of primary dystonias. *Eur. J. Neurol.*, **18**, 5–18.

Ross CA, Tabrizi SJ (2011). Huntingdon's disease: from molecular pathogenesis to clinical treatment. *Lancet Neurol.*, **10**, 83–98.

Saiki S, Sato S, Hattori N (2012). Molecular pathogenesis of Parkinson's disease: update. *J Neurol. Neurosurg. Psychiatry*, **83**, 430–6.

Inherited mitochondrial disorders

Table 5.24 summarizes the major inherited mitochondrial disorders.
- Consider mitochondrial disorders in any patient with multifocal neurological involvement, especially if sensory neural deafness.
- Mitochondrial DNA maternally inherited.
    - deletions, e.g. KSS and CEO, usually sporadic and not transmitted.
    - point mutations, e.g. MELAS, MERRF, LHON, maternally transmitted.
- Nuclear DNA encodes some respiratory chain proteins, e.g. POLGI: variety of phenotypes. AD or AR. Overlapping phenotypes.
    - Alpers syndrome in children—encephalopathy + sensitivity to valproate.
    - Recessive late onset ataxia.
    - Epilepsy.
    - Parkinsonism.
    - Stroke-like episodes.
    - Exercise intolerance.
    - PEO ± myopathy.
    - Ataxic neuropathy.

Investigations
- CK.
- MRI brain (see Fig. 5.25).
- Serum and CSF lactate.
- NCT and EMG studies.
- Blood mt-DNA studies.
- Muscle biopsy:
    - ragged red fibres (not present in all cases);
    - COX-negative fibres;
    - activity of respiratory chain complexes;
    - molecular genetic analysis.

Further reading
Finsterer J, Harbo HF, Baets J, et al. (2009). EFNS guidelines on the molecular diagnosis of mitochondrial disorders. *Eur. J. Neurol.*, **16**, 1255–64.

Table 5.24 Inherited mitochondrial disorders

Syndrome	Phenotype	Inheritance	Mutation
CPEO	Chronic progressive external ophthalmoplegia ± myopathy	AR, AD, maternal	Deletions, point mutations, mtDNA
Kearns–Sayre (KSS)	Ophthalmoplegia, pigmentary retinopathy, cardiac arrhythmia, ataxia, ↑ CSF protein	Not transmitted	Deletions not found in blood; need muscle biopsy
MELAS	Mitochondrial myopathy, encephalopathy, lactic acidosis, stroke-like episodes	Maternal	Point mutation A3243G
MERRF	Myoclonus, epilepsy, ragged red fibres + ataxia, neuropathy, deafness, lipomas	Maternal	Point mutation A8344G
Leber's hereditary optic neuropathy (LHON)	Optic neuropathy. In female carriers: MS-like syndrome	Maternal	Point mutations
NARP	Neuropathy, ataxia, retinitis pigmentosa	Maternal	Missense mutation of ATPase gene
Mitochondrial neuro-gastrointestinal encephalopathy (MNGIE)	Progressive external ophthalmoplegia (PEO), myopathy, neuropathy, GI involvement encephalopathy	AR	Mutation in nuclear genes TYMP
SANDO	Sensory ataxic neuropathy, dysarthria, ophthalmoplegia		POLG deletion

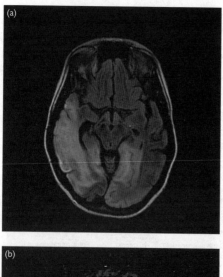

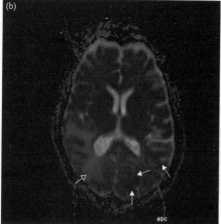

Fig. 5.25 Mitochondrial encephalopathy, lactic acidosis, and stroke-like episodes (MELAS): (a) axial FLAIR; (b) ADC map MRI. Bilateral asymmetric confluent lobar signal abnormality involving both grey and white matter with a typically posterior predilection and failure to conform to vascular territories is the most common presentation. (b) Note the involved parenchyma demonstrating areas of both restricted (hypointense on ADC map (*white arrows*)) and free diffusion (hyperintense on ADC (*open white arrow*)).

Inherited dementias

Alzheimer's disease
- Sporadic AD:
  - no single gene;
  - apolipoprotein E (ApoE) 4 allele × 3 (heterozygote) or × 8 (homozygote) risk of developing AD.
- < 5% AD inherited. Three genes:
  - beta-amyloid precursor protein (APP) (< 5% early-onset AD);
  - presenilin I (50% early-onset familial AD);
  - presenilin 2 (< 1%).
- No specific features to distinguish sporadic from familial apart from early onset.

Frontotemporal dementia (FTD)
- FTD with parkinsonism.
- Gene on chr 17q21 (tau protein).
- Clinical features:
  - behaviour change;
  - parkinsonism;
  - psychotic symptoms;
  - amyotrophy.

Huntington's disease
See 📖 'Inherited movement disorders', pp. 362–3.

Prion diseases
Normal PrP coded by gene on chr 20.

Familial CJD
- Most common point mutation at codon 200.
- Earlier onset than sporadic CJD.
- Otherwise indistinguishable from sporadic CJD.

Gerstmann–Sträussler–Scheinker syndrome
- Point mutation codon 102.
- Onset in third or fourth decades.
- Cerebellar features.
- Dementia.
- Progressive over years.

Fatal familial insomnia
- Onset 20–70 years.
- Progressive insomnia.
- Autonomic features.
- Memory impairment.

Further reading
Burgunder JM, Finsterer J, Szolnoki Z, et al. (2010). EFNS guidelines on the molecular diagnosis of channelopthies, epilepsies, migraine, stroke and dementias. *Eur. J. Neurol.*, 17, 641–8.

Hereditary metabolic diseases

May present in adulthood. See Table 5.25 for a summary.

Table 5.25 Characteristics of hereditary metabolic diseases

Disorder	Clinical features	Investigations
Niemann–Pick type C	Supranuclear gaze palsy, dementia, organomegaly	Bone marrow: foamy storage cells, sea blue histiocytes: NPC1 gene
Abetalipoproteinaemia (X-linked)	Ataxia, head tremor	Acanthocytes, lipoprotein electrophoresis: ↓ cholesterol
Adrenoleucodystrophy	Spasticity, neuropathy, dementia	MRI: leucodystrophy. Very long chain fatty acids. Synacthen test
Fabry's disease	Painful neuropathy, young stroke, skin lesions	Alpha galactosidase deficiency
GM1 gangliosidosis	Extrapyramidal features	Beta galactosidase deficiency
GM2 gangliosidosis	Spasticity, dementia, motor neuropathy/ neuronopathy	Hexosaminidase deficiency
Metachromatic leucodystrophy	Neuropathy, dementia, spasticity	Arylsulphatase A deficiency. MRI: leucodystrophy
Tangier's disease	Neuropathy, orange tonsils	High-density lipoprotein deficiency
Arginase deficiency	Spasticity, dementia	Hyperammonaemia

Further reading

Gray RG, Preece MA, Green SH, Whitehouse W, Winer J, Green A (2000). Inborn errors of metabolism as a cause of neurological disease in adults: an approach to investigation. *J. Neurol. Neurosurg. Psychiatry*, **69**, 5–12.

Viral encephalitis

Infection of the brain parenchyma is usually accompanied by a meningitis producing a meningoencephalitis. The organism is identified in only 30–50% of cases.

Incidence
- Herpes simplex encephalitis (HSV-1) is most frequent cause of sporadic fatal encephalitis: 1 case/million/year (probably underestimate).
- In the Far East Japanese B encephalitis causes 15 000 deaths/year.

Aetiology
See Table 5.27.

Clinical features
- Essential to take a full travel history (e.g. Japanese B encephalitis).
- History of animal bites (e.g. rabies).
- No association between HSV-1 and cold sores.
- Presentation, especially for HSV encephalitis—acute with:
  - headache;
  - fever;
  - focal neurology (e.g. dysphasia);
  - seizures;
  - encephalopathic presentation with confusion, delirium, behavioural changes, and coma.
- Untreated, mortality 70%.
- With aciclovir, still high at 20–30%.

Differential diagnosis
Diffuse encephalopathy
- Liver and renal failure.
- Diabetic coma.
- Anoxic/ischaemic brain injury.
- Systemic infection.
- Toxic drug effects.
- Mitochondrial cytopathies.

Non-viral causes of infectious encephalitis
- Consider NMDA receptor antibody associated encephalitis (see 📖 Chapter 3, 'Anti-NMDA receptor encephalitis', pp. 132–3).
- *Mycobacterium tuberculosis*.
- *Mycoplasma pneumoniae*.
- *Listeria monocytogenes*.
- *Borrelia burgdorferi*.
- Brucellosis.
- Leptospirosis.
- Legionella.
- All causes of pyogenic meningitis.
- Fungal: cryptococcus, aspergillosis, candidiasis.
- Parasitic: human African trypanosomiasis, toxoplasmosis, schistosomiasis.

Table 5.27 Aetiology of viral encephalitis

Worldwide distribution	Geographically specific
HSV-1 and HSV-2	Western equine virus
EBV	Eastern equine virus
CMV	California encephalitis
VZV	St Louis encephalitis
HHV6	Japanese B encephalitis
Non-polio enteroviruses	Tick-borne encephalitis
Mumps	West Nile virus
Rabies	
HIV (at seroconversion)	

Acute disseminated encephalitis (ADEM)

May have a similar presentation but clues include recent vaccination, spinal cord and optic nerve involvement, and widespread white matter involvement on MRI.

Investigations

- Routine blood investigations may reveal a metabolic aetiology.
- CXR to exclude TB, legionella, mycoplasma, and neoplasia.
- Baseline virology serology may later provide evidence of recent infection.
- CT/MRI: gyral swelling and signal abnormality/low attenuation, which is typically bilateral but asymmetric, ± haemorrhage.

EEG

- EEG may be necessary to make diagnosis. Look for diffuse non-specific abnormalities or periodic lateralizing epileptiform discharges (PLEDs).
- In herpes simplex encephalitis PLEDs may be bilateral and evolve with differing periodicity over each lobe.
- If PLEDs occur away from the temporal lobe, interpret with caution.
  - May improve spontaneously and rapidly.

Lumbar puncture

- Lymphocytic pleocytosis 10–200/mm^3.
- Protein, 0.6–6 g/L.
- Rarely, CSF may be normal.
- CSF PCR to detect HSV-1 is 95% specific. Sensitivity if taken 2–10 days after onset is 95%. False-negative results most likely in the first 48 hours and after 10 days.

Management

- Aciclovir (10 mg/kg tds) immediately diagnosis is suspected. Continue for 14 days. It should only be discontinued if an alternative definite diagnosis is made. In immunosuppressed patients treat for 21 days. Note: Renal toxicity may occur and needs to be monitored. 5% of patients may relapse.
- Best predictors of outcome are treatment within 4 days of onset, GCS > 6 at presentation.
- Steroids if there is evidence of raised ICP.
- AED for seizures.
- May need HDU/ITU monitoring.

Further reading

Steiner I, Budka H, Chaudhuri A, et al. (2010). Viral meningoencephalitis: a review of diagnostic methods and guidelines for management. *Eur. J. Neurol.*, **17**, 999–1009.

Neurology of HIV/AIDS: introduction

- HIV infection can affect the whole neuraxis at all stages of the illness.
- Different pathological processes can be present simultaneously.

Basic principles

- 10% of patients may have a neurological disorder at seroconversion:
  - meningoencephalitis;
  - myelitis;
  - GBS;
  - polymyositis.
- Persistent CSF abnormalities, even during the asymptomatic phase, include:
  - mild pleocytosis;
  - ↑ protein;
  - oligoclonal bands.
- To diagnose conditions such as cryptococcal meningitis, specific tests such as the cryptococcal antigen test are required.
- ↓ inflammatory response: a third of patients with cryptococcal meningitis have meningism.
- Low threshold for brain imaging and lumbar puncture required.
- ↓ antibody response: in toxoplasmosis, there is no rise in IgM levels.
- CD4 count is a useful guide to the underlying pathological process:
  - toxoplasmosis, cryptococcal meningitis, progressive multifocal leucoencephalopathy occur at CD4 counts < 200.
  - CMV disease occurs at CD4 counts < 50.

Neurological disorders due to HIV

HIV-associated dementia (HAD)
- Usually occurs late in the disease.
- Symptoms include impaired attention, memory loss, apathy.
- Signs in the early stages include jerky eye movements, brisk reflexes, cerebellar abnormalities.
- Differential diagnoses include metabolic derangement, e.g. hypoxia, recreational drug use, depression.

Investigations to exclude other pathology
- MRI shows atrophy and diffuse white matter changes.
- CSF examination (non-specific cytochemical abnormalities).
- CSF HIV RNA load cannot be used to diagnose HAD.
- Neuropsychological assessment useful—subcortical dementia with abnormalities in the domains of information processing, psychomotor speed, and recall memory.
- Note: there are concerns regarding ongoing cognitive deterioration despite ARV therapy and undetectable viral load. Measurement of CSF viral load may indicate a compartmentalization syndrome with high CSF viral load. This may present with neurological syndromes, e.g., confusion, seizures, ataxia, coma. Requires change to better penetrating ARVs. See Table 5.28.

Vacuolar myelopathy (VM)
- Occurs in conjunction with HIV dementia.
- Signs of a spastic paraparesis without a sensory level.
- Resembles subacute combined degeneration due to vitamin B_{12} deficiency.
- MRI usually normal.
- Check B_{12} level and, if low normal, homocysteine levels.
- Consider checking indicated HTLV-1 serology as co-infection may occur.

Table 5.28 CNS penetration effectiveness (CPE) score

Drug class	4	3	2	1
NRTI	Zidovudine	Abacavir Emtricitabine	Didanosine Lamivudine Stavudine	Tenofovir Zalcitabine
NNRTI	Nevirapine	Delavirdine Efavirenz	Etravirine	
PI	B/Indinavir	B/Darunavir B/Fosamprenavir B/Lopinavir Indinavir	Atazanavir B/Atazanavir Fosamprenavir	Nelfinavir Ritonavir Saquinavir B/Saquinavir B/Tipranavir
Entry/fusion inhibitors		Maraviroc		Enfuvirtide
Integrase inhibitors		Raltegravir		

B = boosted (with ritonavir)

Peripheral nerve syndromes

Distal sensory peripheral neuropathy (DSPN)
- 25% of AIDS patients.
- Occurs late in AIDS.
- Symptoms of paraesthesiae, burning pain, dysaesthesiae.
- Signs: little or no weakness, reduced or absent ankle reflexes. Impaired sensation to pain and temperature (mainly a small fibre neuropathy).
- Neuropathy due to antiretroviral drugs is very similar: ddC, ddI, and d4T.
- Other drugs that may also cause neuropathy include isoniazid, vincristine, thalidomide, metronidazole.

Investigations
- B_{12}, glucose levels, alcohol intake.
- Nerve conduction studies normal or may show an axonal neuropathy.
- Thermal thresholds abnormal.
- Nerve biopsy unnecessary unless abnormal features, such as significant weakness, are present to exclude vasculitis, demyelination, or lymphoma.

Other peripheral nerve syndromes
- Mononeuritis multiplex due to HIV vasculitis and CMV.
- Acute and chronic demyelinating polyneuropathy.
- Diffuse inflammatory lymphocytosis syndrome (DILS) resembles Sjögren's syndrome. Occurs during immunocompetent phases and associated with a high CD8 count.

Polyradiculopathy
- CMV.
- Lymphoma.
- Herpes viruses
- Syphilis.

Myopathy
- Polymyositis occurs in the early stages of HIV infection.
- Zidovudine causes a mitochondrial myopathy.

Opportunistic infections associated with HIV

Toxoplasmosis
- Usually a reactivation in individuals who have been previously exposed and have positive toxoplasma serology.
- Acute or subacute presentation with focal neurological signs or movement disorders such as athetosis, and symptoms and signs of ↑ ICP.
- Imaging: multiple focal enhancing lesions with surrounding oedema.
- Differential diagnoses: primary CNS lymphoma, tuberculoma, or tuberculous abscesses.
- Treatment: see Table 5.29.
- If significant mass effect add dexamethasone 4 mg qds and gradually taper (see Fig. 5.26).

Cryptococcal meningitis
- Acute or subacute presentation with headache, altered mental state, and meningism.
- Imaging: hydrocephalus, cryptococcomas, or dilated Virchow–Robin spaces filled with organisms.
- CSF:
  - opening pressure frequently ↑;
  - pleocytosis, ↑ protein, and ↓ sugar but may be normal;
  - India ink staining positive in 75%;
  - cryptococcal antigen positive in 95%;
  - serum cryptococcal antigen measurement may be a useful screening method in those with mild non-specific symptoms.
- Poor prognostic markers:
  - altered mental state;
  - CSF OP > 20 cm CSF;
  - CSF WCC < 10;
  - hyponatraemia;
  - relapse episode.

Treatment
See Table 5.29.
- In mild cases where none of the poor prognostic markers are present, fluconazole is an alternative drug to amphotericin.
- May require repeated LPs for raised ICP. Consider insertion of a lumbar peritoneal shunt if frequent LPs required.
- Acetazolamide may have an adjunctive role.
- Acute-phase Rx 4–6 weeks or CSF culture negative.

Table 5.29 Treatment of opportunistic infections in HIV/AIDS

Disorder	Acute treatment	Maintenance	Comments
Toxoplasmosis	Pyrimethamine loading dose 100 mg/day PO, followed by 75 mg/day + folinic acid 15 mg/day + sulfadiazine 6–8 g/day IV/PO	Pyrimethamine 25–50 mg/day + sulfadiazine 2–4 g/day + folinic acid 10 mg/day	If allergic to sulpha drugs use clindamycin 2.4–4.8 g/day; maintenance 600 mg/day
Cryptococcal meningitis	Amphotericin, 0.4–1.0 mg/kg/day IV ± flucytosine, 150 mg/kg/day PO	Fluconazole, 200 mg/day/PO	In mild cases fluconazole, 400 mg IV PO may be used

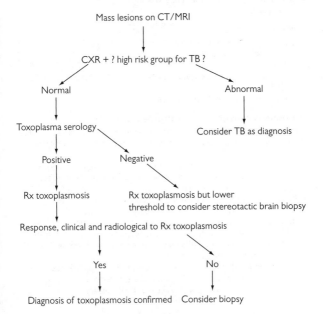

Fig. 5.26 Algorithm for the management of mass lesions (CD4 count < 200/mm³) as detected on CT/MRI (MRI is preferred as more sensitive). If ↑ ICP, treat with dexamethasone 4 mg qds. Once improved, gradually taper. Benefit may be due to ↓ oedema or response if lymphoma. At least 2 weeks may be necessary to assess for a response to anti-toxoplasmosis therapy. In some cases, provided that there is no urgency, one may need to wait 1 month.

Progressive multifocal leucoencephalopathy (PML)

- Caused by reactivation of JC virus, a polyoma virus.
- Subacute presentation with focal signs with no evidence of ↑ ICP.
- Imaging:
  - MRI shows non-enhancing focal white matter lesions with little or no mass effect on T_2-weighted images.
  - T_1-weighted images show discrete low signal changes.
- CSF: JC virus detected by PCR in 75%. Specificity 99%.
- Blood serology unhelpful since 80% of the general population seropositive due to a childhood upper respiratory tract infection.

Treatment

- CART (combined antiretroviral therapy) to improve immune function.
- Various drugs tried but found to be ineffective: cytosine arabinoside, cidofovir, interferon alfa, radiotherapy.
- Anecdotal reports and trials underway for use of mirtazapine and mefloquine.

CMV infection

- May cause a meningoencephalitis.
- Lumbar polyradiculopathy.
- Retinitis.
- Diagnosis: neutrophil pleocytosis in the CSF; CMV isolation in the CSF by PCR.
- Treatment with ganciclovir or foscarnet.

Immune reconstitution syndromes (IRIS)

Definition: 'paradoxical deterioration of clinical or laboratory markers including imaging studies despite a favourable response in the viral load and CD4 count.'

- Introduction of ARV results in recovery of CD4 T-lymphocytes including memory T-cells. Improved immune function results in reaction against active or latent antigens.
- Neurological IRIS described with: *Mycobacteria tuberculosis* causing meningitis and brain abscesses; cryptococcal meningitis; CMV with the development of vitritis, uveitis, and cystoid macular oedema; PML with MRI imaging showing enhancement and biopsies showing inflammatory infiltrates. HIV-associated IRIS may present with a progressive dementia or as an acute encephalitic syndrome.
- Management is difficult—includes treatment of the appropriate organism-specific antimicrobial agents and use of corticosteroids. In life-threatening situations stopping cART may be necessary.

Further reading

Gendleman HE, Grant I, Everall IP, et al. (eds) (2011). *The neurology of AIDS*. Oxford: Oxford University Press.

Johnson T, Nath A (2010). Neurological complications of immune reconstitution in HIV-1 infected populations. *Ann. NY Acad. Sci.*, **1184**, 106–20.

Schouten J, Cinque P, Gisslen M, Reiss P, Portegies P (2011). HIV-1 infection and cognitive impairment in the c-ART era: a review. *AIDS*, **25**, 561–75.

Tan IL, Smith BR, von Geldern G, Mateen FJ, McArthur JC (2012). HIV-associated opportunistic infections of the CNS. *Lancet Neurol.*, **11**, 605–17.

MRI images in infectious diseases

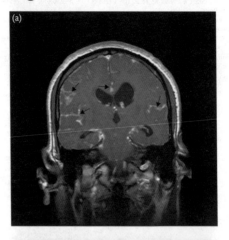

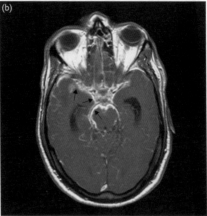

Fig. 5.27 Meningitis: (a) post-contrast coronal MRI; (b) post-contrast axial MRI.

Figure 5.27 (a) shows pneumococcal meningitis: thickening and enhancement of leptomeningeal surfaces over the cerebral hemispheres and Sylvian fissure (*black arrows*); (b) shows tuberculous meningitis: thickening and enhancement of basal meninges in suprachiasmatic and pre-pontine cisterns (*black arrows*). Note that in both cases there is dilation of the ventricles due to communicating hydrocephalus.

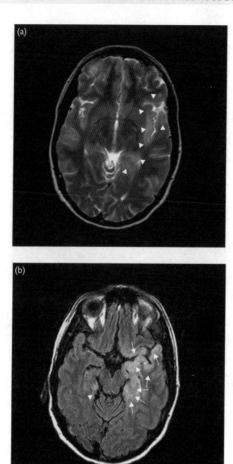

Fig. 5.28   HSV encephalitis. (a) Axial T$_2$W and (b) axial FLAIR MRI.

Figure 5.28 shows ill-defined hyperintensity with gyral expansion involving the anterior and medial aspects of the left temporal lobe, including the amygdala and hippocampus, and the inferior portion of the left frontal lobe and insular cortex ((a) *white arrowheads* and (b) *white arrows*). Asymmetric bilateral temporal lobe involvement is typical. Note the subtle involvement of the right medial temporal lobe ((b) *white arrowhead*). Gyriform enhancement and haemorrhagic change are common.

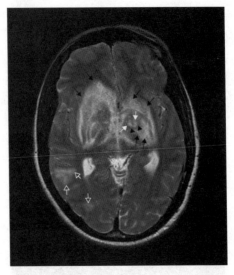

Fig. 5.29 Cerebral toxoplasmosis (axial FLAIR MRI).

Figure 5.29 shows bilateral mass lesions with heterogeneous signal intensity in the deep grey nuclei. Target appearance is shown in the left anterior thalamus with a ring of hypointensity (*black arrowheads*) surrounding an area of hyperintensity (*white arrows*) and central hypointensity. Note also further lesions peripherally at the grey–white matter junction in the right temporo-occipital region (*open white arrows*).

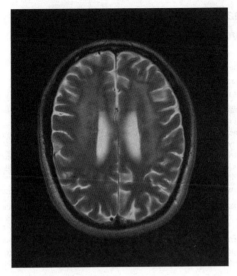

Fig. 5.30 HIV encephalopathy (T$_2$W axial MRI).

Figure 5.30 shows bilateral hyperintensity involving the cerebral white matter in association with volume loss denoted by prominence of the cerebral sulci.

Somatization (or functional or conversion) disorders

Paget's description of hysteria:

> 'They say "I cannot."
> It looks like "I will not."
> But it is "I cannot will."'

Somatization is the condition whereby emotional states are experienced as physical symptoms as a result of:

- expression of a physical aspect of emotion, e.g. palpitations due to anxiety or dizziness due to hyperventilation.
- an attribution or thought arising from a physical symptom implying an illness, e.g. paraesthesiae and multiple sclerosis or muscle twitching and MND.
- underlying psychological distress that the patient is unable to describe.

Processes occur at a subconscious level and therefore are not malingering, which is the invention of symptoms for a specific goal.

Up to 30% of patients presenting to neurologists may have neurological symptoms which remain unexplained after a thorough clinical assessment and all possible investigations including MRI, neurophysiological tests, and invasive tests including CSF examination.

Predisposing factors

- Early life trauma.
- Childhood illness.
- Childhood experience of parental ill health and somatization.
- Potential source of secondary gain, e.g. spousal attention, income benefits.
- History of depression and anxiety.
- Personality dysfunction: antisocial, borderline, and hysterical personality disorders.

Effects

- Causes significant morbidity.
- Risk of drug dependence.
- Occasional suicide.

Clinical presentations

- Non-epileptic seizures.
- Dystonia.
- Mono-, hemi-, or paraparesis.
- Sensory symptoms.
- Movement disorders including tremors.
- Headache.
- Gait disorders.
- Loss of consciousness/coma.

Clinical clues

- Look for 'belle indifference' or an inappropriate manner with excessive joviality out of proportion to the gravity of the symptoms, such as hemiparesis.
- Pseudoseizure (see 📖 'Seizures versus dissociative non-epileptic attack disorder (NEAD) or pseudoseizures', pp. 226–7). Note: frontal lobe seizures can have odd presentations. Some patients have true seizures and non-epileptic seizures. In non-epileptic attacks:
  - eyes tightly screwed up;
  - fighting off help;
  - thrashing of arms and legs;
  - tongue biting rare;
  - urinary and faecal incontinence rare.
- Gross swaying and tendency to fall with Romberg's test.
- Exaggerated arm flailing on tandem gait.
- Useful to get patients with gait problems to illustrate walking forwards and then backwards or side to side—often better!
- Occasionally asking patients to demonstrate their walking before they became ill can be illuminating! (Clinical pearl from Dr Pauline Munroe.)
- In patients with hemisensory loss, testing vibration (using 128 Hz tuning fork) will demonstrate reduced sensation when comparing the left and right forehead. This cannot be explained neuroanatomically as it is the same bone. Similarly, when applied to both sides of the sternum.
- In patients with leg weakness unable to lift either leg ask the patient to sit up. The iliopsoas muscles perform both actions.
- Note: Hoover's sign only indicates inadequate effort. There may be underlying weakness.
- Functional tremors may be 'entrained' by asking patients to perform a rhythmical task with the other hand. The non-organic tremor will adopt the same frequency. Distraction techniques may also be used, e.g. holding a pen in the mouth and asking the patient to draw a circle.
- Sometimes it is worth trying to find an on–off switch by palpating the spine from behind to see if a tremor or movement disorder can be modulated (a clinical pearl taught by the late Professor C.D. Marsden).

Management

- Look on this group of patients as a challenge rather than a nuisance!
- Assess for underlying anxiety or depression and treat. 50% of patients with depression complain of somatic symptoms.
- Adopt a non-confrontational approach allowing the patient to 'save face', especially in the presence of a spouse or family.
- Avoid early psychiatric referral which is likely to alienate patient. Usually no psychiatric disorder is diagnosed.
- Acknowledge the reality of the problem for the patient. Try and identify, in rank order, the symptoms most troublesome for the patient.
- Try and identify emotional and social factors perpetuating the problem.
- After initial clinical assessment, discuss reasons for any investigations (e.g. MRI), making clear the significance of negative test results. Avoid

any further investigations since this will reinforce the patient's idea of an undiagnosed physical disorder.

- After investigations, introduce the concept of the importance of psychological and emotional factors either as maintaining factors or as causally related to symptoms.
- Formulate a plan of management which may include:
  - physiotherapy with a rehabilitation programme;
  - cognitive behavioural therapy;
  - medical follow-up to monitor progress.
- Sometimes it may be helpful to get a second opinion from, but not necessarily transfer care to, another, perhaps more senior, neurological colleague.

Further reading

Brown T (2004). Somatization. *Medicine*, 32, 34–5.

Edwards MJ, Fotopoulou A, Pareés I (2013). Neurobiology of functional (psychogenic) movement disorders. *Curr. Opin. Neurol.*, 26(4), 442–7.

Hadler A, Poole N (2009). A clinical approach to managing somatoform disorders. *Prog. Neurol. Psychiatry*, 13, 4–5.

Hatcher S, Arroll B (2008). Assessment and management of medically unexplained symptoms. *BMJ*, 336, 1124–8.

Price JR (2008). Medically unexplained physical symptoms. *Medicine*, 36, 449–51.

See also ℘ <http://www.neurosymptoms.org/> (a self-help website for patients with functional symptoms).

Lumbar puncture

Indications

- Diagnosis of neurological disorders:
  - infectious meningitis and encephalitis (cytochemical parameters + microbiology + PCR);
  - demyelinating disorders, e.g. MS (oligoclonal bands);
  - inflammatory disorders of the CNS, e.g. sarcoidosis;
  - inflammatory disorders of the PNS, e.g. GBS and CIDP (cytoalbuminaemic dissociation);
  - malignant infiltration (cytology);
  - mitochondrial disorders (CSF lactate);
  - subarachnoid haemorrhage (SAH).
- Measurement of opening pressure, e.g. IIH.
- Treatment of ↑ ICP, e.g. IIH, meningitis due to *Cryptococcus neoformans*.
- Administration of antibiotics and chemotherapy.
- Injection of radio-opaque (myelography) or radio-isotope materials, e.g. leak localization in intracranial hypotension.

Contraindications

- ↑ ICP due to mass lesion or obstructive hydrocephalus.
- Note: in infection a normal CT does not exclude ↑ ICP.
- Local infection at LP site.
- Bleeding diathesis including anticoagulants.

Procedure

- Careful explanation and reassurance.
- Warn about complications of post-LP headache.
- Sedation with 5 mg diazepam may be useful.
- Firm mattress or table essential.
- Maximum one thin pillow.
- Patient lies horizontally in left or right lateral position.
- Neck flexed and knees drawn up in fetal position (see Fig. 5.31).
- Place a pillow between knees.
- Shoulder and pelvis vertical.
- Alternative is to sit patient upright, leaning over bed tray with one pillow.
- Identify L3–L4 interspace—line connecting anterior iliac crests (AICs) (see Fig. 5.31).
- Palpate and mark interspinous space with nail mark or indelible pen.
- Full sterile technique:
  - gloves;
  - clean area extending from each AIC, above and below L3 and L4 interspace, with antiseptic solution starting in middle and cleaning in a circular fashion outwards.
- Infiltrate skin and subcutaneous tissue with small amount of 1–2% lidocaine. Excessive amounts make it difficult to palpate interspace.
- Wait 2–3 minutes.

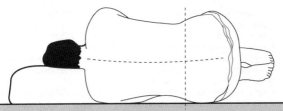

The line connecting the highest points of the crests traverses the L₃–L₄ interspace

Fig. 5.31 Lateral positioning for LP. Reprinted with permission from Sharief M et al. (2004). *Medicine*, 32, 44–7.

- Insert spinal needle with stylet in position between interspace while holding skin taut with index and middle finger of the other hand.
- Aim slightly towards umbilicus.
- Needle passes through interspinous ligaments and resistance as the ligamentum flavum is penetrated.
- Remove stylet to see if CSF drains.
- Measure OP by attaching manometer.
- Ask patient to relax knees a little to obtain accurate OP.
- Watch for respiration-related movement of the CSF column.
- Drain manometer fluid into collection tube.
- Remove manometer avoiding moving needle.
- Collect three or four further tubes at least 3–5 mL each for:
  - protein;
  - microbiology;
  - oligoclonal bands;
  - cytology.
- One further sample for CSF glucose.
- Always take an extra sample if there is a possibility of further tests being necessary. Keep in the fridge or lab.
- Reinsert stylet, remove needle, and apply pressure for 1–2 minutes.
- Apply sterile dressing.
- Allow patient to roll over and back.
- Take blood for glucose and oligobands if necessary.
- Label samples and write out forms yourself.
- Advise flat bed rest for 2–3 hours.

Complications

- Traumatic tap due to vertebral vein puncture. Allow CSF to drain until clear (in SAH, CSF samples uniformly stained); then collect samples.
- Post-LP headache common. Incidence ↓ with smaller gauge needle. Features:
  - postural headache, i.e. ↑ sitting or standing, ↓ lying flat;
  - associated with neck pain;
  - tinnitus;
  - nausea and vomiting.

- Treatment of post-LP headache:
  - reassurance;
  - bed rest and ↑ intake of fluids;
  - caffeine drinks, e.g. coffee, coke, or Red Bull®;
  - very rarely, if symptoms do not settle, consider IV caffeine infusion or autologous blood patch by an experienced anaesthetist.
- Dry tap (failure to obtain CSF). Causes:
  - subarachnoid space not penetrated—try interspace above or below;
  - low CSF pressure due to spinal blockage or intracranial hypotension;
  - adhesive arachnoiditis or malignant infiltration.
- Meningitis or epidural abscess: rare.
- Bleeding (all rare):
  - local extradural;
  - local intradural (subarachnoid);
  - intracranial subdural haematoma (cerebral atrophy risk factor).

Interpreting LP findings

- Characteristics of normal CSF:
  - appearance—clear, colourless;
  - opening pressure 8–16 mm, CSF > 25 definitely abnormal;
  - cells/μL < 5 lymphocytes;
  - protein 0.1–0.45 g/L;
  - glucose > 50% blood glucose.
- Causes of ↑ OP:
  - mass lesion;
  - brain swelling, e.g. meningitis, encephalitis, trauma;
  - idiopathic intracranial hypertension;
  - cerebral venous thrombosis;
  - hydrocephalus (communicating or non-communicating).
- If traumatic tap, subtract one white cell per 500 RBC.
- Causes of xanthochromia:
  - ↑↑ CSF protein;
  - SAH after 12 hours;
  - jaundice;
  - rifampicin.
- Oligoclonal bands present in CSF but not in serum indicative of intrathecal synthesis found in:
  - MS;
  - CNS infections;
  - ADEM.
- See 📖 Chapter 3, 'Meningitis', pp. 122–5, 📖 Chapter 3, 'Acute encephalitis (including limbic encephalitis)', pp. 130–1, and 📖 'Viral encephalitis', pp. 370–2.
- Characteristics of CSF malignant meningitis:
  - appearance, clear or cloudy;
  - opening pressure normal or ↑;
  - cells/μL: < 200, mixed inflammatory and malignant;
  - protein up to 1 g/L;
  - glucose may be < 50% blood level.

Intravenous immunoglobulin (IV Ig)

- Prepared from pooled plasma from > 8000 donors. Therefore batch inconsistencies.
- Blood product—theoretical risk of transmission of (unknown) viruses and prions.
- Contains IgG + traces of IgM, IgA + soluble factors such as cytokines.
- Mechanism of action. Several possible:
  - anti-idiotypic antibodies;
  - ↑ saturation and blockade of Fc receptors on macrophages;
  - modulation of pro-inflammatory cytokines.
- Expensive: approximately £3400 for 5-day course.

Indications

Guillain–Barré syndrome
- Licensed in UK.
- Trials indicate ≡ plasma exchange.
- Dose: 0.4 g/kg/day for 5 days.
- No trial data on initiating treatment after 2 weeks or mild GBS.
- Some patients improve initially but then relapse—reasonable to consider another course.
- If no response, ? further course or PE.

Multifocal motor neuropathy with conduction block
- Treatment of choice.
- Patients may deteriorate with steroids or PE.
- May require regular infusions.

CIDP
- IV Ig ≡ steroids ≡ PE.
- May require regular infusions.

Myasthenia gravis
- Used in myasthenic crises.
- Preoperative prior to thymectomy.

Myositis
- Dermatomyositis—trials support use if steroids fail or inadequate response.
- Inclusion body myositis—no good evidence for benefit.
- Polymyositis—anecdotal evidence for benefit only if steroids fail.

Multiple sclerosis
- ↓ relapse rate in RCTs similar to that with beta-interferons.
- No data in secondary progressive or on disability.

Other disorders (anecdotal evidence only)
- Stiff person syndrome.
- Paraneoplastic syndromes.
- Rasmussen's encephalitis.
- Lower motor neuron syndromes.
- VGKC antibody disorders.

Complications

Usually mild and transient, but caution in patients with renal impairment, cardiac dysfunction, or ↑ viscosity due to ↑ gammaglobulins or ↑ cholesterol. IgA deficiency patients risk an anaphylactic reaction—preparations with low IgA levels available.

- Systemic effects (common): fever, myalgia, headache.
- Cardiovascular: hypertension, cardiac failure, MI, venous thrombosis.
- Renal: acute renal failure.
- Neurological: migraine, aseptic meningitis, stroke, reversible encephalopathy.
- Hypersensitivity reactions: anaphylaxis, haemolytic anaemia, neutropenia, lymphopenia.
- Skin: urticaria, eczema.
- Changes in laboratory results: hyponatraemia (artefactual), ↑ ESR (rouleaux formation), ↓ Hb (dilutional), ↑ LFTs.

Procedure

- Check FBC, renal, liver function, immunoglobulin levels prior to infusion unless extreme urgency.
- Send antibody tests and serological tests.
- Discuss issues regarding blood product and possible complications.
- Obtain consent, especially for unlicensed use.
- Start infusions at slow rate initially.
- Regular monitoring of pulse, BP, and temperature by nursing staff, especially during first infusions.
- Usual dose 0.4 g/kg/day for 5 days. Subsequent doses depend on response and relapse rate. In CIDP and MMN usually every 4–12 weeks.
- Monitor renal function.

Further reading

Elovaara I, Apostolski S, van Doorn P, et al. (2008). Intravenous immunoglobulin: EFNS guidelines for the use of intravenous immunoglobulins in the treatment of neurological diseases. *Eur. J. Neurol.*, **15**, 893–908.

Patwa HS, Chaudhry V, Katzberg H, Rae-Grant AD, So YT (2012). Evidence-based guideline: intravenous immunoglobulin in the treatment of neuromuscular disorders. *Neurology*, **78**, 1009–15.

Diagnosis of brainstem death

Death is defined as 'the irreversible loss of the capacity for conscious-ness, combined with the irreversible loss of the capacity to breathe spon-taneously'. Requisites before assessment of brainstem death are given in Box 5.4.

> **Box 5.4 Requisites before assessment of brainstem function**
> - Known aetiology for the irreversible brain damage.
> - Effects of depressant drugs, hypothermia, and metabolic and endocrine causes of coma should have been excluded.
> - Patient is on a ventilator as spontaneous respiration is inadequate or absent.

Individual examinations should be carried out by two senior doctors after an interval of 24 hours. Staff making the diagnosis should not be involved in potential organ donation.

Criteria for a diagnosis of brainstem death

- Pupils are fixed and do not respond to light.
- Corneal reflex absent.
- Vestibulo-ocular reflex absent (instil 50 mL of iced water into each ear; check tympanic membrane is intact).
- Gag reflex absent and no response to bronchial stimulation by passage of a suction catheter down trachea.
- Motor response: no response within cranial nerve territory to painful stimuli applied to limbs or supraorbital area.
- Respiration: no respiratory movements when disconnected from ventilator. Give 6 L O_2 and ensure PCO_2 rises > 6.5 kPa.
  No further tests, such as EEG, are necessary if all conditions fulfilled.

Further reading

Posner JB, Saper CB, Schiff N, Plum F (2007). *Plum and Posner's Diagnosis of Stupor and Coma* (4th edn), pp. 331–40. New York: Oxford University Press.

Neurology in medicine

Neurological symptoms: cardiac disease 396
Neurological disease: cardiac pathology 400
Neurological features of respiratory disease 402
Respiratory failure in neurology 404
Neurological disorders: gastroenterological symptoms 412
Gastroenterological disorders: neurological presentations 416
Neurology and renal medicine 420
Hereditary disorders of the nervous system and the kidneys 422
Neurology and haematological disorders 424
Neurology and connective tissue disorders and vasculitides 428
Endocrine neuroanatomy 432
Neurology in endocrine disorders 436
Primary pituitary disorders 440
The neuroendocrine syndromes 442
Dermatology in neurology 444
Inherited neurocutaneous syndromes 452
Neurological and neurosurgical issues in pregnancy 456

Neurological symptoms: cardiac disease

Cardiac arrhythmias

- Risk factor for strokes (e.g. AF).
- Paroxysmal arrhythmias should be considered as cause for syncope, collapse, seizures—review ECG, consider 24-hour ECG.
- See Table 6.1 for ECG changes in neurological disease.

Long QT syndrome:

- Potential cause of avoidable sudden cardiac death from ventricular arrhythmias.
- Autosomal dominant with variable expression.
- Prevalence: 1/2000–3000.
- In one series, 39% with long QT were most misdiagnosed as epilepsy.
- Clinical features:
  - cerebral hypoperfusion can manifest as myoclonic jerks or epileptic type movements;
  - vasovagal attacks;
  - exertional syncope (long QT1);
  - syncope during emotional stress (long QT2);
  - sudden syncope at rest (long QT3);
  - rapid recovery;
  - otherwise normal examination;
  - may have family history of unexplained sudden death.
- Numerous drug triggers:
  - antiarrhythmics, e.g. amiodarone, sotalol;
  - antibiotics, e.g. erythromycin, clarithromycin;
  - antihistamines, e.g. ondansetron;
  - antidepressants, e.g. amitriptyline, fluoxetine;
  - antipsychotics, e.g. quetiapine, haloperidol.
- Syncope with long QT on an ECG (> 450 ms in males, > 460 ms in females) in the absence of causative medications or disorders, is suggestive of the diagnosis.
- Automated measurement is frequently inaccurate.
- Manual measurement of QTc using the tangent technique (see Fig. 6.1).

Endocarditis

- Infectious endocarditis, non-bacterial thrombotic endocarditis, Libman–Sacks endocarditis in SLE.
- All are associated with embolic phenomena causing stroke.

Infectious endocarditis

- Neurological complications relatively common.
- Focal:
  - embolism (from valvular vegetations), haemorrhage secondary to rupture of infective arteritis, mycotic aneurysm, cerebral abscess.
- Diffuse:
  - multiple microemboli, DIC, multi-organ failure.

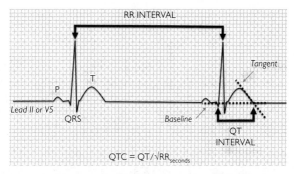

Fig. 6.1 The tangent technique for calculating corrected QT interval. Adapted from Postema PG, de Jong JSSG, van der Bilt IAC, Wilde AAM (2008). Accurate electrocardiographic assessment of the QT interval: teach the tangent. *Heart Rhythm*, 5, 1015–18, with permission.

Non-bacterial thrombotic endocarditis
- Occurs in hypercoagulable states, e.g. advanced malignancies and AIDs.
- Similar presentation to infective endocarditis; haemorrhage less likely.

Cardiac surgery
- Neurological complications either focal or global.
- In order of frequency, the following neurological events are found after cardiac surgery (incidence):
  • persistent cognitive deficits (20–40%);
  • reversible encephalopathy (3–12%);
  • peripheral neuropathies—brachial plexus (1.5–24%), phrenic (10–60%), recurrent laryngeal, sciatic, femoral, saphenous, sympathetic chain;
  • stroke (3–6%);
  • seizures (especially in children) (3%).
- Several proposed mechanisms including embolic (fat, air), cerebral hypoperfusion, metabolic abnormalities, impaired cerebral autoregulation, or systemic inflammatory response.
- Identified risk factors: cross-clamping time, type of surgery (lowest risk in aortic valve replacement), open heart surgery, comorbidities, atherosclerotic ascending aorta disease.

Table 6.1 ECG changes in neurological disease

Condition	Rate & rhythm	Axis	PR duration	QTc	QRS duration	ST segment	T wave	Notes
Subarachnoid haemorrhage	Ventricular/atrial arrhythmias	Varied	Varied	↑	Varied	↑/↓	Inverted	Common within 48 h of onset, lasts up to 6 weeks. Prominent U waves. Most arrhythmias have been described in SAH
Friedreich's ataxia	N	R or L (R > L)	N	N	May be ↑	N	Inversion	Hypokinetic dilated cardiomyopathy. Often inferolateral T-wave inversion
Muscular dystrophies	Onset of arrhythmias with heart block (AF/junctional)	N/L	N/↑	N	May be ↑	↑/↓	Flattened and inverted	Dominant R wave V1, V2. Pseudoinfarction. Anterolateral Q waves. Heart block. Cardiomyopathy
Myotonic dystrophy type I	N*	N	N/↑	N	N	N	N	*Develops heart block severity linked to CTG repeat length
Channelopathies: periodic paralysis								
Hypokalaemic	N/↓	N	↑	N	N	N/↓	Flattened	U waves
Hyperkalaemic	N/ectopic	N	N/↓	N/↓	N/↑	N	Tall/tented	Potassium rarely in cardiotoxic range

								Note
Anderson's syndrome	Often bigeminy	See note	N/absent	↑	N/↑	N	N*	*High incidence of ventricular arrhythmias (torsade/VT/VF) Bidirectional VT (axis switches each beat) unique to subset of patients
Metabolic disorders								
Fabry's disease	N	N	N/↓	N	N	N	N	Pre-excitation LVH
Danon disease (LAMP-2 mutation)	N	N	N/↓	N	N	N	N	Pre-excitation WPW due to myocardial hypertrophy
Lafora disease	N*	N	N/↑	N	N	N	N	May develop heart block
Mitochondrial cytopathies								
Kearns–Sayre syndrome	N*	N/L	↑	N	N/i	N	Normal/inverted	*Complete heart block may develop after ophthalmoplegia
Ocular myopathy	N	N/R	N	N	N	N/↓	Normal/inverted	Cardiac involvement rare
MERFF	N	N/L	N	N	N	N/↓	N	LVH
MELAS	N	N	N/↓	N	N	N/↓	Normal/inverted	WPW LVH
LHON	N	N	N/↓	N/↑	N	N/↓	Normal/inverted	Pre-excitation syndromes (WPW/LGL) LVH (hypertrophic)

N, normal; L, left; R, right; LVH, left ventricular hypertrophy; WPW, Wolff–Parkinson–White syndrome; LGL, Lown–Ganong–Levine syndrome; VT, ventricular tachycardia.

Neurological disease: cardiac pathology

Cushing's response
Bradycardia and hypertension in response to ⇈ intracranial pressure.

See Table 6.2 for neurological diseases associated with cardiac pathology.

Subarachnoid haemorrhage
- ECG abnormalities seen in 80–90% (see Table 6.1); more frequently in severe neurological impairment.
- Onset within 48 hours; may last up to 6 weeks.
- Should not delay surgery unless malignant arrhythmia present or probability of infarction is very high.

Muscular dystrophy
- The muscular dystrophies often have cardiac muscle involvement and can be divided into two groups:

Muscular dystrophy with prominent cardiomyopathy
Becker's muscular dystrophy
- Dilated cardiomyopathy in males aged 20–40 years; later in female carriers.
- May be the first sign in subclinical cases.

Duchenne's muscular dystrophy
- Occurs late in disease; may be under-recognized as patients are less active.
- Mortality from dilated cardiomyopathy 10–15%.
- Serum atrial natriuretic peptide useful for detecting cardiomyopathy and instituting early treatment with beta-blockers plus an ACE inhibitor.

Muscular dystrophy with prominent cardiac conduction disturbance
- Early detection of conduction defects: heart block, AV standstill, severe bradycardia, AF.
- May not be symptomatic and is associated with sudden death. Pacemakers may be life-saving.
- Late-onset dilated cardiomyopathy.

Emery–Dreifuss muscular dystrophy
- Cardiac involvement at any age; may be present at onset.
- Nomal myocardium is replaced by fibro-adipose tissue.
- Inability to pace the atrial paralysis is pathognomonic.

Limb girdle muscular dystrophy
- Neuromuscular symptoms precede cardiovascular symptoms.

Table 6.2 Neurological diseases associated with cardiac pathology

Cardiac pathology	Neurological condition
Long QT syndrome	Periodic paralysis
Cardiac arrhythmia	Epilepsy
	MELAS (WPW)
	GBS
Conduction block	Kearns–Sayre syndrome
	Lafora disease
Ventricular hypertrophy	MELAS (symmetrical)
	MERRF (asymmetrical)
Cardiomyopathy	Muscular dystrophies (dilated)
	Friedreich's ataxia (dilated)
	Glycogen storage disease (dilated/hypertrophic/restrictive)
	MERRF, MELAS (dilated/hypertrophic)

Epilepsy

- Ictal tachycardia: the most common finding (82%).
- Ictal bradycardia: occurs in 3–4% and can cause syncope. Male > female. Most common in temporal lobe seizures.
- Ictal asystole: rare but important finding (temporal and frontal seizures). Possible increased risk of SUDEP; pacemaker should be considered if duration of asystole > 4 seconds.

Guillain–Barré syndrome

- Autonomic dysfunction manifesting as arrhythmias.
- Often tachycardia, though life-threatening brady- and tachyarrhythmias can occur, usually in ventilated patients.

Mitochondrial cytopathies

- Patients with Kearns–Sayre syndrome should be evaluated and monitored for AV conduction disturbances.
- Heart block develops after the ophthalmoplegia. Permanent pacemaker improves survival.
- Patients with MERRF and MELAS should be followed for cardiac hypertrophy and dilated cardiomyopathy.

Neurological features of respiratory disease

Often arise due to changes in PaO_2 and $PaCO_2$, or as a side effect of medication.

Hypoxia (PaO_2 < 10 kPa)

- Symptoms:
    - cognitive dysfunction;
    - confusion;
    - amnesia;
    - behavioural change/aggression;
    - hallucinations;
    - gait disturbance.

Physical signs may include petechial retinal haemorrhages and saccade disruption (seen in altitude sickness).

Hypercapnoea ($PaCO_2$ > 6 kPa)

- Symptoms:
    - drowsiness/fatigue;
    - headaches (especially in morning);
    - episodic confusion;
    - excessive daytime somnolence;
    - impotence;
    - poor concentration.
- Symptoms depend on the rate of CO_2 rise, and can differ between acute and chronic.
- Can arise insidiously in patients with neuromuscular weakness, and so symptoms should be actively sought.
- Neurological signs include tremor (on outstretched hands), papilloedema (which can cause blindness), ↓ GCS, and seizures.
- Can also precipitate ↓ GCS and seizures by over-hyperventilating hypercapnoeic patients.

Hypocapnoea ($PaCO_2$ < 4.5 kPa)

- Symptoms:
    - light-headedness;
    - breathlessness;
    - 'tingling' sensations;
    - headache;
    - palpitations;
    - tetany;
    - tinnitis;
    - chest pain;
    - tremor;
    - visual blurring;
    - transient LOC;
    - unsteadiness.

Respiratory failure in neurology

See Table 6.3 for differential diagnosis and Table 6.4 for central disorders of ventilatory control. See Fig. 6.2 for examples of central respiratory patterns.

Acute respiratory failure

- May be acute presentation or decompensation of a chronic condition.
- In neurological patients consider common causes first, e.g. chest infection, PE, or exacerbation of pre-existing respiratory illness.
- Clues in the background history, tempo of onset, clinical signs, and arterial blood gas (ABG).
- Review medications, especially for opiates, benzodiazepines, and anticholinergics (look for signs of overdose).
- In an acute setting, resuscitate using the ABC approach (Box 6.1).

Chronic respiratory failure

- Often identified by symptomatic hypercapnoea.
- Additional symptoms may include dyspnoea on immersion in water or on lying flat (indicating diaphragm paralysis).
- Paradoxical (inward) inspiratory movement of abdominal muscles indicates a 70% reduction in normal respiratory muscle strength.
- Lying and standing FVC should also be documented as it is often diagnostic.
- Initial non-invasive specialist tests to investigate suspected respiratory muscle weakness include maximal sniff nasal pressure, magnetic/electric phrenic nerve stimulation, and mouth pressure during phrenic nerve stimulation.
- Formal specialist tests required when respiratory muscle weakness cannot be confirmed or refuted on non-invasive tests or if precise sequential measurements are required. These require the placement of oesophageal and gastric balloons.
- Further tests are possible in specific circumstances, e.g. suspected hemi-diaphragm disease.
- Polysomnography is indicated if the patient has:
  - proven severe weakness but denies hypercapnoea symptoms;
  - sleep symptoms without demonstrable severe respiratory muscle weakness;
  - sleep symptoms but fails to meet the British Thoracic Society desaturation criteria for obstructive sleep apnoea.

Respiratory failure: differential diagnosis

The differential diagnosis is shown in Table 6.3.

Central disorders of ventilatory control

Central disorders of ventilatory control are listed in Table 6.4.

Box 6.1 ABC approach

- Secure airway.
- Give high flow oxygen in first instance regardless of cause; adjust according to ABG and clinical response.
- Secure IV access and send bloods for U&Es, bone profile, Mg, CRP, FBC, clotting ± blood cultures.
- ABG (document FiO_2).
- Obtain CXR and ECG.
- Document FVC (if possible).
- Get early anaesthetic support and transfer to ITU if:
  - falling GCS or GCS < 8 (unable to support airway);
  - not responding to initial therapy;
  - becoming progressively exhausted or increasingly shocked despite treatment;
  - FVC < 15 mL/kg (< 1 L).

Table 6.3 Differential diagnosis for respiratory failure in the neurological patient

Neuromuscular junction pathology	Muscular disorder	Peripheral neuropathy	Central causes
Anticholinesterase overdose[A]	Hypokalaemia[A]	GBS (demyelinating & axonal)[A]	Toxic: alcohol, opiates, barbiturates, benzodiazepines[A]
Acute organophosphate poisoning[A]	Periodic paralysis[A]	GBS mimics e.g. HIV, Lyme disease, sarcoidosis, CMV[A]	Pontomedullary SOL[A]: haemorrhage, AVM, tumour, syrinx, etc.
Botulism[A]	Hypo-phosphataemia[A]	CIDP[C] Brachial neuritis[A/C]	Transtentorial herniation[A]
Myasthenia gravis[A]	Acute rhabdomyolysis[A]	Critical illness poly-neuropathy[C]	Bilateral tegmental medullary infarcts[A]
Hyper-magnesaemia[A]	Polymyositis	Toxins: organo-phosphates, thallium, arsenic, lead, gold, lithium[A/C]	Encephalitis[A]
Snake, spider, scorpion bite[A]	Thyroid disease[A/C]	Drugs: vincristine[C]	Cord lesions C3–5 or higher. Either intrinsic (e.g. MS, transverse myelitis) or compressive (e.g. trauma, disc)[A]
Fish, shellfish, crab poisoning[A]	Combined neuromuscular blockade and steroids[A/C]	Lymphoma[A]	Infections, e.g. polio, tetanus, rabies, leptospirosis[A]
Tick paralysis[A]	Barium intoxication[A]	Vasculitis–SLE[A]	Post-polio syndrome[C]
Antibiotic-induced paralysis[A]	Myotonic dystrophy[A/C]	Metabolic–acute intermittent porphyria[A]	

Table 6.3 (*Contd.*)

Neuromuscular junction pathology	Muscular disorder	Peripheral neuropathy	Central causes
Lambert–Eaton syndrome[C]	Limb–girdle syndromes[C]	Hereditary tyrosinaemia[C]	
	Mitochondrial myopathy[C]	Diphtheria[A]	
	Inflammatory myopathy[C]		
	Hereditary myopathy[C] Acid maltase deficiency Carnitine palmityl transferase deficiency		

Superscript indicates usual mode of initial presentation: A, acute (history usually minutes–hours); C, chronic (history longer than several days/detected incidentally). Note that all chronic causes can present as acute on chronic.

Table 6.4 Central disorders of ventilatory control

Disorder	Mechanism	Notes
Cheyne–Stokes respiration	Due to an instability in normal feedback control for respiration	Slow oscillation crescendo–decrescendo hyperventilation followed by apnoea
		May occur due to several factors that cause widespread cortical dysfunction (↑ ICP & metabolic disturbances) which results in ↑ oscillations in blood gas levels
		Causes include heart failure, sleep apnoea, stroke, uraemia
Short-cycle periodic breathing	ICP, lower pontine lesions, and expanding posterior fossa lesions	Similar to Cheyne–Stokes but much faster oscillations (~ 2:4 ratio of hypo- to hyperventilation)
Central neurogenic hyper-ventilation	Infiltrative central tegmental pontine lesion causing stimulation of pontine respiratory group	Definition: hyperventilation that persists during sleep with respiratory alkalosis and absence of another organic cause
		RR: 40–70 breaths/min
		Common lesions: lymphoma, astrocytoma
		If lesion is treatable (very rare), recovery is possible (e.g. lymphatoid granulomatosis)
		Morphine used for palliative symptomatic treatment
Cluster breathing	Lower pontine tegmental lesion	Rapidly alternating hyperventilation followed by apnoeic episodes of variable length
Apneustic breathing	Lesion at dorsolateral lower half of pons	Prolonged inspiratory gasp with pause at full inspiration
Ataxic breathing ('Biot's breathing')	Medullary insult (e.g. poliomyelitis)	Irregular pattern and amplitude
		Combined with bilateral CN VI is warning sign of impending brainstem compression (posterior fossa lesion)

Table 6.4 (*Contd.*)

Disorder	Mechanism	Notes
Ondine's curse	Removal of chemical control of breathing with preservation of voluntary control Lower medullary lesion	Classic syndrome: in children associated with Hirschsprung's disease and GORD; in adults often secondary to trauma High risk of nocturnal sudden death; therefore nocturnal respiratory support required Selected patients benefit from diaphragmatic pacing
Transtentorial herniation	Progressive compromise of respiratory nuclei with breakdown of normal regulatory mechanisms	Cheyne–Stokes ↓ Central neurogenic hyperventilation ↓ Eupnoea (quiet breathing) ↓ Irregular gasping (pre-terminal)
Brainstem/high cervical spine injury	C3–5 and above Loss of voluntary and involuntary control of respiratory muscles	Ventilatory support via tracheostomy Bilateral diaphragmatic pacing may be of benefit if available; only indicated if phrenic nerves are functioning but corticodiaphragmatic is interrupted on cervical magnetic stimulation
Kussmaul breathing	Metabolic acidosis	Deep regular respiration

GORD, gastro-oesophageal reflux disease.

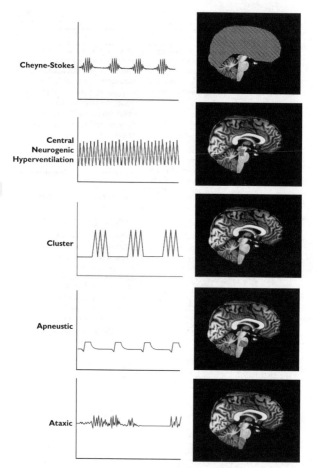

Fig. 6.2 Examples of central respiratory patterns. Graphs represent respiratory pattern (y-axis, tidal volume; x-axis, time). Diagrams indicate the location of the characteristic lesion.

Neurological disorders: gastroenterological symptoms

See Table 6.5 for differential diagnosis.

Dysphagia

- Neurogenic dysphagia suggested by:
  - drooling of saliva;
  - coughing/choking during swallowing;
  - nasal regurgitation.
- May arise from dysfunction at any point in the swallowing pathway. Clues in the history of onset and associated symptoms.
- Assessment should be made with speech and language therapy assessment and videofluoroscopy.

Gastrointestinal motility disorders

Defects in innervation

Achalasia

- Absence of peristalsis with failure of relaxation of the lower oesophageal sphincter (LOS).
- Caused by degeneration of oesophageal myenteric nerves and loss of inhibitory ganglion cells leading to unopposed contraction of the LOS.
- Presents with progressive dysphagia to fluids and solids with regurgitation of undigested food.
- Primary: e.g. triple A syndrome (achalasia, Addison's disease, and alacrima).
- Secondary: uncommon—Chagas' disease, oesophageal cancer, diabetes.
- Diagnosis with oesophageal manometry.

Hirschprung's disease

- Caused by loss of parasympathetic ganglion cells (aganglionosis) from the myenteric and submucosal plexus due to failure of neural migration.
- Always involves the anus and continues proximally for a variable distance.
- Presents soon after birth with constipation and abdominal distension.
- Affected segment is contracted, with colonic dilatation proximally.
- Diagnosis: full-thickness rectal biopsy taken 1.5 cm above dentate line showing aganglionosis with associated increase in acetylcholinesterase staining.

Gastroparesis

- Caused by dysfunction of both the parasympathetic and sympathetic supply of the stomach leading to delayed gastric emptying.
- Presents with nausea, vomiting, reflux, early satiety, abdominal pain, and distension.
- Most common cause: diabetes mellitus.
- Other causes: post-gastric surgery, Parkinson's disease, intestinal pseudo-obstruction, collagen vascular disorders (SLE, scleroderma), stiff man syndrome, CMT, paraneoplastic syndrome.
- Diagnosis: gastric emptying study.
- Treatment: majority respond to prokinetics, e.g. metoclopramide.
- Laparoscopic gastric pacing available for highly treatment-resistant cases.

Table 6.5 Differential diagnosis for lesion of the swallowing pathway

Pathway component	Differential diagnosis
Afferent	Recurrent laryngeal nerve palsy: tumour (neck, lung, mediastinum), surgical trauma (thyroidectomy), aortic aneurysm
	Palatal hypo-aesthesia in Arnold–Chiari type I
Brainstem nuclei	MS, lateral medullary syndrome, Arnold–Chiari type I
Cortical	Stroke (common), MS, PD, PSP, HD, Wilson's disease
Efferent (including NMJ)	GBS, ALS, myasthenia gravis, recurrent laryngeal nerve palsy
Muscle	Polymyositis, dermatomyositis, myotonic dystrophy, muscular dystrophy

Pseudo-obstruction
- Presentation of the signs, symptoms, and radiological appearance of bowel obstruction but with no evidence of an obstructive cause.
- Acute or chronic (rarer, but likely to have neurological aetiology).
- Caused by an imbalance in the autonomic innervation leading to increased sympathetic tone causing inhibition of colonic motility.
- Colon may become massively distended with risk of perforation.
- Broad neurological differential diagnosis, including:
  - Myopathic:
    - NMJ disorder: myasthenia gravis;
    - myopathy: myositis, myotonic dystrophy, muscular dystrophy.
  - Neuropathic:
    - Metabolic: diabetes, porphyria;
    - Infiltrative: systemic sclerosis, amyloidosis;
    - Infection: Chagas' disease, CMV infection;
    - Drugs: anticholinergics, opiates, tricyclic antidepressants, vincristine;
    - Spinal cord injury (trauma, intrinsic/extrinsic lesion, recent surgery);
    - Paraneoplastic (anti-Hu in small cell lung cancer);
    - Primary autonomic failure.
  - Mitochondrial:
    - MNGIE syndrome (mitochondrial neurogastrointestinal encephalomyopathy syndrome).
- Rule out common causes (electrolyte or thyroid abnormalities, sepsis).
- Conservative management initially (NBM and NG decompression).
- Neostigmine can be used if no response to conservative treatment
- Endoscopic/surgical input if failing conservative/↑ risk of perforation.

Examples of neurological associations with common symptoms

Constipation

Parkinson's disease (20 year prodrome before clinical presentation), MS, spinal cord injury, autonomic neuropathy, pseudo-obstruction.

Diarrhoea

Autonomic neuropathy, coeliac disease, Whipple's disease.

Faecal incontinence

Spinal cord lesions, Parkinson's disease, MSA, MS, spinal cord injury, autonomic neuropathy, pudendal nerve injury.

Gastroenterological disorders: neurological presentations

Nutritional deficiency syndromes

Water-soluble vitamins

B_1 (thiamine)

- Often associated with alcohol abuse, but may also emerge in the context of peptic ulcer disease, acute pancreatitis, gastric/oesophageal cancer, anorexia nervosa, bariatric surgery, hyperemesis gravidarum, or starvation.
- Treatment initially with IV thiamine (50–100 mg IV/IM) *before* any IV glucose solutions as this can worsen symptoms. Maintain PO.
- Wernicke's encephalopathy:
  - triad of ocular abnormalities, ataxia (usually gait), and encephalopathy.
  - Ocular findings: ophthalmoplegia (horizontal gaze palsy or gaze paresis), nystagmus (horizontal > vertical); less frequently anisocoria, sluggish pupils, ptosis.
  - Other symptoms: vestibular dysfunction, peripheral neuropathy (↓ proprioception, foot drop), hypothermia, hypotension, coma.
- Korsakoff syndrome:
  - disproportionate impairment in memory relative to other cognitive deficits in an otherwise alert and responsive patient;
  - often follows Wernicke's encephalopathy (Wernicke–Korsakoff);
  - extensive retrograde amnesia, antegrade amnesia (less), confabulation.
- Beri-beri:
  - 'wet' beri-beri—cardiac involvement (high output failure);
  - 'dry' beri-beri—CNS involvement (often Wernicke's ± Korsakoff's); additionally brisk reflexes, polyneuritis (lower limbs > upper limbs), weakness, pain, paralysis, and seizures.
  - cardiac and CNS involvement may present together.

B_3 (nicotinamide):

Pellagra (see 📖 'Dermatology in neurology/Pellagra', pp. 444–50): triad of dementia, diarrhoea, and dermatitis.

B_6 (pyridoxine):

- Very rare; usually a consequence of a genetic enzymatic defect preventing pyridoxine conversion in the liver.
- Seizures, muscle cramps, paraesthesiae.

B_{12} (cobalamin):

- Requires intrinsic factor (IF) for absorption. Due to inadequate intake (e.g. vegetarians), IF deficiency, nitrous oxide abuse, malnutrition, resection of stomach or terminal ileum, terminal ileum disease.
- Often presents with symmetric paraesthesiae (feet > hands) and gait ataxia.
- Sensory: dorsal column involvement (↓ vibration, ↓ proprioception).
- Motor weakness usually lower limb (axonal neuropathy); often hyporeflexic (though may be hyper-reflexic), Lhermitte's sign.

- Autonomic features may also be present.
- Neuropsychiatric features include impaired memory, personality change, hypomania, psychosis, hallucinations, and emotional lability.
- Visual changes: cecocentric scotoma, optic atrophy.
- MRI may show T_2 and FLAIR white matter hyperintensities.
- Measure serum B_{12}: normal value does not exclude deficiency. Measure serum MMA (methylmalonic acid) and homocysteine which are both elevated in B_{12} deficiency, if normal effectively excludes deficiency.
- B_{12}: replacement. Replace *before* starting any folate supplements (to avoid precipitating subacute combined degeneration of the cord). Treat underlying aetiology.
  - Without neurological involvement: hydroxocobalamin 1 mg 3x week, for 2 weeks, then every 3 months.
  - With neurological involvement: hydroxocobalamin 1 mg alternate days until no improvement then 2-monthly.

Fat-soluble vitamins

Can arise from fat malabsorption states such as liver disease, biliary obstruction, pancreatitis, cystic fibrosis, abetalipoproteinaemia (vitamin E), small bowel resection.

Vitamin D:

- Proximal myopathy.

Vitamin E (tocopherol):

- Ataxia, dysarthria, ↓ vibration and proprioception, ↓ deep tendon reflexes, Babinski sign positive, pes cavus, kyphoscoliosis, cardiomyopathy.
- Presentation similar to Friedreich's ataxia.

Other intestinal neurological disorders

Coeliac disease

Neurological features may develop independent of nutritional deficiency (e.g. B_{12}—Ramsay Hunt syndrome).

- Cerebellar ataxia.
- Peripheral neuropathy.
- Dementia.
- Myoclonus.
- Seizures.

Imaging may show cerebellar atrophy or bilateral cortical calcification.

Inflammatory bowel disease (IBD)

- ↑ Thromboembolic disease in both Crohn's disease and ulcerative colitis.
- Myositis seen more commonly in Crohn's disease.
- Neuropathy (more common in ulcerative colitis):
  - Crohn's disease—sensory axonal polyneuropathy;
  - ulcerative colitis—AIDP or CIDP.

Whipple's disease
- Caused by Gram-positive actinomycete *Tropheryma whippelii*.
- Begins as polyarthralgia, chronic diarrhoea, abdominal pain, and weight loss.
- CNS: rhythmic myoclonus, dementia, ophthalmoplegia, neuropsychiatric changes, hypothalamic disturbance (e.g. insomnia, hyperphagia), ataxia.
- Oculomasticatory myorhythmia (pendular convergence nystagmus with palatal, tongue, and mandibular movements) and/or oculofacialskeletal myorhythmia (plus limb involvement) *and* vertical supranuclear ophthalmoplegia are pathognomic. (NB: Movements persist during sleep.)
- CSF: inflammatory (± PAS-containing macrophage). PCR for *T. whippelii*.
- May require gut biopsy to demonstrate PAS-positive macrophages.
- Treatment: chloramphenicol and co-trimoxazole for 1–2 years.

Neurology and renal medicine

Neurological complications may be due to renal failure or the cause of the renal failure, e.g. diabetes, connective tissue disorders.

Uraemic encephalopathy

Consider other causes of encephalopathy: hypertensive encephalopathy, seizures, electrolyte disturbance, sepsis, posterior reversible leucoencephalopathy.

Clinical features

- Conscious level: fluctuating alertness, ↓ concentration, ↑ drowsiness, delirium with visual hallucinations and coma.
- Tremulousness and asterixis (outstretched arms with elbows, wrists, and fingers in extension results in flapping tremor more rapid in flexion due to loss of tone).
- Myoclonus.
- Seizures.
- Brisk reflexes, ↑↑ plantars.
- Autonomic neuropathy.

Investigations

- CSF may be abnormal with a pleocytosis and ↑ protein.
- EEG—diffuse slowing with triphasic waves.
- CT/MRI to exclude other pathology may show oedema, focal infarcts, or haemorrhage.

Uraemic neuropathy

Common in end-stage renal disease. Improves with dialysis. Lower prevalence in patients on peritoneal dialysis than haemodialysis.

Aetiology

- 'Middle molecule (500–12 000 Daltons) hypothesis' less effectively cleared by haemodialysis—controversial.
- ? Parathormone via calcium accumulation in nerves.
- ? Hyperkalaemia.

Clinical features

- Paraesthesias with restless legs syndrome.
- Progressive length-dependent sensory and motor neuropathy usually distal but may in severe cases result in a flaccid quadraparesis.

Investigations

- NCT—axonal neuropathy.

Treatment

- May stabilize or improve with dialysis and renal transplantation.

Complications of dialysis

Dialysis disequilibrium syndrome

- Caused by ↓ blood urea →↓ plasma osmolality → water influx into cells and cerebral oedema.
- Muscle cramps.
- Headache, irritability, and in severe cases coma and seizures.

Subdural haematomas
- May occur in patients on dialysis.

Carpal tunnel syndrome
- Due to B_2 microglobulin amyloid.

Wernicke's encephalopathy (rare)

Dialysis dementia (rare now)
- Related to aluminium accumulation.

Complications of transplantation

Tumours

Common cancers (colon, lung, prostate, breast) ↑ ×2 more frequent; non-Hodgkin's lymphoma (NHL) and non-melanotic melanoma ↑ ×20.
- NHL usually B-cell and related to EBV infection. CNs involvement 25%.
- Primary CNS lymphoma (PCNSL).

CNS infections
- Timing after transplant may give clue to type of infection:
  - *transplant up to 1 month*: CNS infection rare. If present acquired from transplant, related to surgery or present before transplant. Pathogens similar to non-immunosuppressed;
  - *1–6 months*: greatest risk for CNS infection, meningitis, and brain abscesses. Due to immunosuppressive drugs and immunomodulating effect of viruses (CMV + EBV);
  - *after 6 months* due to immunosuppressive drugs.
- Meningitis (acute and chronic): *Listeria monocytogenes*, *Cryptococcus neoformans*, *Mycobacterium tuberculosis*, *Histoplasma capsulatum*, *Nocardia asteroides*.
- Note signs of meningism may be minimal.
- Abscesses: *Aspergillus*, toxoplasmosis, *Nocardia*. Brain biopsy may be necessary for diagnosis.
- PML.

Hereditary disorders of the nervous system and the kidneys

Fabry's disease

X-linked (Xq22 mutation) lysosomal storage disorder due to alpha-galactosidase A deficiency. Most heterozygous females also manifest disease but less severely.

- Progressive renal impairment.
- Painful small fibre neuropathy with severe lancinating pains.
- Autonomic neuropathy (abdominal pain, diarrhoea).
- Cerebrovascular disease (TIA and stroke).
- Angiokeratomas (small, red, vascular skin lesions in bathing trunk distribution).
- Cardiac hypertrophy with conduction defects.

Treatment

Enzyme replacement with recombinant human alpha-galactosidase A.

Von Hippel–Lindau disease

Autosomal dominant due to mutation on chromosome 3p25—a tumour suppressor gene.

- Renal cysts and cancers.
- CNS haemangioblastomas (usually cerebellum, spine).
- Retinal haemangioblastomas.
- Phaeochromocytomas.
- Pancreatic cysts.

Polycystic kidney disease

Autosomal dominant due to mutations on chromosome 16p13.3 (PKD1) and 4q13–q23 (PKD2).

- Hypertension, haematuria, UTIs, progressive renal failure.
- Intracranial aneurysms causing SAH and ICH. No clear guidelines for screening in this group with MRA or CTA.

Neurology and haematological disorders

Iron deficiency anaemia
- Non-specific symptoms—fatigability, tinnitus, headache, syncope.
- Severe anaemia with thrombocytopenia retinopathy with papilloedema, cotton wool spots, and flame-shaped haemorrhages.
- Anecdotal reports of association with IIH and CVT.
- If marked secondary thrombocytosis may present with TIA, cerebral infarction.
- Association with restless legs syndrome and iron supplements may resolve symptoms.

Vitamin B$_{12}$ deficiency

Causes

Autoimmune pernicious anaemia (intrinsic factor and gastric parietal cell antibodies) malabsorption syndromes (e.g. coeliac disease, Crohn's disease), gastric and ileal resections, blind loops, dietary deficiency (vegetarians and vegans), N$_2$O abuse.

Note: all neurological complications may occur with *no* change in blood picture (no anaemia or macrocytosis). Measurement of total homocysteine and methylmalonic acid are better markers of functional B$_{12}$ deficiency.

- Peripheral neuropathy:
  - length-dependent sensory and later motor neuropathy. NCT and nerve biopsy—axonal neuropathy. Usually associated with myelopathy.
- Myelopathy (subacute combined degeneration of spinal cord affecting posterior columns and corticospinal tract):
  - initially paraesthesia and ↓ vibration and ↓ joint position sense in legs later with upper limb involvement including pseudoathetosis. In severe cases spastic ataxic paraparesis with bladder involvement;
  - brisk knee jerks, absent ankle jerks (due to neuropathy), plantars ↑↑.
- Encephalopathy:
  - mood disorders, poor memory, confusion, agitation, delusions, visual and auditory hallucinations;
  - pathology—multiple foci of white matter demyelination.
- Optic neuropathy:
  - painless with centrocaecal scotoma and optic atrophy.
- Treatment: hydroxocobalamin 1 mg IM ×3 a week for 2 weeks, followed by 3-monthly injections.

Folate deficiency
- Affective disorders (usually depression) and encephalopathy most common complications. Myelopathy and peripheral neuropathy unusual.
- Note: do not prescribe folate in undiagnosed megaloblastic anaemia unless B$_{12}$ level is normal as it may precipitate neuropathy. If in doubt give both.

Sickle cell disease (sickle cell disease (Hb SS) and sickle C disease (Hb SC))

Complications arise from insoluble deoxygenated Hb S polymers. There is an associated vasculopathy. In severe hypoxaemia sickle cell trait (HbSA) patients also develop complications.

Causes of crisis
- Hypoxia.
- Dehydration.
- Acidosis.
- Infection.

Neurological complications in Hb SS 25%
- Cerebral infarction.
- Intracranial haemorrhage rare due to posterior circulation aneurysms.
- Vasculopathy and fibrous proliferation result in stenosis of large extracranial and intracranial vessels (moya moya disease).
- Cranial neuropathies, radiculopathy, myeloradiculopathy due to vertebral collapse after bone infarction, optic neuropathy, hypopituitarism.

Leukaemia

↑ frequency of neurological complications related to ↑ survival.

Infiltration
- Meningeal with headache, cranial nerve palsies, radiculopathy, obstructive hydrocephalus. CSF WCC ↑ 90%. Flow cytometry essential to identify leukaemic cells. ↓ glucose and ↑ protein frequent but unreliable. 10% cases repeated CSF normal.
- Parenchymal deposits may occur in any part of the CNS or PNS, e.g. hypothalamic and pituitary syndromes, numb chin syndrome due to mental nerve involvement.
- Extradural spinal deposits present with back pain with progressive quadraparesis or paraparesis.

Leucoencephalopathies
- PML due to immunosuppression.
- IV or intrathecal methotrexate and cranial irradiation. More common in children. Present with agitation, confusion, drowsiness, ataxia, hemi or quadriplegia, dysphasia.

Plasma cell dyscrasias

Multiple myeloma
- Spinal infiltration of vertebrae and extension into extradural space causing spinal cord compression. Lower thoracic cord most common.
- Peripheral neuropathy—paraneoplastic, infiltration with amyloid or myeloma cells.
- Infections due to immune incompetence—pneumococcal infection (meningitis and pneumonia), herpes zoster, cryptococcal meningitis, and toxoplasmosis.

Plasmacytomas

Sclerotic plasmacytomas (usually solitary) associated with demyelinating neuropathy with or without other features of POEMS (polyneuropathy, organomegaly, endocrinopathy, monoclonal gammopathy and skin changes). Papilloedema a feature. Measurement of VEGF (vascular endothelial growth factor) is a useful diagnostic and prognostic marker.

Waldenström's macroglobulinaemia

Production of high concentrations of IgM paraprotein results in:
- Hyperviscosity and bleeding tendency with complications of strokes and haemorrhages in the CNS.
- Sensory-motor neuropathy, some associated with the antibody to myelin associated protein (MAG).

Paraproteinaemias

- Monoclonal gammopathy of unknown significance (MGUS) characterized by low titre (< 3 g/dL) serum monoclonal protein consisting of IgM, IgG, or IgA. Important to exclude myeloma, primary systemic amyloid, or other lymphoproliferative disorder with skeletal survey and bone marrow.
- Risk of progression to myeloma or related disorder is 1% per year.

Neuropathy develops in 5%:
- Anti-MAG neuropathy in IgM cases.
- CIDP.
- Axonal neuropathy.

Neurology and connective tissue disorders and vasculitides

Please see Table 6.6 for a list of the autoantibodies causing neurology and connective tissue disorders and vasculitides.

Table 6.6 Autoantibodies

SLE	ANA + (also 10% normals, low titre 1:10); anti-dsDNA and anti-Sm (Smith not smooth muscle) specific for SLE. Anti-histones + in drug-induced SLE. Other nuclear antigens may be +: anti-Ro (SSA), anti-La (SSB), anti-ribonuclear protein (RNP). Anti-phospholipid (APL) abs—cardiolipin and lupus anticoagulant + 20–40%
Sjögren's syndrome	Anti-Ro, anti-La. ANA + 40%
Rheumatoid	RhA factor + also found in SLE, Sjögren's syndrome
Arthritis	Anti-citrullinated synthetic peptide (anti-CCP) sensitivity 80%, specificity 95%
Scleroderma	Anti-centromere, anti-opoisomerase (Scl-70), anti-polymerase III. Anti-Ro and La + 50%
Wegner's granulomatosis and microscopic polyangiitis	cANCA (myleoperoxidase antigen) and/or pANCA (proteinase 3 antigen) +. pANCA less specific.
Churg–Strauss angiitis	30–50% ANCA +

Systemic lupus erythematosus (SLE)

Central nervous system

- Aseptic meningitis.
- Cerebrovascular disease:
  - ischaemic stroke—APL; non-bacterial endocarditis; vasculitis (rare); ↑ atherosclerosis rate;
  - haemorrhage.
- MS-like syndrome. Relapsing/remitting, multifocal disorder affecting brainstem, optic nerves, spinal cord.
- Myelopathy—acute or subacute, usually thoracic cord.
- Chorea—uni- or bilateral. Sensitive to oestrogen/progesterone levels, e.g. precipitated by COC.
- Migraine in association with APL.
- Seizures due to stroke, APL syndrome. May be presenting feature in 5%:
  - encephalopathy (neuropsychiatric lupus)—memory loss, delirium, depression, anxiety, psychosis. Exclude infections, metabolic disorders, drug side effects.

Peripheral nervous system
- Guillain–Barré syndrome (↑ incidence 1%).
- Mild distal sensory motor neuropathy (epineural vasculitis).
- Vasculitic neuropathy (mononeuritis multiplex)—rare.

Sjögren's syndrome
Central nervous system
- Acute or subacute myelopathy—most common CNS complication.
- Aseptic meningitis—acute, chronic, or recurrent.
- Stroke syndromes due to inflammatory vasculopathy.
- MS-like relapsing/remitting syndrome.

Peripheral nervous system
- Trigeminal neuropathy (sensory not motor, uni- or bilateral, acute or subacute). Common.
- Chronic, sensory motor, axonal neuropathy—nerve biopsy shows vasculitis or perivascular inflammation.
- Sensory neuronopathy (dorsal root ganglionitis):
  • slowly progressive sensory neuropathy affecting small and large fibres;
  • pseudoathetosis, sensory ataxia;
  • areflexia;
  • ↓ or absent SAP on NCT;
  • MRI—T2 high signal in posterior columns;
  • treatment—corticosteroids ± cyclophosphamide; some respond to IV Ig.

Rheumatoid arthritis
Central nervous system
- Cervical myelopathy due to atlantoaxial subluxation and soft tissue pannus. Vertical subluxation → brainstem compression.
  • ↑ risk with longer disease duration.

Peripheral nervous system
- Carpal tunnel syndrome (common).
- Ulnar neuropathy at elbow.
- Common peroneal or tibial neuropathy due to Baker's cyst in popliteal region.
- Vasculitic neuropathy (length dependent or mononeuritis multiplex) rare.

Systemic necrotizing vasculitides
Central nervous system
- Clinical presentation:
  • stroke (ischaemic or haemorrhage);
  • altered mental status (encephalopathy);
  • seizures.
- Aetiology:
  • polyarteritis nodosa (PAN) affects medium-sized arteries. Associated with hepatitis B;

- Wegener's granulomatosis (may also cause a pachymeningitis). Characterized by granulomatous inflammation and vasculitis of small and medium-sized arteries of upper respiratory tract, lungs, kidneys.
- Churg–Strauss angiitis (asthma, eosinophil count > 10%, sinus and lung pathology);
- microscopic polyangiitis.

Peripheral nervous system
- Clinical presentation:
  - mononeuritis multiplex;
  - length-dependent sensory motor neuropathy;
  - Rare—GBS-like syndrome.
- Aetiology:
  - Churg–Strauss angiitis (50–75% of patients);
  - PAN (50%);
  - Wegener's granulomatosis.

Treatment
- Corticosteroids + cyclophosphamide (pulsed IV preferred to continuous oral).

Endocrine neuroanatomy

Hypothalamus

- The hypothalamus is composed of several distinctive subnuclei (see Fig. 6.3 and Table 6.7).
- It regulates and controls the endocrine system through:
  - direct release of hormones into blood stream via posterior pituitary (e.g. ADH);
  - release of hormones into local portal circulation, stimulating the anterior pituitary to secrete specific hormones into the systemic circulation;
  - indirectly through behavioural/autonomic modulation.
- Regulates a range of autonomic functions (BP, electrolyte balance, body temperature, energy metabolism, reproduction, stress response) in addition to circadian rhythms.

Table 6.7 Functions of hypothalamic sub-nuclei

Hypothalamic nucleus	Function
Supraoptic nucleus	Produces antidiuretic hormone (ADH) projecting to the posterior pituitary
Medial preoptic nucleus	Larger in males, involved in sexually motivated behaviour, sleep–wake cycle, parasympathetic functions
Lateral preoptic nucleus	Sleep regulation, thirst
Anterior hypothalamic area	Same as medial preoptic nucleus
Lateral hypothalamic area	Regulation of appetite, body weight, thirst, temperature
Dorsal hypothalamic area	Thermoregulation, cardiovascular regulation, stress response
Posterior hypothalamic area	Autonomic regulation; able to modulate macrophage function
Dorsomedial nucleus	Circadian rhythms (sleep, feeding, locomotion)
Ventromedial nucleus	Glucose sensitive; metabolic regulation
Paraventricular nucleus	Autonomic control, metabolic regulation, appetite, projects oxytocin and ADH to posterior pituitary Synthesizes hormones and projects to anterior pituitary
Periventricular nucleus	Neuroendocrine regulation

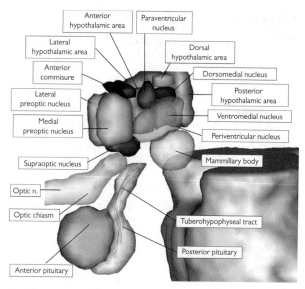

Fig. 6.3 Medial surface of hypothalamus viewed in sagittal section showing hypothalamic sub-nuclei and pituitary gland.

Pituitary

Anterior lobe

- Composed of three subdivisions.
  - Pars distalis: the majority of the anterior pituitary where the hormone secreting cells are located (see Table 6.8).
  - Pars tuberalis: forms a sheath wrapping around the pituitary stalk. High concentration of melatonin receptors, whose activation causes secretion of tuberalin which stimulates pars distalis prolactin secretion.
  - Pars intermedia: thin slice of tissue between anterior and posterior pituitary. No function in humans.

Posterior lobe

- Collection of axonal projections from the supraoptic and paraventricular nuclei, secreting ADH and oxytocin directly into the bloodstream.
- No blood–brain barrier present.

Table 6.8 Hormone-secreting cells of the pituitary

Cell type	Functional subtype	Hormones
Acidophils	Somatotroph (50%)	GH
	Lactotroph (10–25%)	Prolactin
	Mammosomatotroph (> 10%)	GH, prolactin
Basophils	Corticotroph (10–20%)	ACTH
Chromophobes	Thyrotroph (10%)	TSH
	Gonadotroph (10%)	FSH
		LH

Neurology in endocrine disorders

Diabetes mellitus (DM)

- Common; ↑ thromboembolic risk; symptoms of hyper/hypoglycaemia.

See 📖 Chapter 5, 'Diabetic neuropathies', pp. 276–7, for discussion.

Hypoglycaemia
- Produces a rapidly progressive potentially fatal encephalopathy, but easily reversible if identified early and treated promptly.
- Check for in *every* patient with ↓ GCS or encephalopathy.
- Usually due to exogenous insulin in DM. In healthy individuals with fasting hypoglycaemia, consider following causes (EXPLAIN):
  - **EX**ogenous drugs (e.g. insulin, alcohol, quinine sulfate, quinolones);
  - **P**ituitary insufficiency;
  - **L**iver failure/rare enzyme defects;
  - **A**ddison's disease;
  - **I**nsulinoma or immune-mediated (Hodgkin's disease);
  - **N**on-pancreatic neoplasm (e.g. retroperitoneal fibrosarcoma).
- Early symptoms of sympathetic activity (tachycardia, sweating, mydriasis) may be absent in beta-blockade, DM, or other autonomic neuropathy.
- Delirium followed by coma. Progressive rostral–caudal brainstem dysfunction (decorticate → decerebrate → ↓ respiration → hyporeflexia).
- Often associated with partial or generalized seizures.
- **Immediate treatment with 50 mL of 50% glucose IV.**[1]

Hyperglycaemia
- Results in an encephalopathy due to an hyperosmolar, hyperviscous, hypercoaguable state impairing normal brain metabolism.
- Both may present with confusion, ↓ GCS. Seizures or focal neurological signs more commonly associated with HONK. Two forms:
  - Diabetic ketoacidosis:
    - acidosis with ketosis; patient usually younger with type I DM;
    - aggressive fluid resuscitation, insulin sliding scale, determine precipitant, thromboembolic prophylaxis.
  - Hyperosmolar non-ketotic hyperglycaemia (HONK):
    - acidosis absent, blood sugar > 35 mmol/L, high osmolarity > 340 mOsm/kg; patient usually older with type II DM;
    - rehydrate over 48 hours; wait 1 hour before starting insulin; give full heparin anticoagulation.

Thyroid dysfunction

Commonly encountered; if suspected check serum TFTs (TSH, T_3, T_4).

Hyperthyroidism

- General: ↓ weight, diarrhoea, heat intolerance, sweating, ↑ pulse, AF.
- Neurological: tremor (fine), thyrotoxic myopathy (proximal), diplopia, depression, psychomotor agitation, psychosis.

Thyrotoxic storm

- Acute severe hypermetabolic decompensation of hyperthyroidism.
- Symptoms as per hyperthyroidism; may develop seizures and coma.
- Untreated mortality 90%.
- Emergency treatment (get expert help):
  - Hypermetabolic support:
    — fluid resuscitation;
    — active cooling (ice packs, cooling blanket), paracetamol.
  - Treatment of sympathetic decompensation:
    — propranolol—40 mg/8 h PO or 1 mg IV, repeated at 2-min intervals to a maximum of 10 mg.
  - Treatment of hyperthyroid state:
    — carbimazole 15–25 mg/6 h PO/NGT;
    — aqueous iodine oral solution (Lugol's) (to block thyroid hormones) 0.3 mL/8 h PO/NGT. Start at least 1 h *after* carbimazole; continue for 1 week.
  - Other measures:
    — AF may require IV digoxin (500 mg IV loading dose);
    — agitation may require sedation;
    — look for underlying cause (e.g. sepsis).

Hypothyroidism

- General: weight gain, lethargy, constipation, cold intolerance, ↓ pulse.
- Neurological: peripheral neuropathy, carpal tunnel syndrome, myxoedema myopathy (proximal), slow relaxing reflexes, cerebellar ataxia, depression, ↓ cognition, dementia, myxoedema coma.

Parathyroid dysfunction

- Parathyroid hormone acts to ↑ Ca^{2+}, ↓ PO_4^{3-}, ↑ vitamin D activation.
- Assess status with serum PTH, alkaline phosphatase, calcium, and phosphate.
- Neurological sequelae are consequence of calcium and vitamin D levels.

Hyperparathyroidism

- General: dehydration, polyuria, polydipsia, lethargy, abdominal pain.
- Neurological: muscle wasting, proximal myopathy (bulbar sparing), headache, confusion, rarely seizures and coma.

Hypoparathyroidism

- General: nausea, vomiting, abdominal pain.
- Neurological: irritability, delirium, psychosis with hallucinations, tetany (Chvostek's sign), carpopedal spasm, paraesthesiae (perioral, distal!).

Adrenal gland dysfunction

The adrenal cortex produces three classes of steroids in response to pituitary ACTH: glucocorticoids (cortisol), mineralocorticoids (aldosterone), and androgens.

Hypoadrenalism

- Primary adrenocortical insufficiency (Addison's disease) due to autoimmune disease, cancer, infectious destruction (e.g. TB), haemorrhage (Waterhouse–Friderichsen syndrome), or withdrawal from corticosteroids.
- Secondary—impaired ACTH secretion due to pituitary failure.
- Symptoms caused by mineralocorticoid and glucocorticoid deficiency:
  - General: fatigue, ↓ weight, myalgia, hyperpigmentation, nausea, vomiting.
  - Neurological: depression, psychosis, weakness and syncope 2° to ↓ circulatory volume, postural hypotension.
- Addison's crisis:
  - acute decompensated hypoadrenalism, often due to rapid steroid withdrawal or increased steroid demand (e.g. sepsis);
  - may present with hypovolaemic shock or hypoglycaemia;
  - treat hypovolaemia with aggressive fluid resuscitation;
  - take serum cortisol and ACTH but do not wait for result;
  - give 100 mg IV hydrocortisone 6 h and look for cause.

Hyperadrenalism

- Cushing's syndrome: glucocorticoid excess (exogenous/endogenous).
  - General: Cushingoid phenotype, weight gain, gonadal dysfunction.
  - Neurological: proximal myopathy, neuropsychiatric disturbance (depression, anxiety, euphoria, psychosis, delusions, hallucinations), memory impairment, insomnia, ± symptoms of pituitary mass.
- Conn's syndrome: aldosterone excess usually due to adrenal tumour.
  - General: usually asymptomatic; symptoms due to hypokalaemia.
  - Neurological: weakness, hypotonia, cramps, tetany, paraesthesiae.

Phaeochromocytoma

Rare catecholamine-secreting tumours from sympathetic paraganglia cells.
- General: palpitations, nausea, weight loss, abdominal pain.
- Neurological: headaches, seizures, anxiety ('impending doom'), SAH, tremor, weakness, visual disturbance, hypertensive encephalopathy.

Sex hormone dysfunction

Influences a broad spectrum of normal and abnormal neurological functions.

- Migraine: more common in women after puberty. Premenstrual exacerbation (catamenial migraine) linked to decrease in serum oestradiol. May be triggered by oral contraceptive pill.
- Porphyria: oestradiols can precipitate porphyric crisis.
- Catamenial epilepsy: seizures worsen at ovulation or premenstrually.
- Catamenial sciatica: in endometriosis, ectopic endometrium can invade lumbar plexus producing sciatic pain 2–3 days prior to menses.
- POEMS: endocrinopathy often ↑ oestrogen or ↓ testosterone. See 📖 'The neuroendocrine syndromes', p. 442.

Primary pituitary disorders

- From lesions affecting the pituitary gland, stalk, or perisellar region.
- Spectrum of symptoms arising from hormonal hyper- or hyposecretion, or from a mass impinging on local structures.
- Pituitary mass effect—visual field defects (bitemporal hemianopia), headaches, cavernous sinus involvement (palsies of CN III, IV, and VI), CSF rhinorrhoea, insomnia, temperature disturbance. DI may occur.

Hypopituitarism

- Range of presentations from asymptomatic to collapse.
- Hormonal deficiencies:
  - ACTH—hypoadrenalism (see 🕮 'Neurology in endocrine disorders', pp. 436–9);
  - TSH—hypothyroidism (see 🕮 'Neurology in endocrine disorders', pp. 436–9);
  - LH/FSH—hypogonadism;
  - ADH—diabetes insipidus (DI);
  - GH—asymptomatic/fatigue.
- Panhypopituitarism is a deficiency of all anterior hormones.
- Caused by pathology affecting hypothalamus, pituitary stalk, or gland.
- May be affected by tumour, infection (TB, meningitis), inflammation, irradiation, ischaemia or infiltration (e.g. amyloid, haemochromatosis).

Hyperpituitarism

Secretory pituitary tumour (micro- (< 1 cm) or macro-adenoma) causing the following:

Hyperprolactinaemia (PRL)

- Most common (35% of secretory tumours).
- Main features: galactorrhoea, ↑ weight, ↓ libido, amenorrhoea ♀, impotence ♂. May present with mass effect.

Acromegaly (GH)

- Excess growth hormone secretion with high levels of insulin-like growth factor.
- Increased risk of stroke due to ↑ BP and insulin resistance.
- General: acromegalic phenotype (spade-like hands, prominent supraorbital ridge, wide-space teeth, large tongue), ↑ sweating, arthralgia.
- Neurological: headache, carpal tunnel syndrome, peripheral neuropathy, patchy proximal myopathy, mass effect.

Cushing's disease (ACTH)

See 🕮 'Neurology in endocrine disorders', pp. 436–9.

Macro-orchidism (FSH)

↑ FSH. Rare.

Hyponatraemia

Frequently seen post head-injury/pituitary surgery where the distinction between DI, SIADH, or cerebral salt wasting is required. See Table 6.9.

Table 6.9 Hyponatraemia

	Serum [Na]	Serum osmo	Urinary [Na]	Urinary osmo	Urine output	Notes
DI	↑(↓*)	↑	↓	↓↓	↑↑↑	Cranial/renal
SIADH	↓	↓	↑	↑	↓/↔	Hypervolaemic
Cerebral salt wasting	↓	↓	↑	↓/↔	↑	Hypovolaemic Negative Na balance
Primary polydipsia	↓	↓	↓/↔	↓	↑	*Causes ↓ Na in DI

The neuroendocrine syndromes

POEMS syndrome

Polyneuropathy, Organomegaly, Endocrinopathy, M-band, and Skin changes. Constellation always associated with a plasma cell dyscrasia.
- Polyneuropathy: bilateral symmetric motor and sensory, starts distally.
- NCT: demyelination with axonal degeneration.
- Organomegaly: hepatomegaly, splenomegaly, lymphadenopathy.
- Endocrinopathy: most have more than one endocrine abnormality, frequently involving oestrogen/testosterone. All four axes (thyroid, gonadal, adrenal, glucose) may be affected.
- M-Band: usually IgA or IgG.
- Skin changes: hyperpigmentation, scleroderma-like changes, angiomas, nail changes, hypertrichosis.
- Elevated VEGF levels cause increased vascular permeability, detected on fundoscopy with bilateral papilloedema and haemorrhages.

von Hippel–Lindau disease

See 📖 'Inherited neurocutaneous syndromes', pp. 452–4.

Neurofibromatosis

See 📖 'Inherited neurocutaneous syndromes', pp. 452–4.

Dermatology in neurology

- The overlap between neurology and dermatology encompasses a broad and expanding group of heterogenous diseases.
- An approach to narrowing down the extensive differential diagnosis in a patient with a suspected neurocutaneous disorder is provided.
- A symptom-driven classification based on the presenting neurological problem has been used in order to reflect what is commonly encountered when reviewing a patient.
- Many of the diseases listed are covered elsewhere in this book.

For further details, readers are referred to Roach and Miller[1] and Goldsmith et al.[2]

Definitions of dermatological terms and conditions are given in Box 6.2.

Box 6.2 Definitions

- **Angiokeratoma:** Dark red-blue punctuate non-blanching macules or papules. Symmetric, starting at umbilicus and knees → buttocks and scrotum.
- **Buboes:** Swollen lymph glands (plague).
- **Bulla:** As vesicle but > 5 mm diameter.
- **Ecchymoses:** Macular haemorrhage > 2 mm diameter.
- **Erythema migrans:** Growing erythematous lesion.
- **Erythema multiforme:** Symmetric rapidly evolving 'target' lesions, ~ 2 cm diameter, affecting cutaneous and mucous membranes.
- **Erythema nodosum:** Erythematous tender nodules, often on the lower limb, caused by panniculitis.
- **Erythroderma:** Erythema + scaling of most of the cutaneous surface.
- **Ichthyosis:** Persistently dry thickened 'fish-scale' skin.
- **Induration:** Localized oedema.
- **Kaposi's sarcoma:** Reddish-purple maculopapular rash, often with AIDS.
- **Lupus vulgaris:** Cutaneous tuberculosis (apple jelly nodules).
- **Macule:** Localized change in skin colour or texture.
- **Molloscum contagiosum:** Smooth flesh-coloured umbilicated papules.
- **Necrobiosis lipoidica diabeticorum:** Shiny red-brown patches progressing to yellow atrophic plaques. Predominantly pre-tibial region.
- **Nodule:** As papule but > 5 mm diameter.
- **Papule:** Solid elevation in skin < 5 mm diameter.
- **Petechia:** Punctate haemorrhage 1–2 mm diameter.
- **Plaque:** Palpable skin plateau > 2 cm diameter, < 5 mm height.
- **Purpura:** Red discoloration of skin secondary to extravasation of blood.
- **Scale:** Accumulation of thickened keratin, readily shed.
- **Telangiectasia:** Small superficial dilated blood vessels.
- **Vesicle:** Small blister containing fluid < 5 mm diameter.

Diagnostic approach to the neurological patient with skin lesions

- Age of onset:
  - neonatal;
  - childhood;
  - adult.
- Speed of onset?
- Other systems affected? Clinical status of patient?
- Pre-existing medical problems?
- Recent travel?
- Family history?
- Distribution of skin lesions:
  - generalized;
  - dermatomal;
  - photosensitive pattern;
  - peripheral;
  - central;
  - focal;
  - buccal;
  - facial;
  - genital.
- Type(s) of skin lesion?

Associated neurological features:
- Meningitis/meningoencephalitis (see Table 6.10).
- Neuropathy (see Table 6.11).
- Stroke (see Table 6.12).
- Seizures.
- Myopathy (see 📖 Chapter 5, 'Dermatomyositis, polymyositis, . . .', pp. 298–300).
- Psychiatric symptomology.
- Pain (e.g. neuroma, HSV infection).
- Developmental delay/mental retardation (see 📖 'Inherited neurocutaneous syndromes', pp. 452–4).

Additional diagnostic features

Eye involvement
- Iris changes (Lisch nodules in neurofibromatosis type I).
- Ocular telangiectasia (e.g. hereditary haemorrhagic telangiectasia).

Abnormal fundoscopy
- Angioid streak (pseudoxanthoma elasticum).
- Haemorrhages, venous engorgement, exudates (e.g. diabetes, POEMS, vasculitis).
- Retinitis (e.g. CMV retinitis in AIDS).
- Retinitis pigmentosa (e.g. Refsum's disease).

Dental involvement
- Hypo/adontia (e.g. incontinentia pigmenti).
- Dental caries (e.g. Sjögren's syndrome, bacterial endocarditis).

Skeletal involvement
- Examples: POEMS, Refsum's disease.

Table 6.10 Meningitis/meningoencephalitis associated with cutaneous signs

	Erythema nodosum	Erythema multiforme	Hypopigmentation	Hyperpigmentation	Hypohydrosis	Induration	Macular rash	Nodules	Papular rash	Petechiae	Purpura	Ulceration	Vesicles	Notes
AIDS							x	x						Kaposi's sarcoma
Behçet's disease	x								x		x	x		Oral & genital ulcers
Chagas' disease			x											Romaña's sign
Coccidioido-mycosis	x													
H. influenzae						x								Typically single area (face, arm, chest)
Histiocytic reticulosis												x		AR inheritance Neuropathy & jaundice
Leptospirosis							x		x					Jaundice, conjunctival injection
Listeria							x	x						Infants
Lyme borreliosis									x					Erythema migrans ('bull's eye rash')
Meningo-coccaemia											x			Non-blanching
Murine typhus							x							Axillary, shoulders, chest, upper abdomen
Neurocuta-neous melanosis				x										Skin naevi > 20 cm No other melanoma other than CNS Rare
Sarcoidosis	x					x	x		x				x	Cranial neuropathy
Sjögren's syndrome											x			Xerostomia
Syphilis		x					x		x	x		x		Aseptic—2nd stage Late meningovascular syphilis
TB	x	x												Lupus vulgaris
Varicella zoster												x	x	With ataxia
Yersinia pestis		x									x			Also buboes
Leukaemia	x													Painful plaques

Adapted from Hurko O, Provost TT (1999). Neurology and the skin. *J. Neurol. Neurosurg. Psychiatry*, **66**, 417–30, with permission.

Table 6.11 Neuropathy with cutaneous signs

	Alopecia	Erythema nodosum	Hyperpigmentation	Hypohydrosis	Hypopigmentation	Maculo/Papular rash	Nail changes	Photosensitivity	Purpura	Seborrhoeic dermatitis	Telangiectasia	Ulceration	Notes
HIV/AIDS						x				x			Kaposi's sarcoma Molluscum contagiosum
Alcoholism											x		± Ataxia/malar rash
1° amyloidosis	x								x				± Bullae
Arsenic poisoning						x							Dry scaly desquamation Mee's lines
Diabetes mellitus												x	Necrobiosis lipoidica diabeticorum
Dysautonomia				x									Blotchy skin
Fabry's disease				x		x							Angiokeratoma Raynaud's disease
Haemochromatosis			x										'Bronze' pigmentation
Histiocytic reticulosis									x				Jaundice Erythroderma
Leprosy		x	x		x								Skin ulceration
Lyme disease						x							Erythema migrans ('bull's eye rash')
Pellagra	x		x					x					Desquamation, diarrhoea, dementia Glossitis (smooth)
POEMS syndrome			x										Raynaud's disease, angiomas
Refsum's disease													Ichthyosis
Sarcoidosis	x	x			x	x							Lupus pernio
SLE	x					x		x	x			x	Malar rash, discoid lupus
Vitamin B₁₂ deficiency							x					x	Black nail pigmentation Oral ulcers
Werner syndrome (pangeria)	x										x	x	Scleroderma-like skin, premature aging Rare
Xeroderma pigmentosum						x					x		Early-onset skin cancer Atrophy, angiomas

Adapted from Hurko O, Provost TT (1999). Neurology and the skin. *J. Neurol. Neurosurg. Psychiatry*, **66**, 417–30, with permission.

Table 6.12 Stroke associated with cutaneous signs

	Alopecia	Angiomas	Erythema multiforme	Erythema nodosum	Hypopigmentation	Necrotic skin lesions	Petechiae	Photosensitivity	Purpura	Nodules	Telangiectasia	Ulceration	Notes
Behçet's disease				x								x	Genital & oral ulcers
Cerebral cavernous malformation		x											
Diabetes mellitus												x	Necrobiosis lipoidica diabeticorum
Endocarditis							x						Osler nodes, splinter haemorrhages, Roth's spots
Fabry's disease									x				Angiokeratoma
Haemolytic uraemic syndrome						x							
Hereditary haemorrhagic telangiectasia												x	See 📖 'Inherited neurocutaneous syndromes', pp. 452–4
Homocystinuria					x								Malar flush, Livedo reticularis
Hyper-cholesterolaemia													Xanthomas Xanthelasma
Progeria	x												Scleroderma-like skin, premature aging Rare
Neurocutaneous angioma		x											Large irregular haemangiomas
Pseudoxanthoma elasticum										x			Pseudoxanthoma Angioid streaks
SLE	x		x					x	x	x		x	Raynaud's phenomenon
Takayasu's arteritis						x			x				Unequal radial pulses
Werner syndrome (pangeria)	x										x	x	Scleroderma-like skin, premature aging Rare

Adapted from Hurko O, Provost TT (1999). Neurology and the skin. *J. Neurol. Neurosurg. Psychiatry*, **66**, 417–30, with permission.

Seizures associated with cutaneous signs

- Tuberous sclerosis (see 📖 'Inherited neurocutaneous syndromes', pp. 452–4).
- Neurofibromatosis type I (see 📖 'Inherited neurocutaneous syndromes', pp. 452–4).
- SLE.
- Sturge–Weber syndrome (see 📖 'Inherited neurocutaneous syndromes', pp. 452–4).
- Incontinentia pigmenti (see 📖 'Inherited neurocutaneous syndromes', pp. 452–4).
- Porphyria.

Epidermal naevus syndrome
- Congenital skin lesions (raised oval/linear plaques).
- Associated with malformations of the cerebral cortex.

Neurocutaneous melanosis
- Large multiple melanocytic naevi with benign or malignant pigment cell tumors of the leptomeninges.

Hypomelanosis of Ito
- Whorls of pigmentation following Blaschko's lines.
- 40–50% have epilepsy.

Proteus syndrome
- Rare disorder of asymmetrical overgrowth of the trunk, extremities, and digits, bony exostoses, hamartomatous naevi, sole hyperplasia (gyriform).
- Often associated hemi-megalencephaly.

Neuropsychiatric–cutaneous syndromes

Porphyria
- A group of predominantly inherited disorders affecting haem synthesis.
- Those with neuropsychiatric manifestations are all AD inheritance.
- Precipitants include alcohol, physiological stress, menstruation.
- Psychiatric:
  - anxiety, aggression, depression, psychosis, hallucinations.
- Cutaneous:
  - photosensitivity, vesicular rash, bulla.
- Diagnosis:
  - initial screening with urinary PBG (keep sample in the dark);
  - Normally elevated ++ (except for ALA-dehydratase deficiency).

SLE
- Autoimmune disorder causing multisystem microvascular inflammation with immune complex deposition (see *Oxford Handbook of Clinical Medicine* for more details).[3]
- Psychiatric: psychosis (paranoia, hallucinations), delirium.
- Cutaneous: malar rash, photosensitivity, discoid lesions, alopecia, livedo reticularis.
- Diagnosis: serum ANA, anti-dsDNA, and/or anti-Sm.

Pellagra

- Niacin (vitamin B$_3$) deficiency that can lead to multi-organ failure.
- Caused by inadequate dietary intake (alcoholics/malabsorption).
- Psychiatric: aggression, confusion, dementia, insomnia, stupor.
- Cutaneous: dermatitis, fissuring, alopecia, photosensitivity, hyperpigmentation.
- Diagnosis: therapeutic response to niacin replacement. Serum niacin or urinary *N*-methylnicotinamide may be low.

Glucagonoma

- Rare glucagon-secreting tumour. Associated with MEN type I.
- Psychiatric: bipolar disorder, anxiety.
- Cutaneous: necrolytic migratory erythema, ulceration, hyperpigmentation.
- Diagnosis: serum glucagon > 1000 pg/mL.

References

1. Roach ES, Miller VS (eds) (2004). *Neurocutaneous disorders*. Cambridge: Cambridge University Press.
2. Goldsmith LA, Katz SI, Gilchrest BA, Paller A, Leffell DJ, Wolff K (2012). *Fitzpatrick's dermatology in general medicine* (8th edn). New York: McGraw-Hill.
3. Longmore M, Wilkinson I, Davidson E, Foulkes A (2010). *Oxford Handbook of Clinical Medicine* (8th edn). Oxford: Oxford University Press.

Inherited neurocutaneous syndromes

Tuberous sclerosis
- AD.
- Mutation on tumour suppression genes 1 on chr 9q34 or 2 on chr 16p13.3.

Clinical features
- Childhood epilepsy.
- Cognitive impairment.
- Adenoma sebaceum.
- Subungual fibromas.
- Shagreen patches.
- Ashleaf patches (under UV light).
- Risk of malignancy—astrocytomas, cardiac rhabdomyomas, renal angiolipomas.

CT

Shows periventricular calcification, hamartomas.

Neurofibromatosis 1 (NF1)
- AD.
- Mutation of NF1 gene, chr 17q 11.2 (neurofibromin).
- Clinical phenotype:
    - *café au lait* patches, axillary freckling;
    - plexiform neuromas (risk of sarcomatous change);
    - optic nerve and brain gliomas;
    - phaeochromocytoma.
- Diagnostic criteria—two or more of :
    - $\geq$ 6 *café au lait* patches;
    - $\geq$ 2 neurofibromas or one or more plexiform neurofibromas (risk of malignant change);
    - axillary or groin freckling;
    - optic nerve glioma;
    - $\geq$ 2 Lisch nodules (iris hamartomas);
    - dysplasia/absence of sphenoid bone or dysplasia/thinning of long cortex bone;
    - 1° relative with NF1.

Neurofibromatosis 2 (NF2)
- AD.
- Mutation in NF2 gene, chr22 (Schwannomin).
- Clinical features:
    - bilateral acoustic neuromas;
    - meningiomas.
- Diagnostic criteria—bilateral acoustic neuromas or 1° relative with NF2 and:
    - either unilateral vestibular Schwannoma at age ? 30 years;
    - or any two of meningioma, Schwannoma, glioma, posterior subcapsular lens opacity.

von Hippel–Lindau disease
- AD.
- Mutation in VHL tumour suppressor gene.

Clinical features
- Cerebellar haemangioblastomas.
- Retinal angiomas.
- Renal tumours.
- Polycythaemia.
- Phaeochromocytoma.

Screening programme for VHL patient (annual)
- Physical examination.
- Urine testing + 24 hour VMA collection.
- Renal USS.
- Direct and indirect ophthalmoscopy with fluorescein angiography.
- Brain MRI every 3 years.

Sturge–Weber syndrome
- Sporadic occurrence in 1/50 000.

Clinical features
- Port wine stain (V1).
- Buphthalmos.
- Epilepsy developing in first year of life.
- Cognitive impairment in 50%.
- Intracranial calcification.

Ataxic telangiectasia
- AR.
- Mutation 11q22-23.
- Incidence 1/40 000; M = F.

Clinical features
- Often detected between 12 and 36 months when they start walking.
- Gait and truncal ataxia.
- Choreoathetosis.
- Oculomotor apraxia.
- Intellectual lag often develops with time.
- Progressive telangiectasia after the age of 2 years (conjunctiva, face, upper aspect of ears, flexor surfaces).
- Complete or near-complete absence of IgA or IgE combined with impairment of cellular immunity resulting in recurrent sinopulmonary infections and increased risk of cancers (lymphoma, leukaemia).

Incontinentia pigmenti
- X-linked dominant condition.
- Mapped to Xq28 (NEMO gene: NF-kappa beta modulator).

Clinical features

Skin
- Stage I (birth): linear vesicles, pustules and bullae with erythema along lines of Blaschko.
- Stage II (2–8 weeks): formation of warty keratotic plaques.
- Stage III (12–40 weeks): swirled macular hyperpigmentation along lines of Blaschko.
- Stage IV (40 weeks–adult): hypopigmented streaks and/or patches. Cutaneous atrophy.

Ocular features
- Mottled diffuse retinal hypopigmentation pathognomic.
- Abnormal peripheral retinal vessels with hypoperfusion.
- Cataracts.

Dental features
- Hypodontia/adontia with jaw abnormalities.
- May have associated skeletal abnormalities.

CNS features 10–30%
- Developmental delay.
- Microcephaly.
- Ataxia.
- Focal atrophy.
- Seizures.
- Stroke.

Further reading

Ferner RE (2010). The neurofibromatoses. *Pract. Neurol.*, **10**, 82–93.

Ferner RE, Huson SM, Thomas N, et al. (2007). Guidelines for the diagnosis and management of individuals with neurofibromatosis 1. *J. Med. Genet.*, **44**, 81–8.

Ruggiero M, Pascual Castroviejo I, Di Rocco C (2008). Neurocutaneous disorders: phakomatoses and harmatoneoplastic syndromes. New York: Springer.

Neurological and neurosurgical issues in pregnancy

Subarachnoid haemorrhage

- Occurs in 10–20 women/100 000 pregnancies. 5% maternal deaths. Occur in 2nd or 3rd trimester.
- ↑ maternal age and parity ↑ risk. Related to ↑ plasma volume and pregnancy-induced hypertension.
- Presentation and investigations as in non-pregnant patients:
  - urgent CT (with uterine shielding)—radiation dose < 50 mGy no ↑ risk to fetus. MRI an alternative. If CT negative (read by experienced radiologist or neurosurgeon) → LP. If CT or LP positive proceed to 4-vessel angiogram.
- 75% SAH due to ruptured cerebral aneurysm. 6% risk of rupture in 1st trimester, 55% 3rd trimester. 90% of ruptures occur during pregnancy, 8% puerperium, 2% during labour.
- Definitive management for aneurysms—endovascular coiling or surgical clipping depending on expertise available.

Management

- < 26 weeks of gestation → proceed as best for mother.
- 26–34 weeks of gestation—if stable → as best for mother; if unstable → caesarean section followed by aneurysm coiling or surgery.
- > 34 weeks of gestation → caesarean section followed by aneurysm coiling or surgery.

Unruptured aneurysms

International Study on Unruptured Intracranial Aneurysms (ISUIA):

- Asymptomatic, small (< 10 mm), anterior circulation aneurysms risk of treatment greater than non-treatment.
- Annual risk of rupture 0.05%. However, pregnant patients not included therefore extrapolation may not apply.
- Multidisciplinary approach with patient, obstetrician, neuroradiologist, and neurosurgeon necessary to make rational decision.

Arteriovenous malformations (AVMs)

- Overall risk of primary and second haemorrhage in pregnancy 3.5% and 5.8% same as for general population. Greatest risk in 2nd trimester when cardiac output highest.
- Management is as for non-pregnant patients. If AVM bleeds during pregnancy, unlike aneurysms, treatment can be delayed till after delivery unless neurosurgical complications suggest otherwise.
- Treatment options: surgery, endovascular embolization and stereotactic radiosurgery. Endovascular techniques may not completely obliterate AVM and additional radiosurgery may be necessary; may take 1–3 years to work with a small risk of rebleeding during this period.

- Risk of haemorrhage from AVM low with epidural analgesia and assisted 2nd stage. Elective caesarean section advocated for untreated or partially treated AVM especially if it has bled during pregnancy.
- Multidisciplinary approach with obstetrician, neurosurgeon, and neuroradiologist always essential.

Multiple sclerosis

Pregnancy is a relative state of immunosuppression:
- MS and conception: no evidence of physiological effect on fertility although sexual dysfunction may affect conception.
- Pregnancy and relapses—exacerbation rate ↓ 2nd and 3rd trimester. ↑ during the first 3 months following delivery. Therefore no net change in relapses.
- Breastfeeding may reduce postpartum relapse risk.
- Current practice is to treat relapses with IV methylprednisolone (IVMP). Considered safe in terms of fetal risks as largely metabolized by placenta. Postpartum IVMP—only small concentrations excreted in breast milk and has a short half-life.
- Pregnancy and disease progression: few data available but seems that pregnancy has no adverse effect on subsequent disease course.
- Pregnancy outcome: higher risk of caesarean section and slightly smaller babies.
- DMT therapies and pregnancy: current recommendation is to stop DMTs 3 months prior to conception. If conception occurs on DMT recommend stopping as lack of evidence of safety.
- Other issues:
  - UTIs more common during pregnancy and those with neurogenic bladder may require more frequent ISC;
  - immobile patients at greater risk of thromboembolism;
  - no evidence epidural anaesthesia is contraindicated in pregnant MS patients.

Epilepsy

Effects of epilepsy on pregnancy
- ↑ ×3 complications (bleeding, pre-eclampsia, miscarriage and still birth, IUGR, low birth weight, premature labour).

Seizure frequency
- No effect in most patients. ↑ seizures usually in those with severe epilepsy. Causes:
  - hormonal effects (oestrogen may be epileptogenic, progesterone convulsant and anticonvulsant properties);
  - dilutional effect of ↑ plasma volume;
  - ↑ metabolism by liver, fetus, placenta;
  - ↓ drug absorption due to, e.g. antacids, nausea/vomiting;
  - fatigue, sleep deprivation, anxiety.

New-onset seizures in pregnancy

• Incidence of epilepsy at child bearing age 20–30/100 000. Chance development occurs due to factors listed earlier.
• ↑ size of meningiomas, AVM, stroke, SAH, cerebral venous thrombosis.
• CT contraindicated. MRI safe.
• Pre-eclampsia and eclampsia:
  • most common cause of new onset seizures;
  • pre-eclampsia (hypertension, proteinuria, oedema, liver dysfunction, impaired clotting); eclampsia (confusion, focal signs, seizures, coma). May progress to status epilepticus;
  • treatment: magnesium sulfate IV 4g, followed by 10g IM. Then 5g IM every 4 hours as required.

Management during pregnancy

• Measurement of drug levels and dose ↑ as necessary.
• Folic acid 5 mg.

Management during labour

• Continue AED (IV if required).
• If high risk of seizures—clobazam 10–20 mg.
• If seizures occur during labour → caesarean section.

Post partum

• Enzyme inducing AEDs ↓ vitamin K-dependent clotting factors with risk of ICH in neonate.
• Give neonate 1 mg vitamin K at birth and at 28 days.
• Gradually reduce AED levels to prenatal doses.

Migraine

See 📖 Chapter 5, 'Migraine and women', pp. 236–8.

References

1. Ng J, Kitchen N (2008). Neurosurgery and pregnancy. *J Neurol Neurosurg Psychiatry*, **79**, 745–52.
2. Lee M, O'Brian P (2008). Pregnancy and multiple sclerosis. *J Neurol Neurosurg Psychiatry*, **79**, 1308–11.

Chapter 7

Neurosurgery

Cerebral aneurysms 460
Cerebral arteriovenous malformations (AVM) 464
Cavernous haemangioma (cavernoma) and developmental
    venous anomaly (DVA) 466
Dural arteriovenous fistula (dAVF) 468
Hydrocephalus 470
Complications of shunts 473
Intracranial tumours 474
Intracranial tumours: management of specific tumours 478
Imaging of intracranial tumours: examples 484
Imaging of spinal tumours: examples 496
Degenerative spinal conditions: cervical spine 500
Degenerative spinal conditions: thoracic and lumbar spine 504
Imaging of degenerative spinal conditions: examples 508
Developmental abnormalities 512
Imaging of developmental abnormalities: examples 516
Syringomyelia 520

Cerebral aneurysms

Berry aneurysms

Cerebral (berry) aneurysms are highly prevalent 'blow-outs' that occur commonly on the branching points of the cerebral arteries around the circle of Willis in the subarachnoid space.

Incidence and epidemiology

- Prevalence at least 1% in adults in the UK/USA. Increasingly common with age and in females (2:1).
- Aneurysms rarely but classically occur in inherited disorders such as polycystic kidney disease, Marfan's syndrome, pseudoxanthoma elasticum. In countries of high prevalence, e.g. Japan and especially Finland, familial aneurysms are much more common.

Neuroanatomy

Typical aneurysm sites are:
- posterior communicating artery;
- anterior communicating artery;
- middle cerebral branch points, which account for 80% of all aneurysms.
- Cerebral aneurysms are sized as small (< 1 cm maximum diameter), large (1–2.5 cm), and giant (> 2.5 cm). 70% of cerebral aneurysms are small. 20% of cases are multiple.

Natural history

Incidental aneurysms have a haemorrhage rate of < 1% per annum if < 1 cm in diameter. Larger aneurysms and those associated with multiple aneurysms have a higher bleed rate. Risk of bleeding is higher in cigarette-smokers and hypertensives.

Presentation

Cerebral aneurysms present in a variety of ways.
- SAH.
- Incidentally on screening or for unrelated symptoms (e.g. headache).
- Third nerve palsy (usually painful, following rapid expansion of a posterior communicating artery aneurysm).
- Visual failure (with large ophthalmic segment aneurysms).

Treatment

Neurosurgical clipping and neuroradiological coiling are current treatment modalities.
- *Surgical clipping* involves a craniotomy, the microdissection of the blood vessels of the brain, and the passing of a titanium clip across the aneurysm neck. If successful this is a permanent cure with no need for subsequent follow-up.
- *Coiling* has the advantage of obviating the need for a craniotomy. A radiologist passes a catheter endovascularly, similarly to an angiogram, and then delivers a number of platinum coils into the aneurysm itself. In experienced hands this technique probably has less morbidity than neurosurgical clipping. However, there is a slightly higher incidence of long term regrowth of the aneurysm and late re-SAH. Therefore long-term clinical radiological follow-up is advised.

Note: Both techniques need to avoid occluding a cerebral artery or bursting the aneurysm itself. Thus procedural risk is higher in the early period following SAH. Late treatment reduces this risk but increases the risk of re-haemorrhage before treatment, which is highest in the first few days following the initial SAH.

Infectious cerebral aneurysms

Unusual lesions occur most often in the setting of infective endocarditis with septic embolism. Generally occur in the anterior cerebral circulation and are often multiple.

- Pathology: due to acute pyogenic necrosis of arterial wall secondary to vasculitis. Clinically recognized ipsilateral septic thromboembolism precedes haemorrhage in 40% of cases.
- Bacteriology: most frequent causative organisms found in blood culture are Staphylococcus and Streptococcus species.
- Predisposing medical conditions: congenital or acquired cardiac valvular disease, IV drug users, and immunocompromised patients.

Investigations

- High degree of suspicion is required in those high-risk patients who develop neurological symptoms—CT or MR imaging.
- Definitive investigation is four-vessel angiography, where these lesions will be found most commonly in peripheral branches of the middle cerebral artery. Angiography must cover this vascular territory.
- Not uncommon for sequential angiograms to be required to follow the response to antimicrobial treatment if a non-surgical treatment regimen is instituted.

Management

- Some recommend antimicrobial therapy alone to treat infectious aneurysms as in up to 50% of cases such lesions resolve or decrease in size following such treatment.
- Timing of any cardiac surgery is crucial to eliminate the infective focus as a further cause for bacteraemia and emboli.
- Surgery of infectious intracranial aneurysms is technically difficult, but is necessary in selective cases if ↑ size or frank abscess. Excision of the lesion with the involved vessel is required. Neurological deficits may result.

Fungal aneurysms

- Tend to occur more proximally on the intracranial vessels and more frequently involve the large arteries at the base of the brain.
- Occur almost exclusively in immunocompromised patients.
- *Candida albicans* and *aspergillus fumigatus* most common.
- Tend to be more indolent in nature but their management strategies tend to be similar, i.e. persist with antifungal chemotherapy rather than high-risk surgical/radiological interventions unless absolutely necessary.

Traumatic intracranial aneurysms

Unusual condition accounting for < 1% of all intracranial aneurysms. Also known as false or pseudo-aneurysms, which define a tear in the arterial wall, associated with extra-vessel thrombus which constitutes the aneurysm wall.

Aetiologies

- Penetrating injuries such as stab wounds, gunshot wounds.
- Following closed head injury: typically and classically at the distal anterior cerebral artery territory, where an artery is torn against the under edge of the falx cerebri. It may also occur at the skull base where it can cause caroticocavernous fistulae or occlusion.

Clinical presentation

Usually as a delayed cerebral haemorrhage following an otherwise unremarkable recovery from brain injury. A high index of suspicion is required.

Treatment

Neurosurgical excision. Vessel reconstruction is almost never possible and vessel sacrifice or bypass is necessary.

Cerebral arteriovenous malformations (AVM)

Incidence
- 10x less common than cerebral aneurysms.
- Rarely multiple except in hereditary haemorrhagic telangiectasia.
- Congenital in origin.

Pathology
Consist of tangles of pial blood vessels with characteristic early shunting of blood from arteries to veins.

Clinical presentation
- Frequently asymptomatic through life.
- May present with ICH, seizures.
- Unusual manifestations due to development of a vascular steal or venous hypertension phenomenon.

Natural history studies
Inadequate but risk of haemorrhage is 2–4% per annum. Features associated with ↑ risk are:
- intranidal aneurysms;
- venous stenosis;
- ectasia;
- old age.

AVM size is not related to haemorrhagic risk.

Diagnosis

CT
Non-enhanced scan may be normal or show an area of hyperdensity with no mass effect. 25% show calcification. With contrast, avid enhancement and a large draining vein may be visualized.

MRI
Mesh of flow voids, large draining veins. Slow-flow lesions may enhance.

DSA
Defines nidus size and architecture accurately. Identifies feeding arteries, the presence of deep or superficial cortical draining veins, flow rate (important for endovascular planning), intranidal aneurysms (in > 50%), venous stenosis.

Management

- Decisions critically dependent on angiographic findings of size, shape, position, presence of intra- or extranidal aneurysms, patient age, symptoms.
- AVMs are relatively benign in the medium term and bleeding risk is probably not altered by partial treatment.
- Symptomatic treatment (e.g. anticonvulsants) and regular follow-up is an initial option.
- Aim of intervention is complete obliteration. Three treatment options may be used alone or in combination.

Neurosurgery

- Offers the chance of a cure at one operation, but is difficult and has significant morbidity.
- Larger lesions cause normal pressure perfusion breakthrough.
- Surgical risk can be graded between 1 and 5 with the Spetzler–Martin grading system:
  - 1, 2, or 3 points depending on size (< 3 cm, 3–6 cm, > 6 cm);
  - 1 point if deep venous drainage;
  - 1 point if eloquent cortex.
- Preoperative embolization reduces vascularity.
- Significant incidence of residual AVM following surgery.
- Small peripheral AVMs with recent haemorrhage are ideal surgical targets.

Neuroradiological embolization

- Aim is to occlude nidal vessels with glue/onyx.
- Only 10–25% can be obliterated completely.
- Useful adjunct to surgery or radiosurgery.
- Complications due to catheter sticking to fragile vessels, extravasation of glue, infarction, or haemorrhage.

Radiosurgery

- High-dose radiotherapy focused on the lesion using a stereotactic frame and delivered in one treatment session.
- Gamma-knife or Linac-based systems are used to deliver the radiation.
- Advantages: low morbidity, day-case procedure.
- However, obliteration occurs gradually over 2–4 years by progressive endarteritis obliterans. During this period the risk of haemorrhage is not reduced.
- Most suited for lesions < 3 cm.

Cavernous haemangioma (cavernoma) and developmental venous anomaly (DVA)

Cavernomas

- Prevalence: 0.5% (on MRI scans).
- Vascular lesions consisting of large vascular channels with slow blood flow within them.
- Capillary lesions macroscopically resemble blackberries.
- May be located within the brain or spinal cord or cauda equina.
- Familial cases reported (KRIT1 gene).
- May result from trauma or radiation.
- 75% solitary; 25% multiple.
- May enlarge.

Clinical presentation

- Haemorrhage < 1% per annum.
- Epilepsy due to leaching of epileptogenic haemosiderin.
- Progressive neurological deficit especially in the posterior fossa and the spinal cord.

Imaging features (Fig. 7.1)

- CT: normal in 50%. Well defined hyperdense lesion with no oedema ± enhancement unless acute haemorrhage. Occasional calcification.
- MRI: rounded or oval lesion with rim of hypointensity (T_1W and T_2W) results from haemosiderin due to chronic bleeding. Internal heterogeneous signal on T_1W and T_2W represents blood products of various ages. T_2* hypointense (black) lesion.
- DSA usually negative.

Management

- Accessible lesions can be excised.
- Radiosurgery as a treatment option is still controversial.

Developmental venous anomaly (DVA)

- Represent anomalous venous drainage pathways.
- Enlarged white matter, often periventricular; veins radiate around a central vein.
- May be associated with cavernomas and cortical dysplasia.
- Usually asymptomatic lesions found incidentally on CT/MRI.

Clinical presentation

- Rarely haemorrhage except when associated with other vascular lesions.
- Seizures.

Imaging features

- CT and MRI: small linear or stellate enhancing lesions with no mass effect.
- DSA venous phase reveals a 'Medusa head'.

Management

- Now considered benign and left alone.

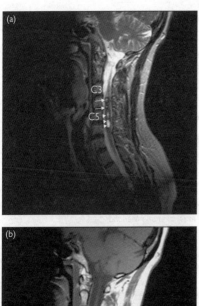

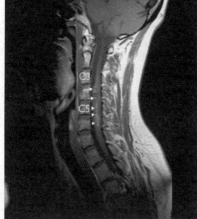

Fig. 7.1 Intramedullary cavernoma. (a) Sagittal T₂W and (b) sagittal T₁W MRI.

Figure 7.1 shows two small focal intramedullary lesions at the level of C4 comprising peripheral haemosiderin rings with haemorrhagic cores (*white arrows*). The spinal cord is mildly expanded and a loculated cavity lies caudally containing haemorrhagic degradation products in keeping with haematomyelia (*white arrowheads*).

Dural arteriovenous fistula (dAVF)

Cranial dAVFs

These occur throughout the neuroaxis. Common sites include anterior fossa floor, adjacent to the major venous sinuses, and the tentorial hiatus.

Clinical features
Presentation is with:
- haemorrhagic stroke;
- progressive neurological deficit due to venous congestion;
- headaches;
- pulsatile tinnitus especially if a bruit is audible;
- seizures.

Imaging
- CT/MRI is usually normal unless there is venous occlusion.
- DSA after haematoma resolution, if acute presentation, defines the location, feeding arteries, and venous drainage.

Grading system according to Djinjian and Merland
- Group 1: blood drains directly into meningeal vein or sinus. Normal direction of flow.
- Group 2: venous reflux into cortical veins.
- Groups 3 and 4: venous reflux is associated with retrograde flow along the venous sinuses.

Group 1 lesions are benign and rarely require treatment to prevent haemorrhage. Other groups are at risk of haemorrhage and warrant intervention.

Treatment
- Require multidisciplinary assessment with neurosurgeon and neuroradiologist.
- Options include occlusion of abnormal fistulous communication between artery and vein by surgery or endovascular techniques using glue occlusion.

Carotid cavernous fistula (CCF)

Subtype of dAVF. Defined as low flow or high flow, traumatic or spontaneous, direct or indirect, aneurysmal or non-aneurysmal.

Clinical features
- Sudden-onset painful pulsatile exophthalmos and ophthalmoplegia.
- Cavernous sinus acts as a barrier and intracranial haemorrhage does not occur.
- High-flow fistulae occur in young males following trauma or a ruptured aneurysm. Result in direct communication between internal carotid artery and the cavernous sinus.
- Low-flow or indirect fistulae occur in older patients with vascular risk factors. Result from dural fistulae within the walls of the cavernous sinus from branches of the internal or external carotid arteries.

Management
- High-flow fistulae rarely close spontaneously. Closure is with endovascularly released detachable balloons or coils.
- Low-flow fistulae tend to obliterate spontaneously. Conservative management by intermittent massage to occlude the internal carotid artery in the neck. Occasionally, partial embolization of external carotid branches, but not internal carotid because of risk of stroke.

Spinal dAVF
- Most common spinal vascular malformation (80%).
- May be acquired secondary to thrombosis of the extradural venous plexus.
- Venous hypertension and engorgement result in a subacute necrotizing myelopathy.

Clinical features
- Presents in middle to older age group with a progressive myelopathy (Foix–Alajouanine syndrome).
- Commonly between T5 and L3.
- Spinal bruit may be heard.
- Diagnosis should be considered in any patient with a cauda equina lesion with a mixture of upper and lower neuron signs + sphincter involvement.

Imaging features
- MRI may be normal or show non-specific abnormalities with intramedullary hyperintensity on T_2W and hypointensity on T_1W.
- Typically involves the conus and lumbar enlargement.
- Specific features are the dilated pial veins along the dorsal surface of the cord best seen on T_2W images as serpiginous foci of flow void against hyperintense CSF. However, may be difficult to differentiate from CSF pulsatile flow.
- Gadolinium may reveal serpiginous areas of enhancement.
- MRA with contrast may demonstrate enlarged intradural veins.
- Spinal angiography is the gold standard for diagnosis, localization, and treatment.

Management
- Endovascular obliteration using liquid embolic agents such as N-butylcyanoacrylate (NBCA) in > 80% of cases.
- Can be performed at the time of spinal angiography.
- Open surgical intervention to divide the fistulous point under a surgical microscope.

Hydrocephalus

- Defined as an excessive accumulation of CSF caused by a disturbance of formation, flow, or absorption.
- Normal CSF production is 500 mL/24 hours.
- Total CSF volume in an adult is 120–150 mL.
- CSF is recycled three times daily.

Types of hydrocephalus

- Communicating hydrocephalus. Enlarged ventricles with preserved CSF flow between ventricles and the subarachnoid space. Impaired CSF reabsorption results in increased CSF pressure and ventricular enlargement.
- Non-communicating hydrocephalus or obstructive hydrocephalus occurs when CSF outflow tracts are obstructed, e.g. exit foraminae of the 4th ventricle (Magendie and Luschka).
- Hydrocephalus *ex vacuo* refers to compensatory ventricular enlargement secondary to brain atrophy.
- Arrested hydrocephalus usually occurs in communicating hydrocephalus due to incomplete obstruction when CSF production is balanced by absorption. The CSF pressure may be normal. However, patients may undergo decompensation spontaneously or after a minor head injury.
- Normal pressure hydrocephalus is a condition with low-grade hydrocephalus with intermittently raised ICP.

Acute hydrocephalus

Aetiology

- Posterior fossa tumours.
- Cerebellar haemorrhage or infarction.
- Colloid cyst of the 3rd ventricle.
- Ependymoma of the 4th ventricle.
- SAH.
- Trauma.
- Acute meningitis.

Clinical features

- Signs and symptoms of ↑ ICP.
- Headache.
- Vomiting.
- Diplopia due to 6th nerve palsies.
- Reduced upgaze.
- Impaired conscious level.
- Occasionally, especially with colloid cyst of the 3rd ventricle, LOC and sudden death.

Chronic hydrocephalus

Aetiology
- SAH.
- Chronic meningitis.
- Slow-growing posterior fossa tumours.
- A third of cases no obvious cause.

Clinical features
- Gait disturbance (apraxia).
- Memory disturbance or dementia.
- Urinary incontinence.
- Symptoms and signs of ↑ ICP.

Imaging features in hydrocephalus
CT/MRI features include:
- ventricular enlargement with ballooning of frontal horns;
- enlargement of temporal horns;
- ballooning of the 3rd ventricle;
- disproportionate enlargement of ventricles compared with sulci (neuroradiological expertise necessary);
- periventricular interstitial oedema;
- thinned or upward bowing of corpus callosum on sagittal MRI;
- a large 4th ventricle implies communicating hydrocephalus or obstruction at the level of the 4th ventricular outflow; a small 4th ventricle suggests aqueduct stenosis.

Congenital causes
May present with acute or chronic hydrocephalus.
- Aqueduct obstruction.
- Arnold–Chiari malformation.
- Dandy–Walker syndrome.
- Benign intracranial cysts.

Management
- Insertion of ventricular peritoneal (VP) shunt via frontal or parietal burr hole. Attached to a combined valve and reservoir connecting to a distal catheter tunnelled under the skin and implanted into the peritoneum.
- Alternative sites: ventriculopleural shunt; (right) ventriculo-atrial (VA) shunt. Both have a higher complication rate than the VP shunt (e.g. pulmonary emboli in VA shunts).
- Programmable shunt valve with variable pressure/flow settings that may be changed by application of magnetic device to skin. Expensive.
- Endoscopic 3rd ventriculostomy: creation of a hole in the floor of the 3rd ventricle allowing CSF to escape from the ventricular system to the basal cisterns. Endoscope introduced into the anterior horn of the lateral ventricle via a frontal burr hole and passed through the foramen of Monro into the 3rd ventricle and a hole punched anterior to the tuber cinereum.

- In communicating hydrocephalus, e.g. due to acute meningitis, serial LP or an external lumbar drain may suffice in the acute period. A CSF protein level > 4 g/L will clog most shunts.

Normal pressure hydrocephalus (NPH)

- NPH is a syndrome of chronic communicating hydrocephalus with normal CSF pressure at lumbar puncture.
- Long-term pressure monitoring reveals intermittently elevated pressures, often at night.
- NPH may follow trauma, infection, or SAH.
- Majority are idiopathic.

Clinical features

Presentation with some or all features of the classical Hakim-Adams triad.

- Gait disturbance: typically the gait is an apraxia, i.e. normal power and sensation, but an inability to lift the legs to walk. However, performance of the bicycling manoeuvre on the bed is remarkably intact.
- Cognitive impairment: gradual slowing of verbal and motor responses, and patients may seem apathetic or depressed.
- Urinary incontinence.

Additional symptoms may include drop attacks and brief episodes of LOC.

Imaging features

- CT. Enlarged ventricles including temporal horns but with normal sulci.
- MRI:
  - no hippocampal volume loss to account for large temporal horns;
  - corpus callosum bowing and accentuation of aqueduct flow void are predictors of a good response to shunting in some studies;
  - presence of periventricular deep white matter lesions indicative of small vessel disease associated with a poor response.
- Isotope cisternography. A tracer injected into the CSF normally fails to enter the ventricles. In patients with NPH, reflux of tracer into the ventricles within 24 hours with retention for 24–48 hours. Usefulness of this technique is controversial.

Management

- There is no gold standard for diagnosis.
- Decision for shunting is based on clinical impression with supportive evidence from radiology and some of the following:
  - timed walking test before and after removing 30 mL of CSF at LP;
  - cranial bolt monitoring over 24–48 hours;
  - measuring the rate of absorption of CSF by infusion of saline into the thecal sac which represents compliance of the CSF compartments. Normal value 5–10 mmHg/mL/min. >18 mmHg/mL/min implies active hydrocephalus.

Complications of shunts

Shunt infection

Usually caused by coagulase-negative *Staphylococcus aureus*. 90% present within 3 months of insertion.

Clinical features
- General malaise.
- Pyrexia.
- Headache, vomiting, meningism.
- Abdominal tenderness or distension.
- Pain and erythema around the shunt.

Laboratory features
- CRP ↑.
- WCC ↑.

Management
- Shunt removal.
- Placement of an external ventricular drain.
- Intrathecal vancomycin for 5–7 days via external ventricular drain (EVD): 5 mg if slit ventricles, 10 mg for normal ventricles, and 15 mg if dilated ventricles daily when CSF draining freely or every 3 days when drain clamped.

Other complications
- Misplacement.
- Haemorrhage.
- Subdural haematomas can occur in the first 6 months especially in the elderly. 10–15% may require surgery.
- Epilepsy. See DVLA regulations. May not drive for 6 months.
- Shunt malfunction:
  - Blockage at ventricular, distal, or valve level. Palpation of the shunt reservoir is unreliable.
  - Underdrainage: symptoms of hydrocephalus persist. Requires placement of a valve with lower-pressure variety.
  - Overdrainage: symptoms of low pressure, i.e. postural headache, dizziness, tinnitus. Imaging reveals slit-like ventricles, subdural fluid collections, dural thickening, and enhancement. Replace with a higher-pressure valve.

Follow-up of patients with shunts
- Baseline CT 6 months after insertion.
- Patient and carers given instructions about symptoms of infection and blockage.
- Documentation about type of valve should be given to the patient.
- Programmable valves may need to be checked for settings after MRI.

Intracranial tumours

Epidemiology
Intracranial tumours are sixth most common neoplasm in adults and the most common solid tumour in children. Incidence of all primary brain tumours is 14–21/100 000/year.

Classification
Tumours of neuroepithelial origin (gliomas)
- Astrocytic tumours:
  - pilocytic astrocytoma, grade I;
  - diffuse astrocytoma, grade II;
  - anaplastic astrocytoma, grade III;
  - glioblastoma, grade IV.
- Oligodendroglioma.
- Ependymoma.
- Choroid plexus papilloma or carcinoma.
- Neuronal and mixed neuronal–glial tumours.
- Pineal parenchymal tumours.
- Embryonal tumours.

Other intracranial tumours
- Tumours of meninges (meningioma).
- Vascular tumours (haemangioblastoma).
- Primary CNS lymphoma (PCNSL).
- Germ cell tumours (germinoma, teratoma).
- Tumours of sellar region (pituitary).
- Tumours of peripheral nerves (neurilemmoma, Schwannoma, neurofibroma).
- Developmental tumours (DNET, craniopharyngioma, colloid cyst, epidermoid and dermoid cysts).
- Metastatic tumours (breast and bronchus most common).

Aetiology
- Majority sporadic.
- Cranial irradiation ↑ risk of meningioma and astrocytoma.
- Immunosuppression (e.g. AIDS) ↑ risk of PCNSL.
- Neurofibromatosis 1 ↑ risk of optic nerve glioma and meningioma. von Hippel–Lindau syndrome associated with haemangioblastomas.
- Tuberous sclerosis associated with giant cell astrocytomas.

Clinical features
- No pathognomonic features of presentation.
- Low-grade lesions present with seizures; high-grade lesions present with raised ICP and a progressive neurological deficit.
- Headache most common presentation but < 1% of patients with headache only have a brain tumour.
  - Frontal headache (supratentorial) or occipital (posterior fossa).
  - Waking in the night or early morning headache.
  - Associated with vomiting.
  - Visual obscurations and papilloedema (late).

- Progressive neurological deficit:
  - hemispheric tumours present with progressive weakness, dysphasia, dyspraxia, visual field deficits;
  - posterior fossa lesions present with ataxia, cranial nerve palsies, and ↑ ICP due to obstructive hydrocephalus;
  - cerebellopontine angle (CPA) lesions (e.g. vestibular Schwannomas) cause progressive deafness, facial weakness and numbness, and ataxia.
- Cognitive and behavioural changes. Usually frontal or subfrontal lesions.
- Seizures are the presenting symptom in 25% of tumours. Usually temporal or frontal lesions. Focal seizures that generalize to tonic/clonic seizures.

Imaging features

- CT ± contrast will identify most gliomas, metastases, meningiomas, and haemangioblastomas. Useful for showing calcification found in oligodendrogliomas.
- MRI ± Gd is more sensitive.
- Contrast enhancement implies BBB breakdown, e.g. in high-grade gliomas, meningiomas, and pituitary adenomas.
- Cerebral angiography can differentiate between giant aneurysm and mimicking lesions and also shows tumours with increased vascularity.

Other investigations

If metastases in differential diagnosis:
- full history and examination including PR;
- CXR;
- mammogram;
- CT chest, abdomen, and pelvis, PET CT scan;
- bone scan;
- germinomas may secrete β-HCG, alpha-fetoprotein;
- CSF cytology (if no ↑ ICP) for lymphoma, meningeal metastases, and ependymoma.

Differential diagnosis

- Infection (pyogenic abscess, tuberculoma, parasitic cysts (e.g. cysticercosis)).
- Vascular lesion (haematoma, infarct with oedema and peripheral luxury perfusion, AVM, giant aneurysm).
- Traumatic haematoma.
- Inflammatory lesions (e.g. tumefactive lesion of MS).

Management

Depends upon:
- patient factors: age, functional status, individual wishes;
- tumour: location, histology, grade.

Biopsy is recommended in almost all cases.

Pre-operative management
- Corticosteroids reduce vasogenic oedema and improve neurological status temporarily.
  - Complications: GI haemorrhage, perforation, immunosuppression, diabetes, osteoporosis.
  - Dosage: loading dose 12 mg dexamethasone IV, followed by 4 mg qds (oral or IV), weaning from postoperative day 2 over 1 week.
- When lymphoma is a differential diagnosis, steroids withheld until biopsy is performed.
- Anticonvulsants rarely used prophylactically as no impact on epilepsy incidence. Treatment instituted following a seizure (except within a few hours of surgery).
- Antibiotics administered for prophylaxis of all intracranial surgery on induction (single dose third-generation cephalosporin, e.g. cefradine 1 g IV).
- Angiographic embolization useful to reduce blood flow in vascular tumours, e.g. glomus jugulare.

Surgical management
Neurosurgical terms
- Burr holes: disc-shaped holes cut in the skull through which a biopsy needle, drain, or electrode is passed.
- Craniotomy: the construction of a bone window that is replaced at completion (now usually with titanium plates and screws). Previously 16 mm burr holes joined by saw, now 1–2 miniburr holes (3 × 5 mm) giving access for a high-speed craniotome drill to cut window.
- Craniectomy: removal of bone to access the cranium. Usually for posterior fossa as dural sinuses limit use of bone flaps.
- Stereotaxy: technique by which a biopsy needle is precisely directed by a frame (attached to the skull) to a predetermined scan target.
- Neuronavigation: method of interactive computer guidance of a surgical instrument displayed on scan during surgery.
- Debulking: subtotal removal of a tumour for diagnosis and relief of mass effect. Usually for high-grade gliomas.
- Excision: complete removal of tumour and site of origin, e.g. meningioma. May be curative for benign lesions.
- Subcapsular removal: internal debulking with preservation of capsule, e.g. vestibular Schwannoma. May be curative, preserving 7th nerve function.

Neurosurgical procedures
- Freehand burr hole biopsy now superseded by guided procedures but used as an urgent procedure when abscess is diagnostic possibility.
- Stereotactic burr hole biopsy provides an accurate and safe method for diagnosis at almost any location. Diagnostic yield 95%; serious complications 2%; mortality 0.5%.
- Open biopsy is used for tumours adjacent to eloquent areas or near major blood vessels (may be image-guided).
- Craniotomy and debulking is the usual procedure for gliomas. Radical removal carries a survival advantage but is not offered if there is a risk of increased neurological deficit. Internal bulking is performed to relieve pressure symptoms and ↓ tumour load prior to radiotherapy.
  - Complications: ↑ deficit and oedema, epilepsy, haemorrhage, infection.

Intracranial tumours: management of specific tumours

Gliomas

Graded histologically from I to IV.

- Grade I (pilocytic astrocytoma usually in children): high cure rate with surgical excision.
- Grade II astrocytoma: median survival 5 years with a subgroup of long-term survivors (30%, 10-year survival).
- Grade III gliomas: median survival 2–4 years.
- Grade IV gliomas: 12–14 months with active treatment.
  Survival is increased by radical resection in all grades.

Radiotherapy

Used as an adjunct for all grade III–IV tumours provided that Karnofsky score > 70.

- Early complications: somnolence, ↑ cerebral oedema, ↑ neurological deficit.
- Late complications: leucoencephalopathy, cognitive decline, parkinsonism, radiation necrosis, ↑ incidence of meningioma and glioma 10+ years after treatment.

Chemotherapy

- Stupp protocol of adjuvant temozolomide with and after DXT now standard for grade IV tumours.
- Recommended for anaplastic oligodendroglioma correlating with 1p and 19q chromosomal losses.

Meningiomas

- Majority are benign—clinically and histologically. Cured by resection.
- 15% have atypical features and adjunct DXT is required for residual tumour.
- < 1% malignant and recur despite resection and DXT.
- Convexity lesions usually completely removed with no residual deficit.
- Parasagittal and parafalcine lesions often involve the superior sagittal sinus. In anterior third sinus may be sacrificed with complete excision. Elsewhere sinus must be reconstructed with vein graft or tumour left *in situ*.
- Suprasellar, tentorial, clivus, CPA, and inner sphenoid wing lesions difficult to excise completely. Remnants need regular MRI or DXT.
- Complications: reactionary haemorrhage and coagulopathy due to DIC-like syndrome, epilepsy, profound oedema, venous infarction.

Primary CNS lymphoma

Extranodal high-grade B cell lymphoma distinct from systemic lymphomas.

Epidemiology

- Sporadic (median age 55 years).
- Immunosuppressed transplant recipients, congenital immunodeficiency, SLE, Sjögren's syndrome, sarcoid, MS patients, HIV infections.

Clinical features

- Brain (50%): patients present with signs and symptoms of ↑ ICP and focal neurological deficit.
- Leptomeninges: cranial neuropathies and rarely hydrocephalus.
- Eye: uveitis, retinal detachment, vitreous haemorrhage, optic neuropathy, and retinal artery occlusion.
- Spinal cord: focal spinal deficit.

Investigations

- CT ± contrast: deep-seated periventricular mass: typically hyperdense but also isodense with marked enhancement and oedema.
- MRI: low-signal lesion on T_1W and high signal on T_2W with homogeneous enhancement with Gd. Multiple lesions seen in immunocompromised and may ring enhance resembling an abscess.
- LP (if no mass lesion): ↑ protein, ↓ glucose, abnormal monoclonal B cells.
- Stereotactic brain biopsy: infiltration with B cells with a dense periventricular pattern. Immunohistochemistry confirms diagnosis, and kappa and lambda stains confirm monoclonality.
  - Note: Steroids must not be given prior to biopsy as enhancement disappears, making targeting difficult, and tumour necrosis precludes histological diagnosis.

Treatment

- Radiotherapy: median survival, 12–17 months; in HIV patients 1.5–4.2 months.
- Chemotherapy: methotrexate induction and maintenance increases survival to 40 months ± DXT.
- In HIV, cART improves survival.

Cerebral metastases

- Most common intracranial tumour (30%).
- Incidence ↑ due to ↑ survival with carcinoma, better imaging, and failure of chemotherapeutic agents to cross BBB.

Aetiology

- Haematogenous spread of carcinoma (lung > breast > kidney > GI > melanoma).
- Spread of primary CNS tumour (high-grade glioma, primitive neuroectodermal tumours (PNETs), ependymoma, pineal tumours).
- Direct invasion from skull or skull base.

Clinical features

- Symptoms and signs of ↑ ICP.
- Focal deficits.
- Seizures.
- Confusion.
- Sudden deterioration due to haemorrhage or vessel occlusion.

Imaging features
- Majority show either ring or solid enhancement.
- Solitary lesion on CT requires MRI (20% multiple).
- Solitary mass with history of carcinoma: > 90% chance of metastasis.
- No history of carcinoma and negative screening < 10% chance of metastasis.
- Solitary lesions in the posterior fossa in the elderly: even in the absence of a known primary, it is likely to be a metastasis.

Management
- Corticosteroids improve symptoms of mass effect.
- Mass lesion primary requires histological diagnosis ± excision.
- If lesion is inaccessible or multiple, stereotactic radiosurgery (SRS) (also known as gamma knife, cyberknife) is an option.
- When lesions are resectable or there are symptoms of mass effect, they should be excised at craniotomy.
- Surgery followed by whole-brain DXT or SRS to residual metastases.
- Chemotherapy may be indicated depending on primary, but BBB penetration is usually poor.

Prognosis
- Untreated: median survival < 3 months.
- Steroids + DXT: survival 3–4 months (most die from cerebral disease).
- Surgical excision, whole brain DXT, SRS, and steroids: survival 12 months (most die from extracranial disease).

Haemangioblastoma

- Benign CNS tumours of vascular origin—usually sporadic single cystic lesions in the cerebellum.
- Multiple in von Hippel–Lindau disease. (See 📖 Chapter 6, 'Inherited neurocutaneous syndromes', pp. 452–4.)

Clinical features
- Female-to-male ratio 2:1.
- Peak incidence 30–60 years.
- Site of lesion: cerebellar > vermis > floor of 4th ventricle > upper cervical cord.

Presentation
- Headache due to obstructive hydrocephalus.
- Cerebellar signs.
- Cervical tumours cause neck pain and posterior column sensory loss.
- Polycythaemia in 20% (↑ erythropoietin secretion).

Imaging features
- CT: hypodense cyst with an isodense mural cyst that enhances. Typically the cyst does not enhance. Occasionally solid mass lesion.
- MRI: cyst hypointense on T_1W; hyperintense on T_2W. Nodule isointense on T_1W; hyperintense on T_2W. Strong nodular enhancement. More sensitive for detecting small tumours.
- DSA: hypervascular nodule with a tumour blush. Occasional AV shunting. It is possible to embolize the lesion preoperatively.

Differential diagnosis
- Adults: metastasis.
- Children: pilocytic astrocytoma.

Management
- Excision for lesions causing symptoms.
- Large solid haemangioblastomas are difficult because of uncontrollable haemorrhage and brain swelling.
- Cervicomedullary tumours removed for progressive neurological deficit or haemorrhage but high risk of postoperative neurological deficit.

Ventricular tumours
- Colloid cysts, usually of the 3rd ventricle; benign cystic tumours filled with jelly.
- Rare: < 1% of intracranial tumours.
- Early recognition is important because of risk of sudden death from hydrocephalus.

Clinical features
- Headaches: may be positional, severe, and recurrent.
- Sudden drop attacks ± headache.
- Sudden leg weakness.
- Progressive cognitive decline.

Imaging features
- Well-demarcated smooth round cystic mass ± hydrocephalus.
- CT: 65% hyperdense; rarely isodense. Usually no enhancement.
- MRI: Variable intensity depending on contents. T_1W isointense or hyperintense. Variable intensity on T_2W.

Differential diagnosis
- Neurocysticercosis: multiple lesions isointense to CSF with enhancing nodule (scolex).
- Large basilar tip aneurysm.

Management
- Small incidental lesions: MRI at regular intervals to monitor size.
- Symptomatic lesions, especially with hydrocephalus, need excision.

Surgical options
- Transfrontal microsurgical excision: curative procedure with good access; 5% epilepsy rate.
- Transcallosal microsurgical excision: curative but with risk of forniceal memory deficit.
- Endoscopic excision: transcortical minimally invasive approach and low morbidity; however, higher technical failure rate and recurrence.
- Stereotactic aspiration: minimally invasive but inevitable recurrence; reserved for elderly and medically unfit patients.

Acoustic neuroma (vestibular Schwannoma)
- Benign tumour arising from the Schwann cells of the vestibular nerve.
- Unilateral tumours are sporadic.
- Bilateral lesions occur in neurofibromatosis 2.
- Malignant transformation is rare.

Clinical features
- Unilateral hearing loss followed by tinnitus, vertigo, unsteady gait, facial numbness, and weakness.
- Late development of hydrocephalus and ↑ ICP.

Investigations
- Audiogram: high-frequency hearing loss with speech discrimination worse than expected for this level; brainstem auditory evoked potential (BSAEP) abnormal.
- CT: usually isointense or rarely hyperintense lesion; enhances with contrast; expansion of the IAC.
- MRI: isointense on T_1W; hyperintense on T_2W. May be confined to the internal auditory canal or emerge like an 'icecream cone'.

Imaging guidelines for screening
- High-resolution MRI of CPA (axial/coronal planes).
- Screen with T_2W images.
- Gd if suspicious lesion.

Differential diagnosis
- Meningioma.
- Epidermoid cyst.
- Aneurysm or vascular ectasia.
- Rarely, arachnoid cyst.
- Metastases.
- Exophytic glomus tumour.

Management

Conservative and interval MRI, especially in the elderly or infirm.

Surgery

- Excision is curative but carries a significant morbidity.
- Possible to preserve hearing with suboccipital/middle fossa approaches.
- Preservation of facial nerve depends on size of the tumour.
- Large tumours with brainstem distortion carry the highest morbidity.
- Translabyrinthine approach (petrous bone hollowed out) for patients already deaf avoids cerebellar retraction.
- Middle fossa approach for intracanalicular lesions.
- Complications: CSF leak; 7th and 8th nerve damage; vertigo; hydrocephalus.

Radiotherapy

- SRS has low morbidity compared with surgery and a high rate of tumour control (> 90% at 10 years).
- Most tumours do not shrink significantly.

Imaging of intracranial tumours: examples

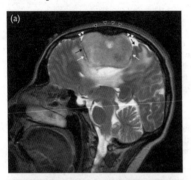

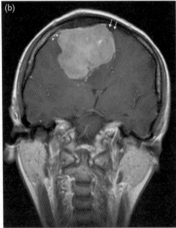

Fig. 7.2 Parafalcine meningioma. (a) T_2-weighted sagittal; (b) post-gadolinium contrast enhanced coronal MRI.

Figure 7.2(a) shows large grey matter isointense extra-axial mass denoted by CSF clefts (*white arrowheads*), displaced cortex (*small black arrow*), and pial vessels (*small white arrows*). Abnormal signal in keeping with vasogenic oedema is demonstrated in the underlying white matter. Note also the focal hyperostosis of the skull vault at the base of the tumour (*open white arrowheads*). (b) The mass enhances homogeneously. Note the CSF cleft (*white arrows*) and small 'dural tail' at the site of attachment (*white arrowheads*). There is significant mass effect with displacement of the midline and effacement of the lateral ventricles.

Figure 7.3(a) shows a large slightly heterogeneous mass expanding the pituitary sella causing depression of the sella floor, mainly on the right with extension into the right cavernous sinus where the right cavernous segment of the ICA is encased (*black arrowhead*). Tumour extends into the supra-sellar space and distorts the optic chiasm mainly on the left (*black arrow*). (b) The mass enhances most avidly in its periphery. The superior aspect of the clivus (the dorsum sellae) is eroded.

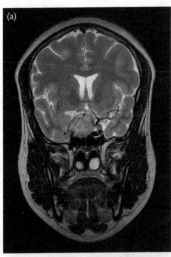

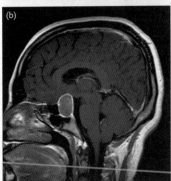

Fig. 7.3 Pituitary macroadenoma. (a) Coronal T_2W and (b) sagittal post-contrast enhanced MRI.

Figure 7.4 shows a large lobulated homogeneously enhancing extra-axial mass (denoted by the CSF cleft (*white arrow*)), in the left CPA cistern extending for a short distance into the internal auditory canal. There is marked distortion of the pons with effacement of the 4th ventricle, mainly on the left (*black arrowheads*). The hyperintensity on T_2W imaging and lack of dural attachment are in keeping with a vestibular Schwannoma rather than a CPA cistern meningioma. Note that effacement of the 4th ventricle has resulted in hydrocephalus with dilatation of the 3rd and lateral ventricles.

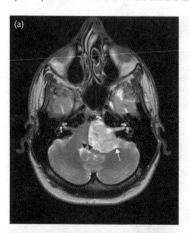

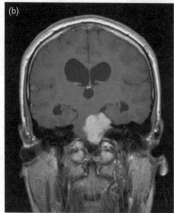

Fig. 7.4 Large vestibular Schwannoma. (a) Axial T_2W and (b) post-contrast enhanced coronal MRI.

Figure 7.5 shows a large mainly solid T_2 hyperintense mass arising from the inferior cerebellar vermis. There are multiple associated cystic components (*white arrowheads*). The tumour extends through the craniocervical junction and a small amount of oedema is shown in the cervical medullary junction ((b) *white arrow*). The brainstem is clearly displaced anteriorly and outflow from the 4th ventricle is obstructed with resulting dilatation of the 3rd and lateral ventricles.

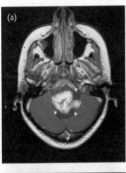

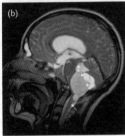

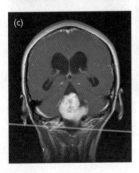

Fig. 7.5 Pilocytic astrocytoma: (a) post-gadolinium enhanced axial and (c) coronal; (b) sagittal T_2W MRI.

Figure 7.6 shows a moderately ill-defined infiltrative mass of homogeneous hyperintensity causing gyral expansion involving the temporal lobe, and extending into the adjacent inferior frontal lobe on the right. No enhancement is demonstrated. Note the mild degree of mass effect with effacement of sulci on the lateral surface of the temporal lobe compared with the contralateral (*small white arrows*).

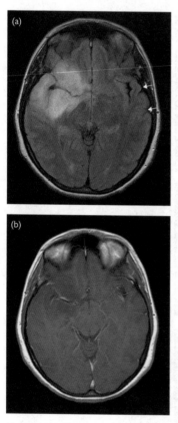

Fig. 7.6 Grade 2 diffuse astrocytoma: (a) axial FLAIR and (b) post-contrast enhanced axial MRI.

Figure 7.7 shows an irregular enhancing heterogenous right parietal mass with surrounding abnormal white matter within which is a second area of enhancing tumour more anteriorly (*white arrow*).

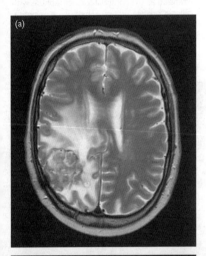

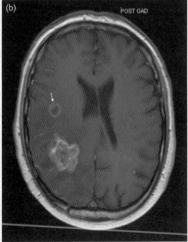

POST GAD

Fig. 7.7 Glioblastoma multiforme: (a) axial T$_2$W and (b) post-contrast enhanced axial MRI.

Figure 7.8 shows diffuse and very ill-defined hyperintensity mainly in the left frontal and anterior portion of the left parietal lobe with loss of grey–white matter differentiation and focal areas of gyral expansion resulting in sulcal effacement. There is extension to the contralateral hemisphere with involvement of the corpus callosum (*white arrows*). There is, as is typical for this diagnosis, the impression of preservation of the underlying cerebral architecture. Post-contrast enhanced images did not demonstrate enhancement.

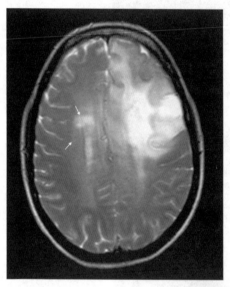

Fig. 7.8 Gliomatosis cerebri: axial T$_2$W MRI.

Figure 7.9 shows a homogeneously enhancing solid mass involving the deep grey structures and with a periventricular location. Surrounding low attenuation denotes vasogenic oedema. Note the mild distortion of the midline. Non-enhanced images revealed a uniformly hyperdense mass.

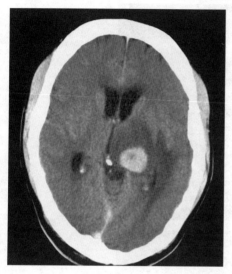

Fig. 7.9 Primary CNS lymphoma (post-contrast enhanced CT).

Figure 7.10 shows the relative T_2 hypointensity and T_1 hyperintensity of this large cerebellar vermian mass which is typical for a melanocytic melanoma deposit. The associated hyperintensity in the surrounding parenchyma denotes vasogenic oedema and there is mass effect on the 4th ventricle.

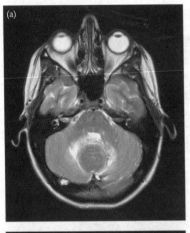

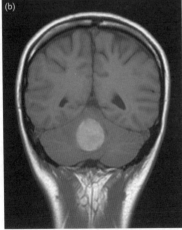

Fig. 7.10 Melanoma metastasis: (a) T_2W axial and (b) T_1W coronal MRI.

Figure 7.11 shows a large well-circumscribed cystic mass with a non-enhancing imperceptible wall ((b) *black arrowheads*) and enhancing mural nodule ((b) *black arrow*). Note the small amount of surrounding low attenuation denoting vasogenic oedema ((a) *black arrowheads*) and effacement of the left side of the fourth ventricle ((a) *black arrow*). There is resulting obstructive hydrocephalus with dilatation of the temporal horns.

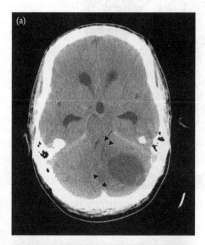

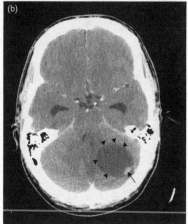

Fig. 7.11 Cerebellar haemangioblastoma: (a) non-enhanced CT; (b) contrast enhanced CT.

Figure 7.12 shows a rounded hyperdense lesion in the anterior aspect of the 3rd ventricle at the site of the foramen of Monro causing subsequent obstructive hydrocephalus with dilatation of the lateral ventricles.

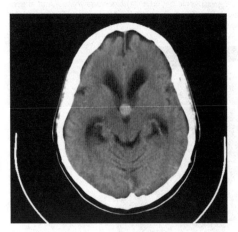

Fig. 7.12 Third ventricular colloid cyst (non-enhanced CT).

Imaging of spinal
tumours: examples

Figure 7.13 shows a large well-encapsulated left-sided extraspinal mass (*black arrows*) extending into the left lumbar intervertebral foramen (*white arrowheads*) causing distortion and displacement of the conus medullaris (*closed white arrow*). There is a small intradural component (*open white arrow*).

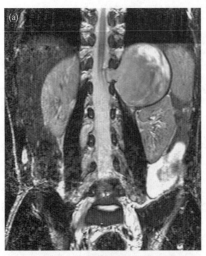

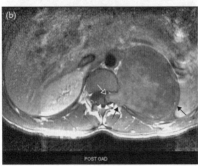

Fig. 7.13 Large spinal neurofibroma. (a) Coronal T$_2$W and (b) post-contrast enhanced axial MRI.

Figure 7.14 shows a homogenously enhancing intradural extramedullary mass at T10 (*closed white arrow*) with a relatively broad dural attachment ((a) *open white arrow*). The spinal cord is compressed and displaced to the posterolateral aspect of the vertebral canal ((b) *open white arrow*).

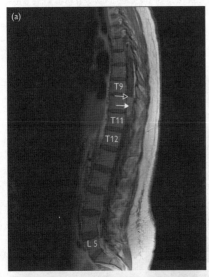

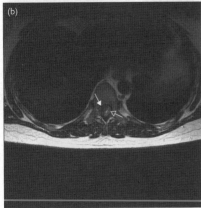

Fig. 7.14 Thoracic spinal meningioma: (a) post-contrast enhanced sagittal and (b) axial T$_2$W MRI.

Figure 7.15 shows an intramedullary heterogeneous signal intensity mass at the C6 and C7 vertebral levels (*white arrow*). Cranially and caudally extending cavities are demonstrated (*open white arrowheads*) and a small area of haemosiderin staining, in keeping with previous haemorrhage, is shown in the dependent portion of the caudal cavity (*closed white arrowhead*). Patchy enhancement following gadolinium administration ((b) *white arrow*) and expansion of the spinal cord from C4 to T2 are typical of an intramedullary tumour.

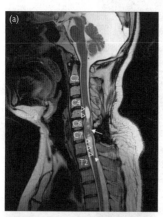

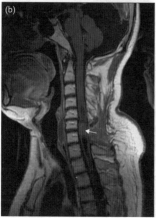

Fig. 7.15 Spinal cord ependymoma: (a) sagittal T$_2$W and (b) post-contrast enhanced sagittal MRI.

Figure 7.16 shows a well demarcated intramedullary mass ((a) *white arrow*) associated with surrounding spinal cord oedema ((a) *black arrowheads*) and expansion ((b) *white arrowheads*). The lesion enhances smoothly after contrast administration ((b) *black arrow*). The patient had multiple systemic and intracranial breast metastases.

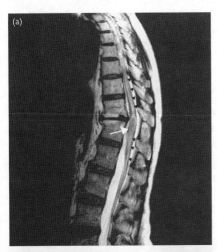

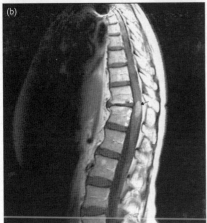

Fig. 7.16 Intramedullary metastasis: (a) sagittal T_2W and (b) post-contrast enhanced sagittal MRI.

Degenerative spinal conditions: cervical spine

Cervical degenerative disease is common but care needs to be taken to distinguish pathological conditions from changes due to ageing.
● > 95% individuals aged > 65 years will have MRI scan abnormalities.

Cervical spondylosis

Non-specific degenerative process resulting in stenosis of the spinal canal and/or root canals. Factors include:
● degenerate disc;
● osteophytes;
● hypertrophy of lamina, articular facets, ligamentum flavum, and posterior longitudinal ligament;
● congenitally narrow canal.

Most common levels affected are C5/C6 and C6/C7.

Mechanical/musculoskeletal neck pain

No root symptoms or signs. Management involves:
● lifestyle and posture changes (occupational therapy);
● anti-inflammatory drugs;
● physiotherapy;
● judicious use of a collar;
● facet joint or epidural injection of LA/steroids;
● surgery rarely indicated.

Radiculopathy

Clinical features
● Referred pain in the arm due to root irritation (brachialgia).
● Initial symptom may be sensory (tingling, burning) in a dermatomal distribution followed by radicular pain (which is in a myotomal pattern).
● Weakness.
● Reflex abnormalities.

See Table 7.1.

Table 7.1 Clinical presentation of cervical radiculopathies

Nerve root (disc level)	Pain	Motor weakness	↓ Reflexes	Sensory disturbance
C5 (C4/C5)	Neck to shoulder and upper arm	Deltoid, supra- + infraspinatus	Supinator	Shoulder, lateral arm
C6 (C5/C6)	Lateral forearm, thumb, and index finger	Biceps and brachioradialis	Biceps	Lateral forearm, thumb, and index finger
C7 (C6/C7)	Posterior arm, dorsum, forearm, middle finger	Triceps, wrist and finger extensors	Triceps	Posterior forearm, middle finger
C8 (C7/T1)	Shoulder, medial forearm, ring and little fingers	Thumb flexor, intrinsic hand muscles		Medial hand, ring and little fingers

Red flags
- Fever, chills.
- Weight loss.
- Relentless nocturnal pain.
- History of cancer.
- Immunosuppression.

Consider infection or tumour.

Imaging studies
- Plain X-rays are of limited use.
- Flexion and extension views may be useful to detect spinal instability.
- MRI is the primary imaging modality.
- CT ± intrathecal myelography is used in those in whom MRI is contraindicated or where there is extensive metalwork. It may also assess the extent of bony spurs and foraminal encroachment.

Non-surgical management
Most patients with acute radiculopathy due to disc herniation improve with conservative measures.
- NSAIDS.
- Hard or soft collar continuously or only at night for 2 weeks.
- Translaminar or transforaminal epidural injections of steroids may be considered. Rare complications include spinal cord infarction. Adequate placebo-controlled trial data are not available.

Surgical management
Surgery indicated for decompression of cervical root:
• profound weakness;
• uncontrollable pain;
• failure of conservative measures for pain after 6–12 weeks.

An **anterior approach** is indicated when pathology extends in front of the root and cord as with a central disc. Procedures include:
• simple discectomy;
• Cloward's procedure, which involves bone grafting into the disc space;
• decompression with plating or synthetic joint insertion.

A **posterior approach** is used when there is lateral canal narrowing. Procedures include foraminotomy, laminectomy, ± laminoplasty.
• Complications are uncommon but include spinal cord injury (< 1%), nerve root injury (2–3%), oesophageal perforation (< 1%), recurrent laryngeal nerve palsy after anterior approach (2%).

Cervical spondylotic myelopathy
This is the most common cause of myelopathy in those aged > 55 years and is due to disc degeneration and osteophytes.

Clinical features
Due to a combination of myelopathy and radiculopathy to varying degrees:
• numb clumsy hands;
• paraesthesiae in hands and feet;
• spasticity of the legs;
• bladder symptoms occur late;
• acute cord syndrome with tetraparesis after a fall in a patient with an already compromised cord (e.g. congenitally narrowed canal).

Differential diagnosis
• MND.
• MS.
• Subacute combined degeneration of the cord due to B_{12} deficiency.

Natural history
Not well defined—disability established early in the disease. Age > 60 years at presentation associated with poor prognosis. Long periods of non-progression may occur.

Imaging
• MRI is modality of choice.
  • low signal change on T_1 may represent poor prognosis;
  • significance of T_2 signal change uncertain;
  • in general, cord changes may be an indication for early surgery.
• Plain X-rays show degenerative change with loss of disc height and osteophytes. However, these are common findings.

Management
Surgical decompression indicated if:
• progressive myelopathy;
• stable myelopathy but as prophylaxis against further deterioration.

Surgery involves enlarging the canal anteriorly with discectomy and/or ver-
tebrectomy at single or multiple levels.
• Posterior decompression involves laminectomy or laminoplasty.
• In general, the outcome is unpredictable. Improvement may occur but
  depends on the severity and duration of symptoms preoperatively.
• If postoperative deterioration occurs, repeat MRI is indicated to assess
  degree of adequate decompression.

Degenerative spinal conditions: thoracic and lumbar spine

Thoracic disc prolapse

Symptomatic disc prolapses are rare: < 1% of all protruded discs. Most common level T11/T12.

Clinical features

- Pain localized to the spine or radicular. Nocturnal recumbent pain typical.
- Sensory symptoms and signs with a sensory level.
- Spastic paraparesis or rarely a monoparesis.
- Sphincter disturbance.
- Rarely, a Brown-Séquard syndrome.

Imaging

MRI for location, severity of cord compression, and associated myelomalacia.

Management

- Radicular pain managed with analgesics and/or local nerve root block. Surgery if intractable.
- Progressive or significant myelopathy or sphincter dysfunction an indication for surgery. If disc is heavily calcified or located midline anterior, transthoracic approach is used. Posterior approach used for lateral and soft anterolateral discs—usually a fusion procedure carried out to ensure spinal stability.

Lumbar intervertebral disc prolapse

- Acute back pain is common but accompanied by sciatica in only 2%.
- L5/S1 disc and L4/5 disc prolapses account for > 95%.

Clinical features

- Acute or gradual onset pain in the back radiating through buttock, thigh, leg to foot. L2 radiculopathy (unusual) causes anterior thigh pain. Triggered by lifting, flexion, or rotation. Dull ache with shooting exacerbations. ↑ with coughing, sneezing, bending, or prolonged sitting.
- Weakness of ankle dorsiflexion, EHL, and inversion (L5).
- Depressed or absent knee jerk (L3, L4); ankle jerk (S1).
- Straight leg raising (Lasègue's sign) causes dermatomal pain.
- Positive femoral stretch test (hip extension with maximal knee flexion) indicates L2, L3, or L4 root pathology. Other causes: psoas abscess or haematoma.
- Cauda equina syndrome (neurosurgical emergency):
  - bilateral leg pain or sensory disturbance;
  - perianal, perineal, and saddle anaesthesia;
  - urinary and/or faecal incontinence;

- low back pain;
- sexual dysfunction;
- bilateral motor and reflex deficits.

Imaging
- MRI is investigation of choice.
- CT or CT myelogram useful alternatives.
- Most commonly a posterolateral prolapse will compress root just proximal to exit foramen, e.g. L4/L5 disc compresses L5 root. However, the L4 root will be affected by upwardly migrated L4/L5 disc fragment or a far lateral disc protrusion.

Management
Acute back pain and 75% of sciatica resolve in 6–8 weeks with conservative treatment. Note: exclude infection and tumour first.
- Initial bed rest, early mobilization.
- Avoid bending, lifting, prolonged sitting.
- Adequate analgesia.
- Muscle relaxants, e.g. diazepam 2–5 mg.
- Consider epidural or nerve root block.

Indications for surgery
- Cauda equina syndrome.
- Significant or progressive motor deficit.
- Severe pain not responding to conservative measures.

Surgery involves microdiscectomy. Recurrent disc herniation rate is 2%. Recurrence of symptoms may also be due to scarring around nerve root. MRI with Gd shows root enhancement.

Lumbar canal stenosis

Narrowing of the spinal canal in the central lateral recesses or interverte-bral foraminae causing root compression. Most common: L4/L5 and L3/L4.

Clinical features
- 'Neurogenic claudication': buttock and leg pain or motor deficit on walking, standing, or lying supine. Alleviated by bending forwards or crouching. Exercise tolerance improved by cycling or pushing a trolley.
- Usually bilateral but may affect only one leg.
- Leg numbness or paraesthesiae.
- Occasionally sphincter dysfunction or impotence.
- Neurological examination may be normal.

Imaging
- MRI investigation of choice: bilateral facet hypertrophy. Lateral recess stenosis results in a trefoil deformity on axial scans.
- CT or CT myelography useful if MRI contraindicated or not available.
- Lateral flexion/extension views indicated to exclude spinal instability as fusion may be necessary at decompression.

Management

Mild symptoms: conservative management.
- Rest.
- Adequate analgesia.
- Lumbar corset.
- Physiotherapy for posture and trunk strengthening.
- Epidural steroid/LA injections reported to result in long-term benefit.
  Surgery indicated if:
- failure of conservative measures;
- pain;
- significant motor deficit;
- sphincter disturbance.

Decompressive surgery consists of variations on lumbar laminectomies.
- If spondylolisthesis (AP slip of one vertebra on another) or instability, variety of fusion procedures performed.
- Complications: dural tear and CSF leakage.

Imaging of degenerative spinal conditions: examples

Figure 7.17 shows multilevel degenerative changes extending from C3/4 to C6/7 with disc osteophyte bars (*open white arrowheads*), which indent the anterior surface of the theca and, together with focal thickening/buckling of the posterior ligamentous structures (*closed white arrowheads*), result in substantial narrowing of the cervical vertebral canal maximally at C4/5 Resultant compression of the spinal cord at this level and intramedullary signal abnormality (*white arrow*). In this case, vertebral alignment is preserved.

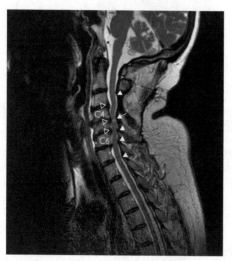

Fig. 7.17 Cervical spondylosis (sagittal T$_2$W MRI).

Although disc osteophyte bars are present in Fig. 7.18, in particular at C4/5 (*open white arrow*), there is a predominantly soft (acute) right-sided disc protrusion ((a) and (b) *closed white arrow*) resulting in marked narrowing of the right C6/7 intervertebral foramen and probable compromise of the right C7 nerve. There is only mild distortion of the spinal cord at this level.

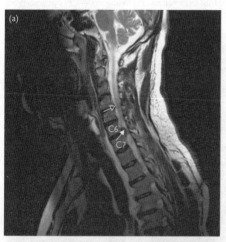

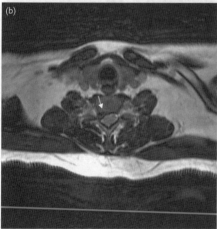

Fig. 7.18 Cervical spondylosis and acute cervical disc prolapse: (a) sagittal T_2W and (b) axial gradient echo T_2W MRI.

Figure 7.19 shows a large cranially migrating left paracentral disc protrusion ((a) *closed white arrow*; (b) *open white arrowheads*) at the L4/5 level. Although the left lateral aspect of the theca is effaced and the forming left L5 nerve is compromised as it exits the theca, the intrathecal nerves in the cauda equina (*white arrow*) are not compressed. The migrating discal component is extradural, elevating and posteriorly displacing the dura ((a) *black arrowheads*). Note the small annular fissure in the L2/3 intervertebral disc ((a) *black arrow*).

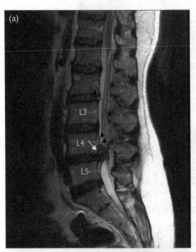

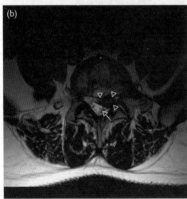

Fig. 7.19 Lumbar disc protrusion: (a) sagittal T_2W and (b) axial T_2W MRI.

In Fig. 7.20 there is mild anterior subluxation of L4 upon L5 (Grade 1 spondylolisthesis). In conjunction with marked facet joint degeneration and thickening of the posterior ligamentous structures ((a) *white arrow*; (b) *white arrowheads*), there is marked narrowing of the vertebral canal at this level ((a) *black arrowheads*) with effacement of CSF and compression of the cauda equina ((b) *closed white arrow*) compared with the normal appearance of the theca (c). The small area of hyperintensity posterior to the theca ((b) *open white arrow*) represents epidural fat rather than residual CSF.

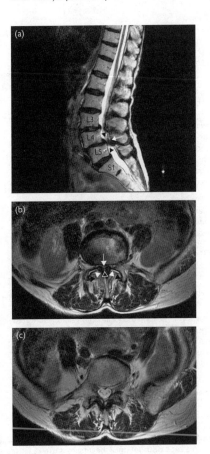

Fig. 7.20 Focal lumbar vertebral canal stenosis: (a) sagittal T_2W MRI; (b), (c) axial T_2W MRI.

Developmental abnormalities

Arachnoid cysts

Congenital CSF-containing cysts developing between arachnoid layers: 50% in the middle cranial fossa, 10% suprasellar, and 10% cerebellopontine angle. Less common sites include quadrigeminal cistern, hemispheric convexity, and the posterior fossa.

Clinical features
- Majority present in childhood:
  - middle cranial fossa—seizures, headache, hemiparesis;
  - suprasellar cysts—hydrocephalus, enlarged skull, developmental delay, visual failure, precocious puberty.
- In adults, incidental finding.

Imaging features
Sharply demarcated cysts, which may have mass effect. May communicate with the subarachnoid space. Walls are indefinable.
- CT: CSF density with no enhancement. Typically, remodelling and scalloping of adjacent walls is evident. Haemorrhage (rare).
- MRI: CSF signal intensity on all images. Null signal on FLAIR. DWI images show free diffusion in contrast to epidermoid cysts, which show restricted diffusion with ↑ signal. Other differential diagnoses: cystic extra-axial tumour (usually has a wall, a solid component with enhancement); cysticercosis; mega cisterna magna in the posterior fossa.

Management
- If asymptomatic, no treatment.
- Symptomatic cysts drained via either a marsupialization into CSF spaces (via a craniotomy or endoscopy) or a shunt to the peritoneum.

Chiari malformation

Syndromes of hindbrain descent. Four subtypes which are probably unrelated. Types 1 and 2 predominate.

Chiari 1 malformation (cerebellar ectopia)
Anatomy
Simple descent of cerebellar tonsils beyond the foramen magnum. Elongated peg-shaped tonsils plug the foramen. Occasionally acquired after LP or LP shunt. Cerebellar descent and arachnoid adhesions interfere with normal transmission of CSF pressure waves across the FM to the spinal reservoir, raising ICP and forcing fluid into the central canal of the spinal cord.

Clinical features
Usually presents in young adults.
- Suboccipital headache. ↑ stooping, straining, coughing.
- Brainstem compression with ataxia, lower cranial palsies, pyramidal weakness.
- Central cord syndrome due to the associated syringomyelia with dissociated sensory loss in a cape distribution. ↓ beating nystagmus.

Management
Foramen magnum (FM) decompression by removal of 3 × 4 cm crescent of bone from the posterior rim of FM. Restores CSF pathway and decompresses syrinx. Complications: aseptic meningitis, CSF leak, hydrocephalus.

Chiari 2 malformation
Anatomy
Congenital hindbrain abnormality associated with spinal dysraphism (myelomeningocele, spina bifida). Descent of cerebellar tonsils, vermis, medulla, 4th ventricle through FM. Associated with hydrocephalus and elongated upper cervical nerves.

Clinical features
Present in infancy with:
• hydrocephalus;
• respiratory distress;
• dysphagia and aspiration pneumonia;
• downbeat nystagmus;
• quadraparesis.
• High mortality from respiratory arrest.

Imaging features
MRI: S-bend medulla, tonsillar descent, large interthalamic connexus, dysgenesis of corpus callosum, hydrocephalus, medullary compression, syringomyelia.

Management
• Insertion of VP shunt for hydrocephalus.
• Posterior fossa decompression.

Dandy–Walker malformation
• Agenesis of the vermis of the cerebellum, resulting in a large posterior cerebellar cyst opening into the 4th ventricle.
• Hydrocephalus is common.
• Associated with agenesis of the corpus callosum, occipital encephalocele, spina bifida, syringomyelia.
• Facial, ocular, and cardiovascular abnormalities.

Management
Insertion of a cyst–peritoneal shunt and/or VP shunt.

Aqueduct stenosis

Congenital aqueduct stenosis presents in childhood with hydrocephalus in the first 3 months of life. Adult forms usually acquired due to inflammation, infection, brainstem tumour, arachnoid cysts.

Clinical features
- Symptoms and signs of ↑ ICP.
- Cognitive impairment.
- Visual field deficit.
- Ataxia.
- Incontinence.

Management
- Insertion of a VP shunt.
- Endoscopic 3rd ventriculostomy (by creation of a hole in the floor of the 3rd ventricle allowing CSF to reach the basal cisterns, bypassing the aqueduct and 4th ventricles).

Spinal dysraphism (spina bifida)

Developmental defects of neural tube closure with a variety of abnormalities:
- Spina bifida occulta. Often clinically insignificant finding of hypoplastic posterior sacral elements with normal dural sac and skin cover. May have skin stigmata: hairy patch, naevus. Associated with intradural lipomas, thickened filum terminale, diastematomyelia (split cord), and dermoid cysts. Cause of tethered cord syndrome:
  - neurogenic bladder;
  - paraparesis;
  - foot deformity.
- Meningocele. Developmental absence of sacral and low lumbar posterior elements with bulging meninges exposed at skin surface. Neurological deficit in 30%.
- Myelomeningocele. Congenital absence of posterior vertebral elements, dura, and maldevelopment of the terminal spinal cord. All have a neurological deficit with hydrocephalus in 80%. Associated with Chiari 2 malformation.

Management

Myelomeningocele requires early closure to ↓ infection rate and protect neural tissue from damage. Hydrocephalus may be apparent after closure and is treated with a VP shunt. With surgery 85% survive infancy, most with normal IQ.

Imaging of developmental abnormalities: examples

In Fig. 7.21 there is marked descent of the cerebellar tonsils below the FM ((b) *black arrows*) to the inferior aspect of C2. The pointed configuration of the tonsillar tips is typical. Note the crowding at the FM with anterior displacement and kinking of the cervicomedullary junction (*white arrowhead*). Some compression and impingement of the upper cervical spinal cord is also demonstrated, with intramedullary signal change at the lower border of C2 (*white arrow*). No definite syrinx or hydrocephalus is shown. The occipito-atlanto-axial osseous configuration is normal in this case.

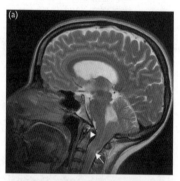

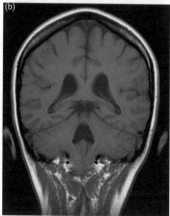

Fig. 7.21 Chiari 1 hindbrain deformation: (a) sagittal T_2W and (b) coronal T_1W MRI.

Figure 7.22 shows typical beaking/tapering of the inferior aspect of the lumen of the aqueduct of Sylvius ((a) *white arrow*) resulting in obstruction to CSF flow and proximal hydrocephalus reflected by dilatation of the superior portion of the aqueduct and of the 3rd and lateral ventricles (b).

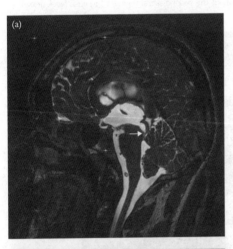

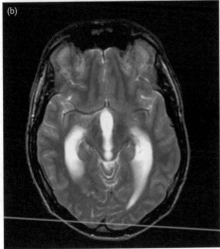

Fig. 7.22 Aqueduct stenosis: (a) thin section T_2W sagittal and (b) axial T_2W MRI.

In Fig. 7.23 the termination of the spinal cord is low-lying at the upper border of L3 (*black arrow*), and an intradural ovoid mass at S1 ((a) *black arrowheads*; (b) *white arrowhead*) contains fatty elements ((b) *white arrow*) representing an intradural dermoid inclusion body. Note deficiency of the posterior elements of the second sacral segment ((a) *open black arrow*).

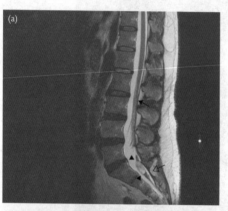

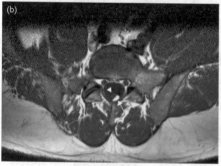

Fig. 7.23 Spinal dysraphism: (a) sagittal T_2W and (b) axial T_1W MRI.

Syringomyelia

Caused by cavitations within the spinal cord with clinical deficits. May coexist with a similar condition, syringobulbia. Due to abnormal CSF circulation resulting from anatomical abnormalities.

Causes
- Cerebellar ectopia (Chiari malformations).
- Intramedullary tumours.
- Trauma.

Clinical presentation
Usually early to middle adult life with:
- cough and positional headache due to pathology at FM;
- lower motor neuron weakness in the hands and arms, e.g. wasted hand + paraparesis of the legs;
- dissociated sensory loss (cape distribution) affecting spinothalamic sensation but sparing posterior columns.

Imaging features
Cranial and spinal MRI + Gd. Assessment of the craniocervical junction; presence of any cord tumours. See Fig. 7.24.

Management
The natural history is unclear. Medical treatment based on physiotherapy, occupational therapy, and pain management.

Surgery
- Decompression of the FM. May arrest and sometimes reverse progression of syringomyelia.
- Syrinx cavity operations consist of a drainage procedure, usually in cases of progressive neurological deficits:
  - syringo-arachnoid shunt;
  - syringo-pleural shunt.

Revision procedures often required.

Figure 7.24 shows a multiseptated centrally located intramedullary long-segment lesion of CSF signal intensity on both T_2W and T_1W imaging which expands the spinal cord and extends into the inferior brainstem as syringobulbia ((a) *white arrow*).

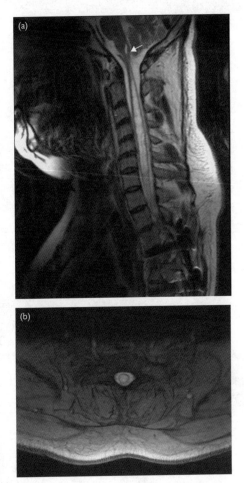

Fig. 7.24 Syringomyelia: (a) sagittal T$_2$W and (b) axial T$_2$W MRI.

Chapter 8

Clinical neurophysiology

Introduction 524
Electroencephalography (EEG): introduction 526
EEG: use and abuse 529
EEG: abnormal rhythms 530
EEG and epilepsy 534
EEG and diffuse cerebral dysfunction 538
EEG in the intensive care unit 540
Technical summary of nerve conduction studies (NCS) 542
Peripheral nerve disorders: NCS abnormalities 544
Technical summary of needle electromyography (EMG) 546
Needle EMG: patterns of abnormality 548
NCS and needle EMG findings in myopathies and motor
    axonal loss 552
NCS and needle EMG findings in Guillain–Barré syndrome 554
NCS and needle EMG findings in neuromuscular transmission
    disorders 556
Small fibre studies 559
Evoked potentials (EPs) 559
Visual evoked responses (VERs) 560
Somatosensory evoked potentials (SSEPs) 562
Brainstem auditory evoked responses (BAERs) 565
Normal values in clinical neurophysiology 566
Suggested reference texts in clinical neurophysiology 568

Introduction

Neurophysiological investigations include the following:

- Electroencephalography (EEG):
  - used in diagnosis and management of epilepsy;
  - combined with video recordings to establish diagnosis of epilepsy;
  - assessment of epilepsy before epilepsy surgery;
  - diagnosis of infective and metabolic brain disorders, e.g. CJD, herpes simplex encephalitis, hepatic encephalopathy.
- Nerve conduction studies (NCS) and needle electromyography (EMG):
  - study of sensory and motor peripheral nerve disorders, e.g. neuropathies, radiculopathies, dorsal root ganglionopathies, and anterior horn cell disorders;
  - neuromuscular junction disorders;
  - skeletal muscle disorders;
  - cranial nerve disorders, e.g. facial nerve, trigeminal nerve.
- Evoked potentials (EPs):
  - study sensory and motor pathways in the peripheral and central nervous systems;
  - useful in investigation of multiple sclerosis, other spinal cord and brainstem disorders, and cranial neuropathies;
  - monitoring of spinal cord function during surgery for scoliosis and of the facial nerve during acoustic neuroma surgery.

The neurophysiological evaluation helps the neurologist by:
- confirming the clinical diagnosis;
- defining type of dysfunction, e.g. axonal versus demyelinating neuropathy;
- excluding certain disorders in differential diagnosis;
- detecting subclinical disease, e.g. optic nerve demyelination or vasculitic peripheral neuropathy;
- defining severity of disease and indicating prognosis, e.g. extent of axonal degeneration in Guillain–Barré syndrome;
- monitoring change in disease over time;
- identifying muscles most suitable for injection with botulinum toxin in treating focal dystonias.

Electroencephalography (EEG): introduction

Conventional EEGs are non-invasive recordings of spontaneous brain electrical activity obtained using scalp electrodes that record fast-changing events. EEG waveforms represent spatiotemporal averages of synchronous excitatory and inhibitory postsynaptic potentials generated by interconnecting cortical pyramidal cells.

EEG electrode placement

Most widely used is the standardized 'International 10/20 system', which uses three anatomical landmarks: nasion, inion, and pre-auricular points. Metal disc electrodes 4–10 mm in diameter are placed on the scalp and held in place by an adhesive conductive paste.

EEG activity

One channel of EEG activity is a plot of the electrical potential between two recording electrodes. The frequency of EEG activity is classified into four bands: delta (0–4/s), theta (4–8/s), alpha (8–13/s) and beta (> 13/s) frequencies. The normal waking EEG (Fig. 8.1) in an adult usually has prominent posterior bilateral alpha activity that is enhanced on eye closure.

EEG display

EEG activity is represented as a graph of voltage (vertical axis) versus time (horizontal axis). Recordings are displayed in various combinations of channels called 'montages'.

EEG recording

The routine EEG is made as follows:
- Usually 21 scalp electrodes are placed, according to the International 10/20 system of electrode placement.
- Simultaneous single-channel ECG recording.
- An eye-movement channel monitors state of alertness or is used to help identify the REM (rapid eye movement) stage of sleep.
  EEG recordings are susceptible to artefacts such as movement or electrical sources, e.g. sudden change in impedance. They are technically difficult to record in young children, uncooperative patients, and in the ICU setting (because of electrical interference).
  Routine EEGs are usually initially recorded in the waking state. The recording room is quiet and dimly lit to allow the patient to become drowsy. Abnormalities can be enhanced by some activation procedures:
- Hyperventilation: vigorous overbreathing for 2–5 minutes, followed by recording for 1 minute. Especially useful in childhood absence epilepsy as lack of epileptiform abnormality virtually excludes the diagnosis in an untreated patient. Can also elicit focal abnormalities. Contraindicated in patients with various cardiac, respiratory, and cerebrovascular conditions.

- Photic stimulation: delivered by a strobe light (flashing light at variable rates) 20–30 cm from the patient's central vision. Flash frequencies are between 1 and 60/s, including during eye closure, in a dimly lit room. Photosensitivity is manifested by generalized self-sustaining epileptiform abnormalities and is associated with forms of primary generalized epilepsy. There is an increased risk of seizures when the generalized epileptiform activity outlasts the duration of a train of photic stimuli.
- Sleep deprivation: usually requires sleep deprivation for up to 24 hours, which may activate epileptiform abnormalities in susceptible patients.

Long-term EEG monitoring

Prolonged simultaneous video and EEG monitoring records behaviour, and can record epileptiform activity during epileptic seizures, often aiding in the classification of a seizure disorder.

- Helps to distinguish epileptic seizures from non-epileptic events.
- Particularly useful in preoperative evaluation to help identify the anatomical site of seizure onset.
- May involve:
  - Additional anterior temporal, sphenoidal, or foramen ovale electrodes;
  - More invasive EEG recordings using subdural strip or intracerebral depth electrodes;
  - Stimulation of underlying cortex by applying electrical current to individual subdural electrodes in the waking state used to map eloquent areas (important for speech) prior to resection;
  - Ambulatory 8- to 32-channel recordings allowing the patient to perform daily activities while clinical events are recorded. Can aid in quantifying seizure burden. They are of value where attacks tend to occur in certain situations. Limited in usefulness because of artefacts and lack of simultaneous video recordings.

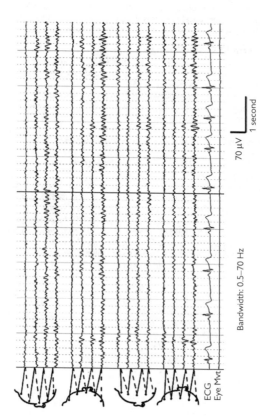

Bandwidth: 0.5–70 Hz

70 μV

1 second

ECG
Eye Mvt

Fig. 8.1 Normal waking adult EEG, longitudinal bipolar montage: ECG, electrocardiogram; Eye Mvt, eye-movement channel.

EEG: use and abuse

EEG abnormalities that indicate definite pathology are:
- epileptiform discharges;
- generalized or focal slowing;
- absence of normal background rhythms—diffuse or focal/unilateral;
- periodic phenomena: relatively stereotyped sharpened complexes that recur in a periodic or quasiperiodic pattern; commonly seen in diffuse encephalopathies.

EEG is useful in the investigation of:
- epilepsy—epileptiform abnormality on EEG is specific, but not sensitive, for the diagnosis of epilepsy as a cause of any paroxysmal event or transient loss of consciousness; in epileptic patients sensitivity is 25–55% and specificity is 80–98%;
- impaired consciousness/coma—to rule out subclinical seizures or non-convulsive status epilepticus;
- toxic confusional states;
- diffuse degenerative disorders, e.g. CJD, Alzheimer's disease;
- metabolic encephalopathies, e.g. hepatic failure, uraemia;
- cerebral trauma;
- parasomnias—episodes of unusual behaviours during sleep such as night terrors, sleepwalking, REM sleep behaviour disorder.

EEG is of less value in the investigation of other disorders such as multiple sclerosis, migraine headache, mental retardation, and psychoses, even though abnormalities, including seizures, can occur in association with these conditions.

EEG should not be used to rule out non-convulsive status epilepticus in patients who are able to answer questions and follow commands.

A normal EEG does not exclude the diagnosis of epilepsy.

EEG: abnormal rhythms

Cortical rhythms are generated locally in the cerebral cortex but are modulated at both thalamic and reticular activating system (brainstem) levels.

Periodic phenomena

Periodicity refers to repetitive discharges reflecting diffuse dysfunction of grey and white matter.

- Periodic lateralized epileptiform discharges (PLEDs) (see Fig. 8.2(a)):
  - Confirm local pathology but are not specific. Most commonly seen in acute cerebral infarctions (35%). May also be seen in other mass lesions (e.g. metastases), or infections (such as HSE), cerebral abscess, anoxia.
  - May be associated with subtle and transient focal clinical events.
  - Tend to resolve after 1–2 weeks, even when underlying lesion is progressive.
  - May occur independently bilaterally (BIPLEDs) in association with hypoxic/ischaemic encephalopathy; indicates poor prognosis.
  - See 📖 Chapter 5, 'Viral encephalitis', pp. 370–2.
- Generalized periodic discharges occur in:
  - Hypoxic/ischaemic encephalopathy.
  - Subacute sclerosing panencephalitis (SSPE): simultaneous bilateral complexes of slow and fast components, repeating at 4–20 second intervals.
  - Sporadic CJD (Fig. 8.2(b)): discharges at 1–2 second intervals; may be confused with ECG pickup on scalp, and simultaneous ECG channel is important.
  - In SSPE and CJD: progressive loss of cortical rhythms until repetitive complexes occur on a silent background.

Pathological slow waves

- Slowing of underlying posterior dominant activity: occurs in hypoxia, hypoglycaemia, cerebrovascular disease, dementia, and metabolic encephalopathies.
- Focal voltage attenuation can suggest grey matter dysfunction and can also be associated with regional fluid collections (subdural, epidural).
- Focal theta/delta slowing aids localization of cerebral dysfunction; focal delta waves are hallmark of electrically silent mass lesions such as tumours, infarctions, and abscesses (Fig. 8.2(c)).
- Focal slowing can also occur in patients with focal seizure disorders.
- Seizure activity (see 📖 'EEG and epilepsy', pp. 534–7).

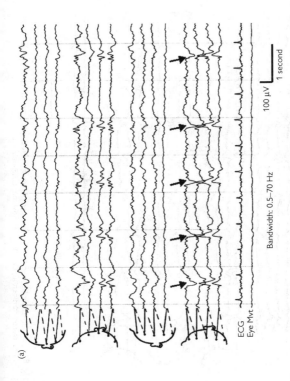

Bandwidth: 0.5–70 Hz

Fig. 8.2 (a) Right-sided periodic lateralized epileptiform discharges (PLEDs), indicated by arrows, in an elderly drowsy patient 2 days after right-sided cerebral infarction; ECG, electrocardiogram; Eye Mvt, eye-movement channel.

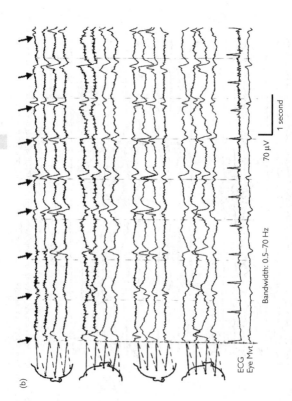

Bandwidth: 0.5–70 Hz

ECG
Eye Mvt

70 μV

1 second

Fig. 8.2 (b) Generalized periodic sharp wave complexes, indicated by arrows, in an adult patient with CJD. ECG, electrocardiogram; Eye Mvt, eye-movement channel.

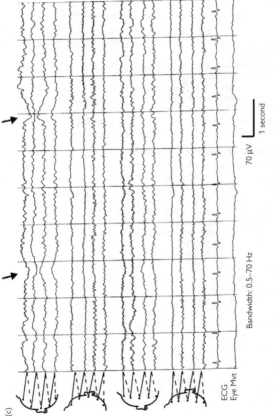

Fig. 8.2 (c) Left temporal focal delta rhythms, indicated by arrows, in a waking adult patient who had a left-sided subarachnoid haemorrhage 2 years previously; ECG, electrocardiogram; Eye Mvt, eye-movement channel.

Bandwidth: 0.5–70 Hz

70 µV

1 second

ECG
Eye Mvt

(c)

EEG and epilepsy

Epileptiform activity
The hallmarks are:
- spikes with 20–70 ms duration;
- sharp waves, with 70–200 ms duration;
- spike and slow-wave activity or sharp and slow-wave activity;
- electrographic seizures, with or without clinical correlates.

Similar patterns can occur in the normal EEG, but are recognized by the characteristic waveforms, topography, and circumstances of occurrence. Examples of benign EEG variants:
- rhythmic bursts of 6/s and 14/s positive spikes occur in adolescents and young adults during drowsiness and light sleep;
- benign epileptiform transients of sleep (BETS);
- rhythmic midtemporal discharges (psychomotor variant);
- bifrontal slow-wave activity elicited in children by hyperventilation;
- rare 6/s bilateral spike and slow wave discharges in anterior regions of waking males or in the occipital region of drowsy females.

Diagnostic strategy in epilepsy
- Misinterpretation of non-epileptiform features is an important cause of false-positive EEG reports. Prevalence of rigorously defined epileptiform discharges is 0.5–2% in normal adults.
- A normal EEG does not exclude a diagnosis of epilepsy.
- 33% of epileptic patients exhibit interictal epileptiform discharges in waking EEGs (Fig. 8.3(a)); 16% never do. Probability of interictal epileptiform abnormality in a patient with epilepsy in a 30-minute waking recording is 1 in 3.
- Repeated waking EEGs can increase detection rate of interictal epileptiform abnormality in patients with epilepsy; epileptiform discharges are recorded on the first EEG in 30–50% of patients with epilepsy, and in 60–90% by the third EEG.
- Sleep EEG, particularly following sleep deprivation (Fig. 8.3(b)), increases yield to 80%; hyperventilation and photic stimulation also increase the probability of focal or generalized epileptiform abnormalities; drowsiness and sleep increase probability of focal interictal epileptiform abnormalities.
- If interictal EEG is persistently normal, consider long-term video–EEG monitoring.
- There is no relationship between presence or absence of interictal epileptiform abnormality on EEG and seizure frequency or response to medication.

EEG and seizure classification
- EEG findings, combined with patient's clinical history, support distinction between focal and generalized seizures. This will guide therapy. Identification of focal elements at onset of seizures is important, as focal events can rapidly propagate to secondarily generalized discharges.

- Focal asymmetry, slowing, or generalized abnormalities may assist in differentiation.
- Photosensitivity occurs in 5% of epileptic patients, especially in juvenile myoclonic epilepsy. See Fig. 8.3(c).

EEG and discontinuation of treatment

The EEG can be a useful guide as persistent epileptiform abnormality may indicate a high risk of relapse in some patients if discontinuation of treatment is being considered.

(a)

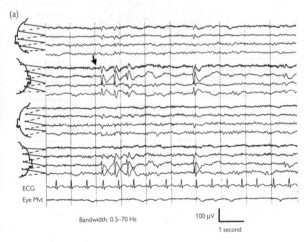

Bandwidth: 0.5–70 Hz   100 μV

1 second

Fig. 8.3 (a) A burst of focal subclinical epileptic activity, indicated by the arrow, in the right centrotemporal region of a waking adult patient: ECG, electrocardiogram; Eye Mvt, eye-movement channel.

(b)

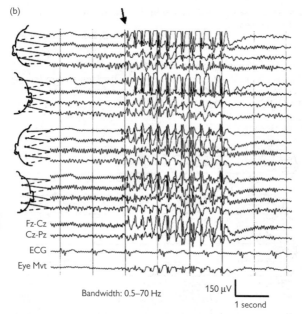

Fz-Cz
Cz-Pz
ECG
Eye Mvt

Bandwidth: 0.5–70 Hz

150 µV

1 second

Fig. 8.3 (b) A burst of generalized subclinical spike/polyspike and slow-wave activity, indicated by the arrow, in a waking adult patient following sleep deprivation. A previous waking EEG had been normal. The patient had one generalized seizure: ECG, electrocardiogram; Eye Mvt, eye-movement channel.

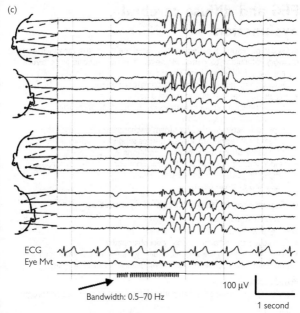

Fig. 8.3 (c) A burst of generalized subclinical spike/polyspike and slow-wave activity in a waking adult patient elicited by photic stimulation. The arrow indicates the photic stimulation markers: ECG, electrocardiogram; Eye Mvt, eye-movement channel.

EEG and diffuse cerebral dysfunction

EEGs can be helpful in patients with altered mental status, ranging from mild memory difficulties to coma. However, it is non-specific as to aetiology. Useful in the following clinical situations:

- Detection of seizure activity in a comatose patient.
- Suggesting aetiology in undiagnosed coma:
  - may reveal focal abnormalities in setting of intracerebral space-occupying lesions;
  - periodic lateralized epileptiform discharges (PLEDs) over the temporal region can suggest herpes simplex encephalitis (HSE).
- Diagnosing diffuse degenerative conditions, e.g. CJD, SSPE.
- Help in identification of psychogenic coma or locked-in syndrome.
- Prognostic guide after anoxic brain injury.
- Evaluation of brain death.

EEG patterns in diffuse cerebral dysfunction

Generalized slowing

See Fig. 8.4.

- Can suggest toxic or metabolic encephalopathy.
- Sensory activation using visual, auditory, tactile, or painful stimuli important, as reactive EEG activity implies a better prognosis.

Periodic spiking

Occurs in post-anoxic encephalopathy and is associated with a poor prognosis.

Alpha coma

Non-reactive 8–12/s activity associated with a poor prognosis.

Burst suppression

- Bursts of high-amplitude slow and sharp activity alternating with periods of attenuation of background EEG activity.
- May occur after severe anoxic brain injury, general anaesthesia, hypothermia, and barbiturate overdose.
- Used as a marker of adequate barbiturate dosage in status epilepticus treatment.

Triphasic waves

Can occur in:

- metabolic conditions—hepatic, uraemic, and anoxic encephalopathy;
- CJD;
- post-ictal state.

Periodic complexes

- PLEDs occur in destructive lesions: ischaemic stroke, intracerebral haemorrhage, encephalitis.
- Generalized or asymmetrical periodic sharp waves often found in sporadic CJD at some stage of the illness; do not occur in vCJD or familial CJD.
- Generalized periodic stereotypic complexes occur in SSPE and correlate with myoclonic jerking.

Epileptiform patterns
- Non-convulsive status epilepticus.
- Post-ictal.

Normal EEG
- Locked-in syndrome with lesion in pontine tegmentum.
- Psychogenic unresponsiveness.

Electrical inactivity
- Absence of brain waves > 2 μV amplitude.
- In brain death, severe poisoning, general anaesthesia, hypothermia.

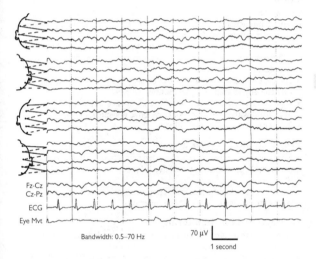

Fz-Cz
Cz-Pz
ECG
Eye Mvt

Bandwidth: 0.5–70 Hz   70 μV
                            1 second

Fig. 8.4 Diffuse symmetrical theta and delta slowing in a waking adult with Lewy body dementia: ECG, electrocardiogram; Eye Mvt, eye-movement channel.

EEG in the intensive care unit

- Clinical neurological assessment is limited in the unconscious or paralysed and ventilated patient. EEG can help by demonstrating a response to stimulation of the limbs or the cranial nerve territories.
- EEG can provide important information about cerebral function, particularly in detecting potentially treatable disorders. EEG activity generated by cortical pyramidal neurons is sensitive to hypoxia/ ischaemia.
- EEG abnormalities need to be distinguished from the effect of sedatives and anaesthetic agents.

Coma

See Fig. 8.5.

Changes in reactivity, variability, and wake–sleep state in the EEG can suggest certain aetiologies of coma.

- Focal repetitive periodic lateralized discharges typically occur in HSE.
- Diffuse slow waves: metabolic encephalopathy, anoxic brain injury, drug overdose.
- Spindle or beta coma patterns can be seen in overdoses with tricyclic agents, benzodiazepines, barbiturates.
- Alpha coma, characterized by diffuse unreactive alpha activity, is typically associated with severe hypoxic/ischaemic encephalopathy.
- Non-convulsive status epilepticus.

Prognosis after cardiac arrest

- Recovery of continuous activity within first 4 hours correlates with good recovery. In contrast, the predictive value for recovery of EEG is poor at 48 hours.
- Isoelectric and burst suppression patterns not caused by drugs or hypothermia also indicate a poor prognosis.

Continuous EEG monitoring

- Used to detect seizures in patients with status epilepticus who are paralysed and ventilated.
- Used to assist management of sedation and raised ICP in ventilated patients following severe head injury.
- Used in assessment and early identification of hemispheric infarctions; EEG changes occur within minutes of ischaemia.
- Used in detection of arousals.
- Used in assessment of prognosis of sepsis-associated encephalopathy by monitoring severity scores based on EEG features.

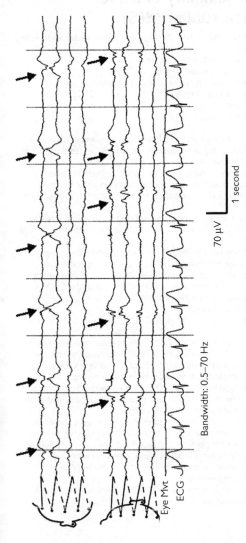

Bandwidth: 0.5–70 Hz

Fig. 8.5 Loss of normal background rhythms and bilateral independent periodic lateralized epileptiform discharges (PLEDs), indicated by arrows, in an adult comatose patient following hypoglycaemia: ECG, electrocardiogram; Eye Mvt, eye-movement channel.

Technical summary of nerve conduction studies (NCS)

Standard NCS assess function of the large myelinated motor and sensory fibres (see Table 8.1).

- NCS depend on many technical factors:
  - subject's age, gender, and height;
  - skin temperature must be controlled or a correction applied; conduction velocity varies by 2.4 m/s/°C from 29°C to 38°C;
  - recording equipment;
  - operator experience.
- NCS are:
  - orthodromic where direction of propagated potentials is the same as normal physiological conduction in the nerve, e.g. sensory nerve distal-to-proximal;
  - antidromic where studies are in the opposite direction to normal physiological conduction, e.g. sensory nerve proximal-to-distal.
- Conduction velocity (CV) reflects the velocity of the fastest conducting nerve fibres.
- Durations of the nerve action potential (NAP) or compound muscle action potential (CMAP) waveforms reveal the spectrum of CV in large nerves (Fig. 8.6).
- Motor conduction velocity (MCV) in metres/second is calculated by dividing the distance (millimetres) between two separate points of stimulation (one close to muscle being recorded, the other more proximal) by the difference between onset latencies of the CMAP waveforms elicited proximally and distally by separate supramaximal stimulation (milliseconds).
- Compound muscle action potentials (CMAPs) are recorded from the skin overlying a muscle in response to stimulation of the motor nerve to that muscle. Onset latency, amplitude, area, and duration are measured.
- Sensory nerve action potentials (SNAPs) are recorded from a nerve in response to supramaximal stimulation of the nerve at another site. Onset latency, amplitude, area, and duration are measured.
- Sensory conduction velocity (SCV) is calculated by dividing the distance (millimetres) between stimulation and recording electrodes by the onset latency of the SNAP waveform (milliseconds).
- F wave: supramaximal distal stimulation of a motor nerve also elicits an impulse that travels antidromically to the axon hillock region of the spinal cord where it elicits further motor fibres that propagate back to the muscle. Only explores 1–3% of motor axons in a nerve.
  - Gives information on conduction over the whole length of motor nerve, including proximal sections.
  - Frequency of occurrence out of 20 stimuli, minimum latency, and range of latencies are recorded.

Table 8.1 Most common nerves studied by NCS

	Motor	Sensory
Head and neck	Facial	Trigeminal
Upper limb	Median	Median
	Ulnar	Ulnar
		Radial
Lower limb	Tibial	Sural
	Peroneal—deep	
	Peroneal—superficial	Peroneal—superficial

- H reflex:
  - measures conduction through afferent and efferent fibres in a monosynaptic reflex arc;
  - usually recorded from calf muscles in response to submaximal stimulation of Ia afferents in the tibial nerve at the knee;
  - usually equivalent to eliciting ankle deep tendon reflex;
  - absent if F wave and other NCS are abnormal.

Evaluation of proximal nerve conduction

Indirect studies
- F wave.
- H reflex.

Direct studies:
- Needle EMG of paraspinal muscles.
- Nerve root stimulation by:
  - high-voltage surface electrical stimulation;
  - monopolar needle electrode stimulation;
  - magnetic stimulation.

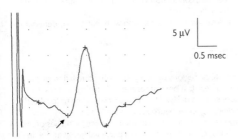

5 µV

0.5 msec

Fig. 8.6 Sensory nerve action potential. The ulnar sensory fibres were stimulated at digit V using surface electrodes and the recording electrodes were placed over the ulnar nerve at the wrist. Arrow indicates 1st positive peak, used in this example to calculate sensory conduction velocity (in this case, 57 m/s). The amplitude (14 µV) was measured between the negative (upward) peak and the 2nd positive (downward) peak. Ten waveforms were averaged. Supramaximal stimulation rate, 1/s.

Peripheral nerve disorders: NCS abnormalities

NCS will help classify a peripheral nerve disorder into the following categories:
- sensorimotor;
- pure sensory or pure motor;
- axonal, demyelinating, or mixed;
- generalized, multifocal, or length dependent.

Demyelinating neuropathies

Characterized by ↓ conduction velocities with preserved SNAP and CMAP amplitudes.
- Abnormalities supportive of demyelinating neuropathy include:
  - ↓ CV < 70–80% of lower limit;
  - ↑ F wave latencies > 130% lower limit of normal;
  - ↑ distal sensory and motor latencies > 130% lower limit of normal;
  - ↓ CMAP amplitude from proximal stimulation compared with distal stimulation (motor conduction block).
- In many hereditary demyelinating neuropathies, abnormalities tend to be diffuse and to a similar degree in all nerves.
- In acquired demyelinating neuropathies:
  - focal slowing;
  - temporal dispersion (↑ duration of action potentials);
  - regions of conduction block.
- Needle EMG studies can show abnormalities indicating denervation and reinnervation, depending on severity and chronicity.

Axonal neuropathies

Characterized by:
- ↓ or unrecordable SNAPs and CMAPs.
- With severe axonal loss, conduction velocity may be reduced as result of loss of fast-conducting fibres.
- Needle EMG confirms axonal degeneration with features of denervation and reinnervation.

Focal neuropathies

See Fig. 8.7.
- Lesions may cause focal regions of demyelination. Stimulation of the nerve distal to lesion elicits a normal response. Proximal stimulation produces a response with delayed latency corresponding to localized conduction slowing, e.g. ulnar neuropathy at the elbow.
- Focal lesion may result in conduction block at the site of the lesion. For example, with neuropraxia of the common peroneal nerve at the fibular head resulting in foot drop, distal response may be normal but proximal stimulation may not elicit a response because of conduction block.
- Focal lesion may also cause axonal degeneration distal to site of lesion. This can result in reduced amplitude of SNAPs and CMAPs.

(a)   (i) Ulnar nerve   (ii) Deep peroneal nerve

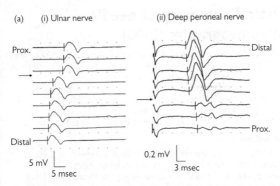

Fig. 8.7 (a) Localization of focal ulnar and peroneal neuropathies using inching studies. (i) Recording from abductor digiti minimi muscle, demonstrating ulnar motor slowing (arrow) localized to the region of the medial epicondyle. Supramaximal stimuli over the nerve at 2 cm intervals, proximal-to-distal. (ii) Recording from extensor digitorum brevis muscle, demonstrating deep peroneal motor slowing and partial motor conduction block (arrow) localized to the region of the head of fibula. Supramaximal stimuli over the nerve at 2 cm intervals, distal-to-proximal.

(b)

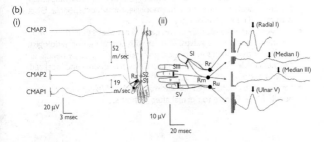

Fig. 8.7 (b) Localization of focal median neuropathy in the right hand of a patient with carpal tunnel syndrome, using surface electrodes. (i) Conduction studies of median motor fibres. CMAP1, CMAP3, CMAP3: compound muscle action potentials elicited by supramaximal stimulation of the median motor nerve at palm, wrist, and elbow (S1, S2, and S3 cathode stimulation sites), respectively, recorded from the thenar muscles. Ra, active recording electrode (Ambu® Blue Sensor NF electrode (44 × 22 mm); distal motor latency of CMAP2, 5.2 msec; skin temperature, 33°C; bandwidth, 0.02–10 kHz. (ii) Conduction studies of median sensory fibres: filled arrows indicate sensory nerve action potentials (SNAPs) recorded at the wrist elicited by supraximal stimulation of the radial fibres from digit I, the median fibres from digits I and III, and the ulnar fibres from digit V (conduction velocities, 56, 34, 25, and 59 m/sec, respectively, using latency to first positive peak). SNAPs recorded by: Ambu® Blue Sensor NF electrode (44 × 22 mm) placed over the wrist at Rr, Rm, and Ru sites for radial, median, and ulnar fibres, respectively. SI, SIII, and SV: sites of stimulating cathodes on digits I, III, and V respectively. Stimulating–recording electrode distances, 135 mm; skin temperature, 33°C; bandwidth, 0.002–10 kHz.

Technical summary of needle electromyography (EMG)

Needle EMG involves extracellular recording of muscle action potentials using either monopolar or concentric needle electrodes. This is a qualitative assessment, and therefore is operator dependent.

- The motor unit refers to the motor neuron cell body, motor axon, and all innervated muscle fibres. The motor unit potential (MUP) is the sum of activity from muscle fibres of one motor unit.
- Transection of a motor nerve is followed by regrowth at 1–2 mm/day.

Technical aspects

- A needle electrode is inserted into the belly of the muscle at rest.
- Insertional activity is assessed. Normally no other activity at rest.
- Subject is asked to activate muscle voluntarily. MUPs are studied and reflect synchronous discharge of muscle fibres in a motor unit.
- With minimal effort, a few motor units fire initially at 5–7/s. With more effort, more motor units, of higher amplitude and faster firing frequencies, are recruited.
- Recruitment and interference pattern of MUPs assessed at increasing levels of contraction and at maximal voluntary effort.

Notes

- Needle EMG may be contraindicated in patients with coagulopathies, e.g. anticoagulant medication, haemophilia, thrombocytopenia. Discuss with clinical neurophysiologist.
- Transient bacteraemia may occur, causing endocarditis in those with prosthetic or diseased valves. Discuss with clinical neurophysiologist.
- Muscle biopsy findings in a muscle previously examined by needle EMG can yield misleading information due to muscle trauma and localized inflammation.
- Serum creatine kinase (CK) levels may rise by 150% of normal after needle EMG. Return to normal after 48 hours.

Needle EMG: patterns of abnormality

Spontaneous activity at rest

Fibrillations and positive sharp waves

See Fig. 8.8(a).
- Generated by individual muscle fibres.
- Reflect ↑ excitability of muscle cells due to alteration in resting membrane potentials.
- Occur in:
  - recent denervation;
  - myopathic processes.

Fasciculation potentials
- Result from spontaneous discharges of a group of muscle fibres from all or part of a motor unit.
- May result from pathology in the anterior horn cell, motor root, or more distal motor nerve.

Myotonia

See Fig. 8.8(b).
- Characterized by rhythmic discharges triggered by insertion of EMG needle into muscle. Waveforms resemble positive sharp waves or fibrillations. Discharges wax and wane in amplitude, producing a noise resembling a decelerating motorcycle.
- Occurs in:
  - myotonia congenita;
  - myotonic dystrophy;
  - paramyotonia congenita;
  - hyperkalaemic periodic paralysis.
- Electromyographic, as opposed to clinical, myotonia is also seen in:
  - polymyositis;
  - hypothyroidism;
  - acid maltase deficiency, typically in the paraspinal muscles.

Complex repetitive discharges
- Have a uniform shape, frequency, and amplitude. Have abrupt onset, mimicking the sound of a machine gun, with a frequency of 5–100/s.
- Represent a group of muscle fibres firing in near synchrony.
- Occur in:
  - myopathies, e.g. polymyositis, Duchenne muscular dystrophy;
  - chronic denervation, e.g. radiculopathy, spinal muscular atrophy, hereditary neuropathies.

Neuromyotonia
- Characterized by spontaneous and continuous rhythmical discharges at high frequencies.
- Represents single-fibre or motor unit discharges and originate from a distal motor axon.
- Occurs in conditions associated with continuous muscle fibre activity, e.g. stiff person syndrome, encephalomyelitis with ridigity, Isaac's syndrome.

(a)

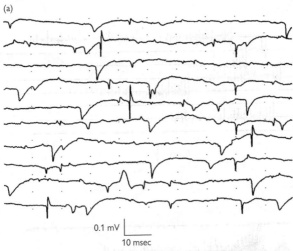

0.1 mV
10 msec

Fig. 8.8 (a) Concentric needle EMG recording of fibrillations and positive sharp waves (downgoing) at rest indicating recent denervation of the muscle.

Myokymia
- Consists of repetitive discharges of one or more motor units, usually in complex bursts.
- Occurs in chronic neuropathies and represents a non-specific response to injury.
- Occurs in radiation plexopathies.
- Can be recorded in facial muscles in patients with multiple sclerosis or pontine glioma.
- May be exacerbated by hypocalcaemia, e.g. hyperventilation-induced.

Neurogenic processes (affecting motor axons)
- Denervation results in fewer motor units that can be activated voluntarily.
- Acute denervation changes recorded from a muscle at rest initially include spontaneous fibrillations and positive sharp waves.

Reinnervation results in denser motor units that contain increased number of fibres manifesting as long-duration MUPs and increased fibre density. With ongoing reinnervation, MUPs are unstable (Fig. 8.8(c)).

(i)

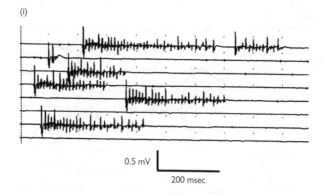

0.5 mV

200 msec

(ii)

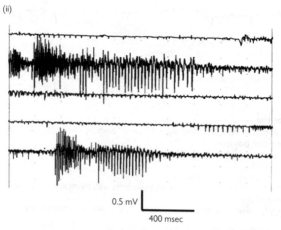

0.5 mV

400 msec

Fig. 8.8 (b) Concentric needle EMG recordings of myotonia from two adult patients with myotonic disorders: (i) paramyotonia congenita; (ii) myotonia congenita.

(c)

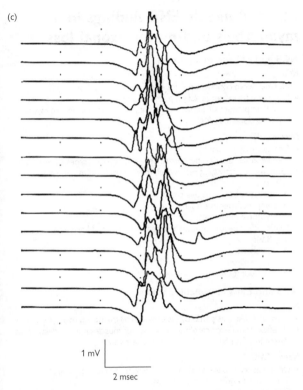

1 mV

2 msec

Fig. 8.8 (c) Concentric needle EMG recording, in raster display, of a triggered unstable and irregular motor unit potential, indicating recent reinnervation.

Myopathic processes

- Excessively full interference pattern so that baseline is obliterated at earlier effort than in normal muscle.
- Low amplitude and short-duration MUPs.
- Complex or polyphasic MUPs due to variation in diameter of pathological muscle fibres.
- Fibrillations and positive sharp waves at rest.
- Unstable MUPs, indicating a recent or active process.
- Stable late potentials in long-standing myopathic disorders.

NCS and needle EMG findings in myopathies and motor axonal loss

NCS and EMG in myopathies

NCS
- Normal nerve conduction velocities.
- Normal sensory nerve action potential amplitudes.
- CMAP amplitudes of motor nerves may be reduced in severe myopathy involving distal muscles.

Needle EMG
- Changes may be patchy.
- Needle EMG cannot differentiate between different types of myopathy.
- Spontaneous activity at rest, which may be confined to paraspinal muscles:
  - fibrillations and positive sharp waves;
  - complex repetitive discharges;
  - myotonic discharges.
- MUPs reflecting loss of muscle fibres and increased fibre type variation (Fig. 8.9):
  - polyphasic;
  - low amplitude;
  - short duration.

NCS and EMG in radiculopathies

NCS
- Normal SNAPs, as pathology is proximal to the dorsal root ganglion.
- H-reflex from flexor carpi radialis or soleus muscles may be delayed or absent in C7 or S1 radiculopathies respectively.

Needle EMG
- Denervation of paraspinal muscles helps to differentiate root lesions from more peripheral nerve lesions.
- Evidence of denervation is required in at least two muscles innervated by each motor root.
- Needle EMG of adjacent myotomes determines extent of involvement.

NCS and EMG in motor neuron disease (MND)

MND can be difficult to diagnose in the early stages especially in bulbar onset cases or if confined to one limb.
- Normal sensory NCS.
- Normal motor conduction velocities.
- CMAPs may be reduced.
- Important to rule out motor conduction block.
- Needle EMG: active denervation with partial reinnervation involving different roots and nerves corresponding to different spinal and bulbar segments.
- Progression can be monitored by repeated measurement of CMAPs.

(i)

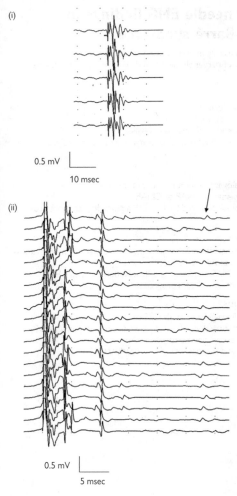

0.5 mV

10 msec

(ii)

0.5 mV

5 msec

Fig. 8.9 Concentric needle EMG recording, myopathic patterns: (i) raster display of a triggered low-amplitude polyphasic stable motor unit potential; (ii) raster display of a triggered polyphasic motor unit potential associated with late (satellite) potentials (arrow).

NCS and needle EMG findings in Guillain–Barré syndrome

- Motor nerves usually more involved than sensory nerves.
- Large number of nerves should be studied as involvement may be patchy.

Early

- Studies may be normal.
- Delayed distal motor latencies.
- Reduced frequency and delayed F waves.
- Early reduction of F wave frequency may indicate proximal conduction block.

Late

- Widespread slowing in sensory and motor nerves.
- Temporal dispersion of NAP or CMAP.
- Conduction block detected by ↓ CMAP amplitude with more proximal stimulation.

Needle EMG

- Evidence of denervation 2–3 weeks after onset indicates motor axonal loss in addition to demyelination.
- Degree of ↓ CMAP amplitude and denervation on needle EMG indicates severity and guides prognosis.

GBS subgroups

NCS and EMG findings can classify GBS subgroups.

- Acute inflammatory demyelinating polyradiculoneuropathy (AIDP).
- Acute motor axonal neuropathy (AMAN).
- Acute motor and sensory axonal neuropathy (AMSAN).

NCS and needle EMG findings in neuromuscular transmission disorders

Classified into:

- postsynaptic, e.g. myasthenia gravis;
- presynaptic, e.g. Lambert–Eaton myasthenic syndrome, botulism.
  Note: it is important to study clinically affected muscles.

Myasthenia gravis

- Normal sensory nerve conduction studies.
- Amplitude of CMAP from affected muscle may be ↓ due to motor endplate destruction with normal motor conduction velocities.
- Needle EMG: no evidence of denervation or reinnervation.
- Repetitive nerve stimulation (RNS) (see Fig. 8.10(a)):
  - slow rate of repetitive supramaximal stimulation (1–3/s) results in 'decrement', i.e. > 8% ↓ amplitude of 5th CMAP compared with 1st CMAP;
  - maximal voluntary contraction of the muscle for 20 seconds or a train of high-rate stimulation (10–50/s) may result in some ↑ in CMAP amplitude, but < 200%, i.e. post-activation potentiation due to transient ↑ in acetylcholine release.
  - degree of decrement correlates with clinical severity.
- Single-fibre EMG (SFEMG) (see Fig. 8.10(b)).
  - Studies transmission in individual motor endplates.
  - Performed if RNS is negative.
  - Reveals subclinical neuromuscular transmission defects.
  - ↑ jitter found in extensor digitorum communis muscle in all cases of moderate or severe generalized MG and 96% of mild cases. In ocular MG, ↑ jitter of frontalis muscle found in 89%.

(a)

(i)

2 mV/D   21.0 mA   2 ms/D
                0.2 ms
                3 Hz

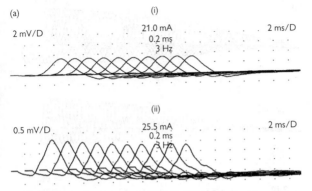

(ii)

0.5 mV/D   25.5 mA   2 ms/D
                0.2 ms
                3 Hz

Fig. 8.10 (a) Repetitive nerve stimulation at 3 Hz, recorded from nasalis muscle: (i) normal (2 mV/D); (ii) 15% decrement in a myasthenic patient (0.5mV/D).

(b)

(i)

1 mV/D   0.5 ms/D   (ii)   0.5 mV/D   0.5 ms/D

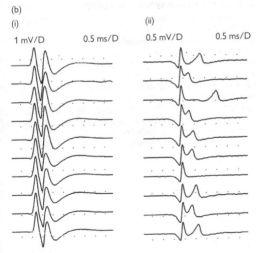

Fig. 8.10 (b) Single-fibre EMG: (i) normal jitter; (ii) increased jitter and blocking in a myasthenic patient.

(b)

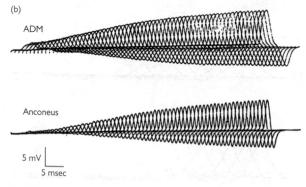

Fig. 8.10 (c) Increment in a patient with Lambert–Eaton myasthenic syndrome (LEMS). Repetitive nerve stimulation at 20 Hz, recorded from abductor digiti minimi (ADM) and anconeus muscles.

Lambert–Eaton myasthenic syndrome (LEMS)

- Sensory nerve conduction studies usually normal unless associated with a paraneoplastic neuropathy.
- CMAP amplitudes are absent or ↓, especially from foot muscles. Normal motor conduction velocities.
- No evidence of denervation or reinnervation on needle EMG.
- RNS (see Fig. 8.10(c)):
  - slow rate of repetitive supramaximal stimulation (1–3/s) elicits a decrement > 8%, similar to myasthenia gravis.
  - maximal voluntary contraction for 20 seconds or high rate of RNS (10–50/s) results in > 200% of CMAP post-activation potentiation due to transient ↑ release of acetylcholine.
- SFEMG: ↑ jitter in clinically-affected muscles.

Small fibre studies

Pain and temperature perception

Peripheral small fibre neuropathies cause pain (burning or stinging) or electric shock sensations, particularly in the feet. The most common cause is diabetes mellitus.

The most common diagnostic studies are:

- skin biopsy to assess intra-epidermal nerve fibre density;
- quantitative sensory testing—measurement of warming, cooling, heat pain and cold pain thresholds.

Autonomic function

Autonomic nerve dysfunction represents a type of small fibre neuropathy.

The most common diagnostic studies are:

- R–R interval response to deep breathing;
- blood pressure response to standing from the recumbent position;
- sympathetic skin response.

Evoked potentials (EPs)

Evoked potentials are elicited by external stimuli to sensory systems (visual, auditory, or somatosensory). They consist of complex waveforms with positive and negative components.

Visual evoked responses (VERs)

VERs are recorded from the scalp and are averaged from the EEG background of the occipital cortex. They reflect the integrity of the central visual field from retina, optic nerve, and cortex.

- The full field VER is elicited by stimulating each eye while the subject fixates on the stimulus. Sensitive to lesions of the optic nerve and anterior chiasm.
- Pattern-reversal stimulation usually used.
- Hemifield stimulation helpful in assessment of retrochiasmatic lesions. May be difficult to interpret.
- Pattern reversal electroretinography (ERG) can be recorded simultaneously with VERs; enables retinal abnormalities to be excluded as a cause of abnormal VERs.

The P100, the most consistent waveform, is a large positive deflection at approximately 100 ms latency, maximal in the occipital midline.

- Latency most consistent parameter.
- Amplitude varies amongst normal individuals.
- Elicited by the following:
  - luminance change, i.e. flash VER;
  - contrast change with repeated reversal of a black-and-white checkerboard pattern (pattern-reversal VER) (Fig. 8.11(a)).

Applications

Most commonly used for detection of asymptomatic lesions in MS (Fig. 8.11(b)).

- 90% of patients with a history of optic neuritis have abnormal pattern-reversal VERs.
- 70% of patients with definite MS and no history of optic neuritis have delayed VER.
- Unilateral delay suggests impaired conduction in visual pathway anterior to the optic chiasm.
- Site of abnormality cannot be localized when delay is bilateral and equivalent from each eye.
- Normal pattern-reversal VERs do not exclude retrochiasmal lesions. Possible to have recordable VERs with cortical blindness.
- Malingering: normal VER latencies make lesions of the optic nerve or anterior chiasm very unlikely as the cause of subjective visual loss.

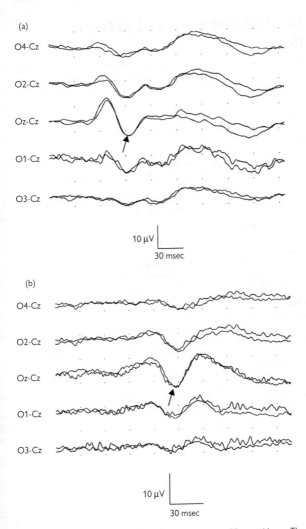

Fig. 8.11 (a) Normal pattern-reversal VERs recorded from a 25-year-old man. The midline P100 latency (indicated by arrow) was 100 ms. (b) Delayed pattern-reversal VERs recorded from a 48-year-old man with multiple sclerosis. The P100 latency indicated by the arrow was 143 ms. (Visual acuity was 6/9.)

Somatosensory evoked potentials (SSEPs)

SSEPs are time-locked responses following stimulation of afferent peripheral nerve fibres from the upper and lower limbs. They enable study of the integrity of the large fibre sensory pathways in peripheral nerves, spinal cord, and brain.

Upper limb SSEPs

- Stimulation of median nerve at wrist (Fig. 8.12(a)).
- Recordings from:
  - Erb's point (N9, generated by brachial plexus);
  - upper cervical cord (P/N13, generated by postsynaptic activity in central cord grey matter at the cervicomedullary junction/upper cervical cord);
  - scalp over hand area of contralateral somatosensory cortex (N19, thalamus; P22, parietal sensory cortex).

Lower limb SSEPs

- Stimulation of tibial nerve at ankle (Fig. 8.12(b)).
- Recordings from:
  - T12/L1 (N20, cauda equina potential);
  - scalp over foot/leg area of contralateral somatosensory cortex in midline (N/P37, parietal sensory cortex).

Notes

- Lesions alter SSEPs by delaying or abolishing component waveforms. Waveform amplitude is less reliable than latency.
- Lower limb SSEP latencies are proportional to standing height.
- Differentiate between central and peripheral causes of large fibre sensory dysfunction.
- SSEPs enable study of proximal peripheral nerves when standard sensory NCS are normal.
- Used to monitor integrity of spinal cord during risky spinal surgery.
- Confirmation of non-organic peripheral sensory loss.

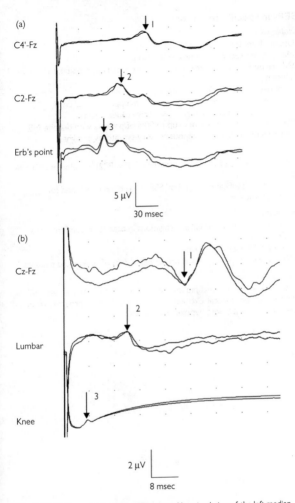

Fig. 8.12 (a) Normal upper limb SSEPs elicited by stimulation of the left median nerve of a 34-year-old woman at the wrist: standing height, 173 cm. Arrow 1, cortical (N19) waveform; arrow 2, cervicomedullary (N13) waveform; arrow 3, brachial plexus potential. (b) Normal lower limb SSEPs, elicited by stimulation of the left tibial nerve of a 36-year-old woman at the ankle: standing height, 180 cm. Arrow 1, cortical (P37) waveform; arrow 2, lumbar (N20) waveform; arrow 3, peripheral nerve waveform recorded at the popliteal fossa.

SSEPs in specific conditions

Multiple sclerosis

- Usually ↑ central sensory latencies.
- May indicate second asymptomatic lesion.
- Where peripheral sensory conduction is normal it is possible to localize a lesion:
  - above cervicomedullary junction;
  - at region of cervicomedullary junction/upper cervical cord;
  - below upper cervical region but above cauda equina.
- SSEP abnormalities present in up to 90% of patients with definite MS and 50% of MS patients without sensory symptoms or signs.

Coma

- Bilateral absence of the thalamocortical (N19–P22) waveforms indicates poor prognosis.
- Prognostic classification based on SSEPs has been developed for post-hypoxic coma.

Brain death

- Role of neurophysiological investigations in brainstem death remains controversial.
- Absent N19–P22 waveforms.
- P/N13 waveform complex is preserved in 70% of brain-dead patients.

Cortical myoclonus

Using back-averaging techniques, abnormally large cortical waveforms reflect enhanced cortical excitability conditions such as progressive myoclonic epilepsy, CJD, post-hypoxic myoclonus.

Brainstem auditory evoked responses (BAERs)

BAERs (Fig. 8.13) are elicited by clicks presented to the ear by a headphone. Recorded between disc electrodes placed on the scalp at vertex and mastoid of the ear being studied. Normally six or seven waveforms are recorded. Latencies for waveforms I, III, and V are the most consistent and clinically useful.

- Wave I: generated in auditory nerve near cochlea.
- Wave III: generated in superior olivary nucleus.
- Wave V: generated in the lateral leminiscus/inferior colliculus, i.e. upper pons/lower midbrain.
- Most sensitive measure is the wave I–wave III interwave latency difference.

Indications

- Identifying hearing impairment in infancy or in patients who have difficulty cooperating with conventional audiography.
- Determining nature of hearing loss.
- Helping diagnose acoustic neuroma: 98% with acoustic neuroma have abnormal BAERs; 33% have unrecordable BAERs.
- Aiding diagnoses of MS: abnormal in 20–50% of patients who have no brainstem symptoms or signs.
- Aiding localization of brainstem pathology: delayed or absent wave V with normal wave III indicates abnormal conduction in the auditory pathways in the region of the pons.

Note: BAERs are normal in cortical deafness.

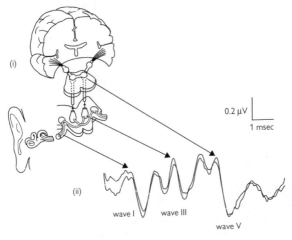

Fig. 8.13 BAERs: (i) schematic diagram of the auditory pathways and the origin of the BAER waveforms; (ii) example of normal BAER waveforms elicited by click stimulation to one ear of a 36-year-old woman.

Normal values in clinical neurophysiology

- Nerve conduction and evoked potential data are influenced by many subject variables including age, height, skin temperature, and sex.
- They can also be affected by technical factors such as electrode specifications, stimulating and recording parameters, recording equipment, and the person carrying out the study.
- Specific factors exist for particular studies, such as the importance of visual acuity, check size, and luminance for pattern-reversal VERs and hearing threshold for BAERs.

It is an important principle that, where possible, individual departments should collect normal data using the same methods that are employed in the routine clinical work of that laboratory.

The normal limits in Tables 8.2–8.4 are approximate for adults and should only be used as a general guideline.

Table 8.2 Motor nerve conduction studies (surface electrodes)

	Median nerve	Tibial nerve
Muscle recorded from	Abductor pollicis brevis	Abductor hallucis brevis
Distal motor onset latency (ms)	≤ 4.0	≤ 6.2
Amplitude (mV)	≥ 5.0	≥ 5.5
Conduction velocity (m/s)	≥ 50 (elbow–wrist)	≥ 40 (knee–ankle)
F-wave latency (ms)*		
Minimum of 20	≤ 30	≤ 58
Interside difference	≤ 2.5	≤ 3.5
H-reflex minimum latency (ms)		≤ 33

*It is particularly important to take subject's height into account.

Table 8.3 Sensory nerve conduction studies (surface electrodes)

	Median nerve	Sural nerve
Conduction velocity (m/s)	≥ 50 (digit III–wrist)	≥ 40 (calf–ankle)
Amplitude (µV)	≥ 10	≥ 6

Table 8.4 Evoked potential latencies

Median SSEPs	Erb's point	N13	N19	N13–N19	
Normal range (ms)	≤ 11	≤ 16	≤ 21	≤ 7	
Tibial SSEPs	N20	P37	N20–P37		
Normal range (ms)*	≤ 22	≤ 40	≤ 20.5		
Pattern-reversal VER	P100	Inter-eye difference			
Normal range (ms)	≤ 120	≤ 11			
BAER	Wave I	Wave III	Wave V	Wave I–III	Wave III–V
Normal range (ms)	≤ 2.2	≤ 4.5	≤ 6.5	≤ 2.5	≤ 2.4

*It is particularly important to take subject's height into account.

Suggested reference texts in clinical neurophysiology

General

Aminoff MJ (ed) (2012). *Aminoff's Electrodiagnosis in clinical neurology* (6th edn). Philadelphia, PA: Elsevier Saunders.

Daube JR, Rubin DI (eds) (2009). *Clinical neurophysiology* (3rd edn). Oxford: Oxford University Press.

Cooper R, Binnie C, Billings R (eds) (2003). *Techniques in clinical neurophysiology: a practical manual.* Philadelphia, PA: Elsevier Churchill Livingstone.

Liveson JA, Ma DM (1999). *Laboratory reference for clinical neurophysiology.* Oxford: Oxford University Press.

Yamada T, Meng E (2011). *Practical guide for clinical neurophysiology testing.* Philadelphia, PA: Lippincott Williams & Wilkins.

Electroencephalography

Ebersole JS, Pedley TA (eds) (2003). *Current practice of clinical electroencephalography* (3rd edn). Philadelphia, PA: Lippincott Williams & Wilkins.

Osselton JW, Binnie CD, Cooper R, et al. (eds) (2002). *Clinical neurophysiology: electroencephalography, pediatric neurophysiology, special techniques and applications.* Elsevier Health Science Division.

Schomer DL, Lopes da Silva F (eds) (2011). *Niedermeyer's Electroencephalography: Basic Principles, Clinical Applications and Related Fields* (6th edn). Philadelphia, PA: Lippincott Williams & Wilkins.

Nerve conduction studies and electromyography

Binnie CD, Osselton JW (eds) (1995). *Clinical neurophysiology: EMG, nerve conduction and evoked potentials.* Oxford: Butterworth Heinemann.

Dumitru D, Amato AA, Zwarts MJ (eds) (2002). *Electrodiagnostic medicine* (2nd edn). Philadelphia, PA: Hanley & Belfus.

Kimura J (2013). *Electrodiagnosis in diseases of nerve and muscle: principles and practice* (4th edn). Oxford: Oxford University Press.

Lee HJ, DeLisa JA (2000). *Surface anatomy for clinical needle electromyography.* New York: Demos Medical Publishing, 2010.

Stålberg E, Trontelj J, Sanders D (2010). *Single fiber EMG* (3rd edn). Edshagen.

Stewart JD (2010). *Focal peripheral neuropathies* (4th edn). JBJ Publishing.

Evoked potentials

Chiappa KH (ed) (1997). *Evoked potentials in clinical medicine* (3rd edn). Philadelphia, PA: Lippincott–Raven.

Chapter 9

Neuroradiology

Techniques in diagnostic radiology 570
Cerebrovascular disease 576
Subarachnoid haemorrhage 580
Intracerebral haemorrhage 582
Guidelines for head injury 583
Imaging strategies for cervical spine trauma 584
Guidelines for the neuroradiology of tumours 586
CNS infections 588

Techniques in diagnostic radiology

Plain radiography

- Limited contrast resolution and risk of ionizing radiation.
- Pregnancy is a contraindication as is lack of menstruation within previous 10 days.
- Skull X-ray (SXR) used occasionally for penetrating head injury, characterization of skull vault bone lesions, and assessment of shunt tubing.
- Spinal X-ray indicated in trauma, characterization of bone lesions in haematological disorders (skeletal surveys), flexion/extension views for assessment of stability of cervical spine (e.g. rheumatoid arthritis) and lumbar spine (e.g. pars defects).

Computed tomography (CT)

- CT employs a highly collimated X-ray beam that is differentially absorbed by various tissues depending on their density. Thinner slices (< 2 mm) increase spatial resolution.
- Usually used for the evaluation of bones, e.g. spine and base of skull.
- Contrast enhancement with non-ionic iodinated IV contrast, which appears as higher density, is used to opacify blood vessels and reveal blood–brain barrier (BBB) breakdown: tumours, infection, inflammation.
- Rapid administration of IV contrast (using a pump injector) can be combined with early arterial phase thin-slice CT to generate angiographic images (CTA) of neck vessels and circle of Willis (e.g. in SAH) and perfusion data (CTP) of the whole brain (e.g. in acute stroke imaging).
- Multidetector CT allows coverage of the whole brain with images of < 1 mm slice thickness in just a few seconds.

Dose issues

- Essential to limit number of studies.
- Thinner slices increase dose.
- CT head/cervical spine not contraindicated in pregnant women—extremely low risk over background radiation. A lead apron over the abdomen can be psychologically beneficial.
- CT of thoracic and lumbar spine contraindicated in pregnancy unless life-threatening condition.

Ultrasonography (USS)

Operator-dependent—requires skill and experience.

Carotid artery Doppler

Indications

- History of TIA/stroke in anterior circulation.
- Asymptomatic carotid bruit.
- Preoperative evaluation before major cardiovascular surgery.
- Post-endarterectomy follow-up.
- Arterial dissection.

Imaging signs

- Visual characterization of atheromatous plaque at bifurcation of common carotid artery (CCA) and in proximal internal carotid artery (ICA): calcification/plaque size/degree of stenosis/plaque ulceration.
- May be difficult to distinguish occluded from near-occluded vessel.
- Sensitivity 95%; specificity 85–99%.
- In dissection: intimal flap/double lumen/intramural thrombus/vessel tapering.
- Assessment of vertebral arteries limited to gross patency and direction of flow.

Transcranial Doppler

Performed with a high-frequency probe over the thin portion of the temporal bone using it as an acoustic window.

Indications

- Intracranial stenoses.
- Occlusions (e.g. middle cerebral artery (MCA)).
- Cross-flow through anterior and posterior communicating arteries.
- Monitoring of emboli.
- Vasospasm in SAH.
- Detection of supratentorial haematomas, aneurysms, AVM.

Magnetic resonance imaging (MRI)

- Success of technique is based on its sensitivity to protons in water, which constitutes 70–90% of body tissues.
- Content and properties of water are altered in disease processes, providing MRI with diagnostic opportunity.
- MRI has superior contrast resolution, especially of soft tissues, and is safe with no ionizing radiation.

Contraindications

- Pacemaker.
- Ferromagnetic implants (aneurysm clips, cochlear implants).
- First trimester pregnancy.
- Large metallic spinal fixation devices make interpretation difficult.
- Claustrophobia (10%)—consider sedation or, in essential cases, anaesthesia. Open MRI may be an alternative in some cases.

Different imaging sequences

Increased resolution.

- T_1-weighted spin echo (SE) (T_1W). White matter gives higher signal than grey matter; fat, gadolinium, melanin, proteinaceous fluid and many blood breakdown products are hyperintense.
- T_2W SE. Grey matter gives higher signal than white matter; fluids (including CSF), oedema, and to a lesser extent fat are hyperintense.
- Gradient echo (GE), also known as T_2*. Low signal with air, blood products (deoxy-, met-haemoglobin and haemosiderin), Ca^{2+}, Fe^{2+}, surgical metalwork, and bone. Susceptibility weighted MRI (SWI) is exquisitely sensitive to these products.
- Fluid-attenuated inversion recovery (FLAIR): suppression of fluid signal.

- Contrast-enhanced MRI. Gadolinium is a strongly paramagnetic metallic element injected IV. Rapidly distributed, excreted renally with a half-life of 1.5 hours. Results in enhancement (hyperintensity) on T_1W images where there is BBB breakdown or in vascular tumours and slow-flow vascular malformations.
    - Contraindications: if severe renal impairment (relative contraindication if eGFR is < 30 due to the risk of nephrogenic systemic fibrosis (NSF)—this risk is largely mitigated by administering multicyclic gadolinium agents); lactating mothers (no breastfeeding for 24 hours); known allergy.

Magnetic resonance angiography (MRA)

In conventional MRI, flowing blood alters signal intensity by the 'time of flight' and 'phase-shift effect'. Time-of-flight (TOF) angiography uses GE sequences; fast-flowing blood is hyperintense. Two-dimensional TOF is MRA of choice for neck arteries and three-dimensional TOF for the circle of Willis.

Problems
- Blood products are also high signal.
- Insensitive to slow flow: overestimates degree of vessel stenosis; cannot distinguish between occlusion and near occlusion.

Phase contrast (PC) MRA
Useful for assessing dural venous sinuses.

Contrast-enhanced MRA
Uses gadolinium and is independent of flow dynamics and TOF effects.

Diffusion-weighted MRI (DWI)

Acute infarction, amongst several other applications, is high signal. Perfusion-weighted MRI (PWI) measures volume of blood flow to that tissue over time. The combination is under investigation to identify patients with stroke who may have salvageable tissue.

Magnetic resonance spectroscopy (MRS)

Provides information on the relative concentrations and distribution of compounds and ions (^1H, $^{32}P32$, and ^{23}Na). N-acetyl aspartate (NAA) is a marker of neuronal integrity and ↓ concentration indicates neuronal loss, e.g. in neurodegenerative disorders, stroke, and MS. Lactate levels are ↑ in anaerobic metabolism, e.g. stroke. Myoinositol (MI) is a breakdown product in Alzheimer's dementia and tumours.

Functional MRI (fMRI)

Used in the evaluation of physiological alterations that occur in brain tissue during normal and abnormal activity, e.g. epilepsy and migraine.

Clinical applications
- Epilepsy surgery planning.
- Determination of language and memory lateralization (alternative to Wada test).
- Defining the proximity of eloquent areas in surgery planning, e.g. tumours, AVM.

Catheter angiography

Indications

- Characterization of vascular lesions (e.g. tumours, aneurysms, and AVM) prior to surgery or endovascular therapy.
- Investigation of SAH.
- Neck vessels, cerebral and spinal circulation.
- Follow-up on endovascular or operative interventions.

Pre-procedure

- Informed consent is mandatory.
- Check clotting. Contraindicated if INR > 1.3 or platelet count < 100.
- Check renal function.
- IV access necessary.

Contraindications

- Uncooperative patient with no anaesthetic cover.
- Contraindication to contrast:
  - history of contrast reaction;
  - severe renal impairment (but not on dialysis);
  - asthma without steroid prophylaxis unless life-threatening indication—hayfever is not a contraindication.

Note: Patients with DM on metformin must stop the drug for 2 days after contrast study and have renal function checked prior to restarting it.

Procedure

- Catheter angiography is usually performed by the transfemoral approach.
- A Seldinger technique is used to introduce a catheter into the aorta, and iodinated contrast is injected into the arterial circulation during image acquisition.
- Background structures are digitally subtracted (digital subtraction angiography (DSA)) to leave only vessels.
- Patient cooperation and lack of movement (including breath-holding for cerebral DSA) are essential.
- Sedation or anaesthesia may be required.

Complications

Related to puncture

- Groin haematoma, iliac artery dissection, pseudoaneurysm, and a ruptured vessel may require urgent repair.
- Failure to gain access.
- Multiple puncture attempts may lead to AV fistula or distal embolic shower ('trashed foot').
- Vasovagal episodes, especially if puncture is difficult.

Related to angiography:

- 1% risk of stroke, usually temporary. The risk of thromboembolic events is related to duration of procedure and technique. These are determined by level of experience.
- Spinal cord ischaemia due to radicular artery occlusion or embolus in spinal angiography (risk 1–2%).
- Arterial dissection may be a source of emboli.

Related to contrast:

- Mild reaction (vomiting and urticaria).
- Moderate and severe bronchospasm, facial and laryngeal oedema, hypotension, bradycardia, pulmonary oedema, and seizures.

Myelography

Indications

- Patients not suitable for MRI.
- Confirmation of equivocal MRI findings, e.g. nerve root compression.
- Dural fistula.
- Traumatic nerve root avulsion.

Pre-procedure

- Informed consent.
- Check clotting and renal function.

Contraindications

- Raised ICP.
- Pregnancy.
- Previous contrast reaction.
- Clotting abnormality or thrombocytopenia.

Procedure

A maximum of 3 g of iodinated non-ionic contrast is administered intrathecally under fluoroscopic guidance via a standard LP at L3/4. A cervical puncture at C1/2 can be performed if the lumbar approach is unsuccessful.

Complications

- Post-LP headache.
- SAH or extradural haemorrhage.
- Pain.
- Instillation of contrast into subdural or extradural space.
- Infection.
- Contrast reaction including seizures (rare with non-ionic contrast).

Nuclear isotope studies

PET (positron emission tomography)

Uses elements emitting positrons; ^{18}F-labelled deoxyglucose (FDG) most commonly used. This identifies areas of increased glucose metabolism.

Indications

- Distinguishing between radionecrosis and glioma.
- Epilepsy surgery planning.
- Localization of neoplasms in paraneoplastic syndromes.

SPECT (single-photon emission computed tomography)

Uses ^{99m}TC or iodinated (^{123}I) tracer mainly to study blood flow. Thallium SPECT is used to differentiate between abscesses and tumours such as primary CNS lymphoma (PCNSL) and toxoplasmosis in HIV/AIDS patients.

Interventional neuroradiology

Increasingly used in the management of vascular lesions previously only treated by surgery.

- Aneurysm occlusion with endovascular coiling.
- Parent vessel occlusion for giant aneurysm.
- AVM or AVF embolization, both intracranial and intraspinal.
- Hypervascular tumour embolization, e.g. meningioma and glomus tumour.
- Internal carotid and vertebral artery stenting.
- Super-selective intra-arterial or venous sinus thrombolysis.
- Caroticocavernous fistula occlusion.
- Petrosal sinus venous sampling.

Cerebrovascular disease

Ischaemic stroke

CT scan

- CT should be performed as soon as possible, especially if thrombolysis is being considered.
- May detect other unexpected lesions, e.g. tumours.
- If thrombolysis is being considered, haemorrhage and large infarct (> 1/3 MCA territory) are contraindications.
- Contrast not indicated and can be misleading.
- CT in acute stroke will differentiate infarct from haemorrhage for up to 5 days.
- A normal scan excludes haemorrhage but not infarct.
- Small haemorrhages lose their high density (white), become isodense and then hypodense, and therefore may be indistinguishable from infarct: in small haemorrhages by 7–10 days, and in larger haemorrhages by 2–3 weeks.
- Small infarcts less likely to be visible than large ones. 90% of large infarcts are visible at 48 hours compared with 40% of lacunar or small cortical infarcts.
- Large infarcts may show subtle changes by 3 hours (low density and swelling)—depends on expertise of interpretation. Between 10 days and 3 weeks infarcts become isodense and difficult to define ('fogging').
- After 2–3 months they are more visible as same density as CSF and associated with parenchymal volume loss.

MRI

- Shows ischaemic lesion more often than CT and therefore useful in those with CT-scan-negative infarcts.
- However, because of infarct evolution, 'fogging' also occurs with routine MR imaging (T_2, proton density, and T_1) and it may not show lesions.
- FLAIR (fluid-attenuated inversion recovery) sequences increase sensitivity but will reveal additional incidental lesions, making interpretation more difficult.
- Diffusion-weighted imaging (DWI) is very sensitive but not specific for infarction. Encephalitis, demyelinating plaques, and tumours all show increased signal.
- DWI most useful in identifying minor cortical or lacunar strokes, or, in patients with a previous stroke and deteriorating signs, it may show the development of a new lesion.
- Salvageable territory requiring intervention, such as thrombolysis denoted by mismatch of PWI relative to DWI, may be more available in the future.
- GE and especially SWI sequences are sensitive to acute blood products. They are at least as accurate at detecting acute haemorrhage in the acute stroke setting as CT.
- FLAIR allows discrimination of DWI positive acutely infarcted tissue within 3–6 hours from longer than 6 hours of onset of ischaemia and hence potentially aid in selecting patients for thrombolysis presenting with strokes of unknown onset.

Imaging of atheromatous extracranial vessels

Doppler USS

The simplest, safest, and quickest method of assessing carotid (high sensitivity but moderate specificity) and vertebral arteries to detect stenosis or dissection. Very operator-dependent.

DSA

Whilst DSA (conventional catheter angiography) will identify stenosis severity and differentiate between complete occlusions and almost occluded vessels, the risk of stroke (0.3–1%) and cost against the improved reliability and availability of non-invasive techniques means this is rarely undertaken.

CTA and MRA

- Good correlation between normal MRA and CTA and absence of disease.
- Multidetector CT (MDCT) and contrast enhanced MRA (CEMRA) have superseded time-of-flight MRA (non-enhanced technique).
- Both techniques give good morphological assessment but CEMRA may still not differentiate between occlusion and very slow flow ('flow gap').

NASCET

NASCET is the consensus method for measuring internal carotid artery stenosis.

Arterial dissection

- CT scan can be (rarely) diagnostic. Expanded mixed-density carotid artery at the skullbase.
- MRI with fat-suppressed T_1W axials recommended as first choice for suspected carotid dissection. Less reliable for vertebral arteries:
  - 'fried egg appearance'—eccentrically located narrowed lumen within an expanded artery;
  - lumen may be patent (flow void), reduced flow (isointense), or occluded/very slow flow (hyperintense);
  - surrounding crescent of intramural haematoma (hyperintense on T_1W axials with fat suppression after 2–3 days especially).
- Doppler ultrasound may demonstrate an intimal flap, a double lumen, and intramural thrombosis.

If MRI is not diagnostic, CTA or MRA may show lesions. DSA now rarely required.

Venous thrombosis

Difficult diagnosis to make clinically and radiologically.

- CT scan reveals:
  - Local or diffuse swelling.
  - Hyperdense venous sinuses and cortical veins.
  - Parenchymal lesions—often multiple low-attenuation lesions with oedema and haemorrhage (high density). Thalami and basal ganglia involved if internal cerebral veins thrombosed. SAH may be present.
- Contrast-enhanced CT: enhancement of dural sinuses around non-enhancing expanded thrombus ('delta sign').

- CT venogram demonstrates filling defects and expansion of thrombosed sinuses.
- MRI shows:
  - Absent flow void in dural sinus. Rarely, in the acute setting, a T_2W hypointense thrombosed sinus may be mistaken for a patent flow-void.
  - Parenchymal lesions are hyperintense on T_2W/FLAIR with oedema ± haemorrhage ± enhancement ± swelling (local or diffuse).
  - SWI may demonstrate a thrombosed superficial cortical vein.
- MRV shows loss of flow, or irregularity, or severe narrowing, indicating thrombus. However, slow (but normal) flow or a hypoplastic sinus can mimic thrombosis.
- CT venography is often more reliable—especially for the major dural sinuses. DSA very rarely required.
- Multiple modalities may be required to make a diagnosis:
  - prominence of oedema prior to and around haemorrhages suggests venous hypertension;
  - degree of normal variation in the size of the lateral sinuses and cortical veins makes interpretation difficult.

Cerebral vasculitis

- Typically, the appearances are non-specific with periventricular subcortical white matter hyperintensities with or without evidence of cortical infarcts and haemorrhagic foci.
- Intracranial MRA and CTA can give good visualization of first and second order branches of the circle of Willis arteries.
- Catheter angiography is the most sensitive modality with multiple luminal irregularities, narrowings, occlusions, and sometimes aneurysms. Generally reserved for CTA negative cases and appropriate level of suspicion. Often prior to biopsy.

Subarachnoid haemorrhage

Diagnosis of SAH

Non-enhanced CT positive in 95% within the first 24 hours. Sensitivity decreases with time so that at 1 week < 50% positive. Imaging features include the following:

- Blood (high density) in subarachnoid space ± intraparenchymal ± subdural space.
- Distribution of blood indicates site of aneurysm:
  - predominant Sylvian fissure ± temporal lobe = MCA;
  - symmetric distribution or marked involvement of anteroinferior interhemispheric fissure or medial frontal lobe = ACom artery;
  - lateralization in suprasellar, prepontine, ambient cisterns ± tentorial subdural component = PCom artery;
  - prepontine and 4th ventricle = PIC artery;
  - interhemispheric subdural = pericallosal artery;
  - perimesencephalic haemorrhage, i.e. blood in prepontine, interpeduncular, and ambient cisterns = venous aetiology.
- Early communicating hydrocephalus is typical.
- Low-attenuation areas may indicate ischaemia from vasospasm.

MRI

T_1W and T_2W are relatively insensitive; FLAIR is the best sequence with hyperintensity in the subarachnoid space. Hypointense on T_2^*.

Differential diagnosis

- Leptomeningeal infection.
- Inflammation.
- Infiltration.
- Propofol anaesthetic/100% oxygenation.

Investigation of cause of SAH

- MRA and CTA detect aneurysms > 3 mm.
- Negative in 15–20% of cases of aneurysmal SAH.
- Aneurysms are multiple in 20% and these modalities should provide information on which is responsible as well as vasospasm.
- Phase contrast MRA removes effect of T_1 shortening of blood.
- DSA remains the gold standard:
  - greater sensitivity for aneurysms < 3 mm;
  - largest aneurysm with irregular contour ('nipple') will typically be responsible for the SAH;
  - DSA identifies vasospasm accurately;
  - however, negative in 7–10%.

Guidelines for imaging for SAH

- If non-enhanced CT positive or LP positive → CTA (or DSA).
- If CTA positive → surgery or DSA + endovascular coiling.
- If CTA negative → DSA.
- If DSA positive → surgery or endovascular coiling.

- If DSA negative → may be due to vasospasm or large haematoma → consider repeat DSA after an interval.
- If no vasospasm, probable perimesencephalic bleed requiring no further investigation, provided typical distribution of SAH.

Saccular aneurysms

- These are well defined extra-axial lobulated lesions that may present as a result of an SAH or size.
- On CT, if patent, show up as hyperdense to brain tissue and enhancing with or without intramural calcification. If thrombosed, hyperdense lesion with calcification commonly.
- MRI shows variable signal due to slow or turbulent flow. 50% have flow void. Thrombosed lesions often hyperintense on T_1W and hypotense on T_2W images.
- Further investigation is with MRA or CTA or DSA.

Differential diagnosis

- Meningioma, especially in suprasellar region.
- Macroadenoma/suprasellar mass (especially hyperintense on T_1W).
- CP angle AICA or PICA aneurysm.
- 3rd ventricular mass (basilar tip aneurysm).

Note: Differentiating an unruptured aneurysm from a mass, particularly if thrombosed, can be difficult. Aneurysm should always be considered in the differential diagnosis of a mass in the classic sites.

Intracerebral haemorrhage

Guidelines

Non-enhanced CT and then:

1. If haematoma location and history typical of hypertension, i.e. striatocapsular (65%), thalamus (20%), pons and cerebellum (10%), no further radiology necessary.
2. If atypical contrast-enhanced MRI, T_2* (or SWI) may give evidence of previous haemorrhagic lesions. Also consider MRV or CT venography.
3. If there is suspicion of an underlying vascular abnormality or an aneurysm, perform a DSA.
4. If initial investigations are unhelpful, repeat delayed MRI or DSA as the acute haematoma can obscure features.

Serial imaging features

Hyperacute (< 6 hours)

- Presence of oxyhaemoglobin, mass effect, and oedema.
- CT: hyperdense with low density elements.
- MRI: T_1W isointense, T_2W variable, T_2* heterogeneous or hypointense.

Acute (6 hours to 3 days)

- Presence of deoxyhaemoglobin, mass effect, and oedema.
- CT: hyperdense.
- MRI: T_1W isointense, T_2W hypointense, T_2* hypointense.

Early subacute (3 days to 1 week)

- Presence of cellular methaemoglobin, mass effect, and oedema.
- CT: hyperdense.
- MRI: T_1W hyperintense, T_2W hypointense, T_2* hypointense.

Late subacute (1 week to 1 month)

- Free methaemoglobin, minimal mass effect, and oedema.
- CT: isodense with hypodense rim.
- MRI: T_1W hyperintense, T_2W hyperintense, T_2* hypointense.

Chronic (months)

- Presence of haemosiderin. No mass effect or oedema.
- CT: hypodense.
- MRI: T_1W, T_2W, and T_2* hypodense.

Note

Coagulopathy and severe anaemia result in isodense acute haematoma on CT. Rapidly accumulating haematomas may have fluid levels and swirls.

Guidelines for head injury

- No indication for SXR unless there is a penetrating injury (or if suspected non-accidental injury in children).
- Non-enhanced CT ± bone windows indicated if:
  - GCS < 15;
  - open, depressed, or skull base fracture;
  - retrograde amnesia;
  - seizure or focal neurological deficit;
  - persistent headache and/or vomiting;
  - patients > 65 years of age or with coagulopathy.
- However, 5% of patients with GCS = 15 and no other abnormality will have an abnormal scan. There is pressure to perform CT in all cases of head injury.
- Brain imaging should be carried out early, especially to manage mass lesions.
- Have a low threshold for re-imaging as intra- and extra-axial mass lesions may expand rapidly or insidiously.
- MRI is more sensitive for intrinsic and shallow extra-axial collections as well as diffuse brain injury.
- Consider cervical spine injury and appropriate imaging in all head injury patients.

Imaging strategies for cervical spine trauma

- MRI has revolutionized the diagnostic evaluation of spinal injuries.
- Plain radiography and CT remain the most practical and cost-effective methods of investigation in the acute situation.
- Early surgical intervention is aimed at stabilization of the vertebral column and decompression of the spinal canal.
- Appropriate imaging is critical.
- MR examination in the acute period is indicated in any patient who has a persistent neurological deficit after spinal trauma.
- Some centres perform cervical spine MRI in any unconscious patient with normal X-ray and CT to exclude ligamentous and disc injury.

Figure 9.1 gives an algorithm for the use of imaging in cervical spine trauma.

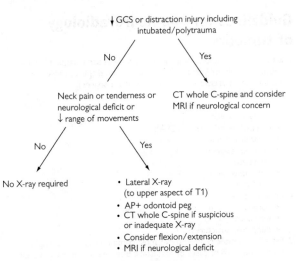

↓ GCS or distraction injury including
intubated/polytrauma

No / Yes

Neck pain or tenderness or   CT whole C-spine and consider
neurological deficit or   MRI if neurological concern
↓ range of movements

No / Yes

No X-ray required

- Lateral X-ray
  (to upper aspect of T1)
- AP+ odontoid peg
- CT whole C-spine if suspicious
  or inadequate X-ray
- Consider flexion/extension
- MRI if neurological deficit

Fig. 9.1 Algorithm for the diagnosis of cervical spine trauma.

Guidelines for the neuroradiology of tumours

1. Is the lesion extra-axial or intrinsic? Extra-axial compartment involves extradural, sub- or intradural, and subarachnoid spaces (which also include the basal cisterns and intraventricular spaces).
- Extra-axial lesions:
  - pineal;
  - intraventricular;
  - cerebellopontine angle (CPA);
  - parasellar region;
  - foramen magnum;
  - skull base;
  - cavernous sinus;
  - meninges.
- Intrinsic lesions:
  - corpus callosum;
  - mainly cortex;
  - deep grey structures.
2. Establish multiplicity. Metastases most common cause of multiple lesions, but 50% of cases of metastatic disease present with a solitary lesion.
3. Evidence of mass effect. May be subtle with effacement of sulci or interhemispheric hemisphere, gyral, or parenchymal distortion. Lesions other than tumours can cause mass effect:
  - acute ischaemic infarcts;
  - acute haematomas;
  - inflammatory masses;
  - demyelinating lesions ('tumefactive').
4. Other imaging characteristics:
  - surrounding oedema;
  - degree of definition;
  - presence of calcification (CT may be necessary);
  - degree and pattern of enhancement;
  - hetereogeneity;
  - necrosis.
5. Consider alternative diagnoses—clinical input essential.
  - Multiple areas of abnormality can be due to encephalitis, multifocal glioma, or acute embolic infarcts.
  - Differential diagnoses for ring-enhancing lesion: tumour, abscess, haematoma, aneurysm, or inflammatory lesion.
  - Remember lymphoma as a differential diagnosis.

CNS infections

Meningitis (acute viral, bacterial, or granulomatous (e.g. TB))

Suspected cases do not require imaging routinely unless:
- reduced level of consciousness;
- symptoms and signs of raised ICP;
- focal neurological signs;
- seizures.

Imaging features

CT and MRI may be normal.
- CT may reveal ventricular enlargement, effacement of the basal cisterns, high-density subarachnoid space exudate. With contrast exudates may be more prominent and may show pial enhancement.
- MRI may show leptomeningeal enhancement. Other complications of meningitis include hydrocephalus, ventriculitis (ependymitis), abscess, or empyema formation. Vasculitis and venous thrombosis may sometimes be evident.

Differential diagnosis of meningeal thickening
- Metastatic disease including lymphoma.
- Sarcoidosis.
- Post-LP or shunting.

Encephalitis (herpes simplex)

Usually involves the limbic system: temporal lobe/insula/subfrontal region and cingulate gyrus.

Imaging features

CT and, less so, MRI may be normal, at least initially.
- CT: grey matter + white matter, low attenuation with mass effect ± patchy enhancement.
- MRI more sensitive with bilateral changes detected earlier. Cytotoxic oedema ↓ T_1W and ↑ T_2W. Haemorrhage and necrosis later.

Differential diagnosis
- Infarction.
- Tumour.
- Limbic encephalitis (paraneoplastic).

HIV infection

HIV encephalopathy

Characterized by atrophy and ill-defined white matter hyperintensity on T_2W images. Usually bilateral; commonly frontal with no enhancement or mass effect. Differential diagnosis is PML or CMV encephalitis.

Opportunistic infections and tumours

Toxoplasmosis

Most common cause of mass lesions in HIV-infected patients. Ring-enhancing mass lesions with mass effect usually involving the basal ganglia and at the grey/white matter interface. Rarely, haemorrhagic. Differential diagnosis:
- primary CNS lymphoma (PCNSL);
- tuberculous abscesses or tuberculomata;
- fungal mass lesions.

Cryptococcal infection
- *Cryptococcus neoformans* is most common cause of meningitis in HIV patients.
- Imaging studies may be normal or show nodular leptomeningeal enhancement, basal ganglia hyperintensities (gelatinous pseudocysts), cryptococcomas (small parenchymal mass lesions), and hydrocephalus (see Fig. 9.2).

CMV
- Typically results in an ependymitis with nodular enhancement and periventricular oedema.
- Also causes a lumbosacral polyradiculopathy with nodular enhancement of the nerve roots.
- Differential diagnoses:
  - lymphoma;
  - neurosyphilis.

Progressive multifocal leucoencephalopathy (PML)
- Typically involves the parieto-occipital lobes with discrete white matter lesions ↓ T_1W and ↑ T_2W images.
- Little or no enhancement or mass effect. CT reveals low-attenuation white matter lesions.

Immune reconstitution syndrome

Reconstitution of the immune system following the introduction of combination antiretroviral therapy (cART) can cause the development of complex brain appearances. Lesions with enhancement, oedema and mass effect are typically observed.

Parasitic infections—cysticercosis
- Imaging appearances vary with the stage of cyst formation with some individuals showing lesions of differing ages.
- Although usually multiple, solitary in 40%.
- Brain parenchymal lesions more common than intraventricular.
- Subarachnoid lesions in 10%. Grape-like clusters of cysts ('racemose') may mimic a tumour.

Cysts can be classified as follows:
- Vesicular: thin-walled cyst of CSF density on CT and MRI. Mural nodule represents the scolex. No enhancement or oedema.
- Colloidal vesicular: hyperdense cyst with enhancement and oedema on CT. On MRI, cyst is iso/hyperintense on T_1W and hyperintense on T_2W images.
- Granular nodular: involuting cyst is isodense on CT with calcifying scolex hyperdense. Reducing oedema and enhancement. On MRI isointense on T_1W and hypodense on T_2W.
- Nodular calcified: small calcified nodules on CT with no oedema or enhancement.

Other complications include obstructive hydrocephalus and meningitis.

Tuberculosis

TB meningitis
- CT scan: iso- or hyperdense exudates in the subarachnoid spaces with avid enhancement with contrast. Hydrocephalus common.
- MRI: basal cistern exudates are isointense on T_1W, hyperintense on T_2W. Thick nodular enhancement with gadolinium. Additional pathology such as arteritis causing ischaemic changes may also be seen.

Tuberculoma
- CT scan: solitary or multiple lesions of variable density develop from areas of low-density cerebritis. Calcification uncommon (< 20%); implies old lesions. With contrast the 'target sign' = central enhancement with enhancing rim and a non-enhancing intervening portion and surrounding oedema.
- MRI: T_2W hyperintense centre with hypointense rim, nodular enhancement, and oedema.

Differential diagnoses
Abscesses, metastases, granulomatous lesions, e.g. sarcoidosis.

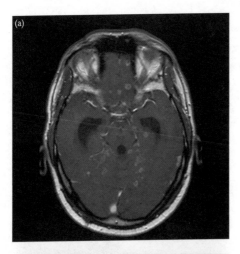

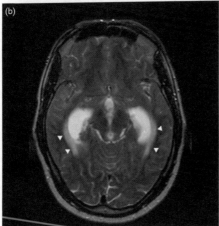

Fig. 9.2 Parenchymal TB. Axial (a) post-contrast-enhanced and (b) T_2-weighted MRI. Multiple ring enhancing nodules in infra- and supratentorial compartments with surrounding white matter vasogenic oedema. Note meningeal involvement with obstructive hydrocephalus and periventricular transependymal interstitial oedema lateral to the grossly dilated temporal horns ((b) *white arrowheads*).

Appendices

1 Neurological disability scales *595*
2 Clinical pearls *599*
3 Neurological eponyms *603*
4 Useful websites *611*

Appendix 1

Neurological disability scales

Box A1.1 Kurtzke expanded disability status scale (quantifies disability in multiple sclerosis)

1.0	No disability; minimal signs in one FS (functional system)
1.5	No disability; minimal signs in more than one FS
2.0	Minimal disability in one FS
2.5	Mild disability in one FS or minimal disability in two FS
3.0	Moderate disability in one FS, or mild disability in three or four FS; fully ambulatory
3.5	Fully ambulatory but with moderate disability in one FS and more than minimal disability in several others
4.0	Fully ambulatory without aid; self-sufficient; up and about some 12 hours a day despite relatively severe disability; able to walk without aid or rest some 500 metres
4.5	Fully ambulatory without aid; up and about much of the day; able to work a full day; may otherwise have some limitation of full activity or require minimal assistance; characterized by relatively severe disability; able to walk without aid or rest some 300 metres
5.0	Ambulatory without aid or rest for about 200 metres; disability severe enough to impair full daily activities (e.g. work a full day without special provisions)
5.5	Ambulatory without aid or rest for about 100 metres; disability severe enough to preclude full daily activities
6.0	Intermittent or unilateral constant assistance (cane, crutch, brace) required to walk about 100 metres with or without resting
6.5	Constant bilateral assistance (canes, crutches, braces) required to walk about 20 metres without resting
7.0	Unable to walk beyond approximately 5 metres even with aid; essentially restricted to wheelchair; wheels self in standard wheelchair and transfers alone; up and about in wheelchair some 12 hours a day
7.5	Unable to take more than a few steps; restricted to wheelchair; may need aid in transfer; wheels self but cannot carry on in standard wheelchair a full day; may require motorized wheelchair
8.0	Essentially restricted to bed or chair or perambulated in wheelchair, but may be out of bed itself much of the day; retains many self-care functions; generally has effective use of arms
8.5	Essentially restricted to bed much of day; has some effective use of arms; retains some self-care functions
9.0	Confined to bed; can still communicate and eat
9.5	Totally helpless bedbound patient; unable to communicate effectively or eat/swallow
10.0	Death due to MS

Table A1.1 Barthel Index for chronic neurodisability[*]

Parameter	Finding	Points
Controlling bowels	Independent. Patient is able to control bowels and have no accidents	10
	Patient may occasionally have an accident or may require a suppository or enema	5
	Cannot meet defined criteria	0
Controlling bladder	Independent. Patient is able to control bladder day and night	10
	Patient may occasionally have an accident or cannot wait for a bedpan or is unable to get to the toilet in time	5
	Cannot meet defined criteria	0
Getting on and off toilet	Independent. Patient can get on and off toilet, adjust clothing, use toilet paper, and keep clothes from becoming soiled. The patient can use an object for support if needed	10
	With help	5
	Cannot meet defined criteria	0
Feeding	Independent. Patient can feed self if food is placed within reach. The patient may use an assistive device if needed. Eating needs to be accomplished within a reasonable time	10
	Some help is needed such as cutting up food	5
	Cannot meet defined criteria	0
Moving from wheelchair to bed and return	Independent in all phases of the activity	15
	With some minimal help or some supervision	10
	Requires assistance	5
	Cannot meet defined criteria	0
Walking on level surface	Independent. Patient can walk at least 50 yards without help or supervision	15
	With help	10
	Unable to walk but can propel a wheelchair independently	5
	Unable to walk and unable to propel a wheelchair	0
Dressing	Independent	10
	With help	5
	Cannot meet defined criteria	0

Table A1.1 (*Contd.*)

Parameter	Finding	Points
Ascend and descend stairs	Independent. Patient is able to go up and down a flight of stairs safely without supervision or help	10
	With help	5
	Cannot meet defined criteria	0
Grooming	Patient can wash, comb hair, and brush teeth. Men can shave themselves and women can apply make-up	5
	Cannot meet defined criteria	0
Bathing self	Patient may use a bath tub or shower, or take a complete sponge bath unassisted	5
	Cannot meet defined criteria	0

* Barthel Index = sum of points for all 10 items (minimum score 0, maximum 100).

Table A1.2 Modified Hoehn and Yahr scale

Stage of disease	Description of severity of disease
1	Unilateral involvement only
1.5	Unilateral and axial involvement
2	Bilateral involvement without impairment of balance
2.5	Mild bilateral involvement with recovery on pull test
3.0	Mild to moderate involvement; some postural instability but physically independent
4.0	Severe disability; able to walk and stand unassisted
5.0	Wheelchair-bound or bedridden unless aided

Table A1.3 Rankin stroke disability scale

Scale	Description of severity of disease
1	Able to carry out all activities of daily living; almost no disability
2	Slight disability; self-caring; may not be able to carry out all activities of daily living
3	Moderate disability; able to walk without an assistant or with a stick; requires some help in daily tasks
4	Moderately severe disability; needs an assistant to walk; needs help with toileting and other activities
5	Severe disability; bedbound and incontinent, requiring continuous nursing care

Appendix 2

Clinical pearls

These are useful clinical vignettes that have been collected on ward rounds and at clinical meetings, but never seem to enter the textbooks. The following are personal favourites (HM and AW).

- *Absent ankle jerks, extensor plantars*
  Causes:
  - B_{12} deficiency;
  - Friedreich's ataxia;
  - HIV (neuropathy + myelopathy);
  - spinal AVM;
  - cervical and lumbar spondylosis;
  - syphilis (taboparesis).
- *Beevor's sign:* movement of the umbilicus on attempting to sit up indicates weakness of the abdominal muscles away from direction of movement. Causes:
  - muscular dystrophy;
  - thoracic radicular muscle weakness.
- *Cluster headache*
  - Patients are restless and walk around, whereas migraine sufferers prefer to lie still.
  - May experience unilateral photophobia ipsilateral to headache.
- *Downbeat nystagmus:* usually evident on lateral gaze. Causes:
  - foramen magnum lesion;
  - Arnold–Chiari malformation;
  - tumour;
  - syringobulbia/myelia;
  - cerebellar degeneration.
- *Dropped finger* when hands held outstretched and pronated. Causes:
  - anterior horn cell disease (MND, syringomyelia);
  - multifocal motor neuropathy with block;
  - transiently in brachial neuritis;
  - ruptured tendon as in rheumatoid arthritis.
- *Foot drop*
  Causes:
  - common peroneal nerve lesion (inversion preserved);
  - L5 root lesion (inversion affected);
  - cortical lesion (extensor plantar);
  - cord lesion;
  - sciatic nerve lesion (common peroneal nerve fibres selectively affected);
  - rarely, myopathic cause, e.g. IBM or MG;
  - consider dystonia if no weakness.

- *Functional coma or status epilepticus*
  - Elevate one arm over the face and drop. In patients with retained consciousness the arm will fall to one side missing the face. In true coma the arm will fall onto the face.
  - Insert a vibrating tuning fork gently into one nostril. Very unpleasant and unexpected stimulus and will wake most non-organic patients.
- *Headache*
  Red flags suggesting serious underlying disorder:
  - systemic symptoms: fever, weight loss;
  - risk factors: HIV, cancer;
  - focal neurological signs;
  - sudden onset (thunderclap);
  - age > 50 years (giant cell arteritis);
  - previous headache with change in character, severity, or resistant to therapy.
- *Head thrust test (Halmaygi)*
  If positive indicates lateral semicircular canal dysfunction.
- *Hoover's sign*
  When assessing hip flexion on one side, test for counterextension on the contralateral side. If absent, indicates inadequate effort.
    Please see 🖱 <http://www.neurosymptoms.org/> (a self-help website for patients with functional symptoms).
- *Internuclear ophthalmoplegia*
  Causes:
  - MS;
  - pontine stroke;
  - MG (pseudo-INO);
  - Wernicke's encephalopathy.
- *Jaw supporting sign*
  Indicative of neck flexion weakness especially in MG.
- *Lhermitte's sign*
  Neck flexion results in paraesthesiae down the spine or arms.
   Causes:
  - MS;
  - cervical spondylosis (occasionally, reversed with neck extension);
  - B_{12} deficiency;
  - cervical cord tumour;
  - cisplatin.
- *Lumbar canal stenosis*
  Patients can cycle for miles but develop pain and weakness after walking a few yards. In the flexed trunk position the AP diameter is increased.
- *Lumbar puncture*
  Technically this is much easier to perform with the patient sitting and leaning forward over a bed tray/trolley with pillows. However, this position is not suitable if it is necessary to measure the opening pressure.

- *Neck flexion extension weakness*
  Causes:
  - myopathy;
  - MG;
  - MND;
  - myotonic dystrophy;
  - Guillain–Barré syndrome.
- *Parkinson's disease*
  Reconsider diagnosis if:
  - early falls, especially backwards (PSP);
  - early dysarthria and dysphagia (PSP);
  - early autonomic dysfunction (MSA);
  - marked antecollis (MSA);
  - rapid decline—'wheelchair sign';
  - early cognitive dysfunction (DCLB);
  - apraxia, myoclonus (CBD).
- *Sensory levels*
  May be inaccurate in spinal cord lesions, e.g. cervical myelopathy may be
  result in thoracic sensory level.
- *Shoulder shrug*
  In hemiplegic or hemirigid (as in parkinsonism) patients, a weak or
  delayed shrug implies intracerebral lesion rather than spinal cord lesion.
  Innervation of upper trapezius fibres located C1–C5, and are rarely all
  involved in cervical cord lesions.

Appendix 3

Neurological eponyms

Adie pupil: large pupil reacting slowly to light and accommodation. W.J. Adie, English neurologist.

Alzheimer's disease: most common cause of dementia. A. Alzheimer, German neurologist who collaborated with Nissl, Erb, and Kraepelin.

Anton's syndrome: visual anosognosia. G. Anton, Austrian neurologist.

Argyll Robertson pupil: syphilitic pupil that 'accommodates but doesn't react'. D. Argyll Robertson, Scottish physician and golfer.

Arnold–Chiari syndrome: congenital inferior displacement of cerebellar tonsils. J. Arnold/H. Chiari, German/Austrian pathologists.

Babinski sign: stroking lateral aspect of sole resulting in plantar extension of big toe. J. Babinski, Polish neurologist, pupil of Charcot.

Bassen–Kornzweig disease: ataxia, retinitis pigmentosa, abetalipo-proteinaemia. F. Bassen/H. Kornzweig, US physician/ophthalmologist.

Battle's sign: bruising over mastoid suggesting fractured base of skull. W. Battle, English surgeon.

Becker muscular dystrophy/myotonia congenita. P. Becker, German geneticist.

Beevor's sign: excessive displacement of umbilicus on attempted sit-up due to weakness of abdominal musculature. C. Beevor, English neurologist.

Bell's palsy: idiopathic lower motor neuron paralysis of facial nerve. C. Bell, Scottish surgeon, accomplished artist, founder of the Middlesex Hospital.

Benedikt's syndrome: ipsilateral oculomotor palsy with contralateral ataxia. M. Benedikt, Austrian physician and soldier.

Berry aneurysm. J. Berry, English surgeon.

Binswanger's dementia: widespread cerebral small vessel disease. O. Binswanger, German psychiatrist.

Bourneville's disease: tuberous sclerosis. D. Bourneville, French neurologist.

Broca's aphasia: expressive aphasia. P. Broca, French surgeon and Darwinist.

Brodmann areas: cytoarchitectural map of the brain. K. Brodmann, German neurologist.

Brown-Séquard syndrome: hemitransection of the cord leading to ipsilateral paralysis and impairment of light touch, joint position, and vibration sense with contralateral impairment of temperature and pinprick sensation. C. Brown-Séquard, Mauritian neurologist, peripatetic, with eccentric ideas about testicular extracts.

Canavan's disease: infantile dysmyelination with macrocephaly. M. Canavan, US pathologist.

Charcot–Marie–Tooth disease: peroneal muscular atrophy/HMSN. J. Charcot, French neurologist. Described multiple sclerosis, MND, and ankle clonus. Taught P. Marie, Babinski, and Freud. P. Marie, French neurologist. H. Tooth, English physician, keen musician, and carpenter.

Cheyne–Stokes breathing: alternating hyperpnoea and apnoea. J. Cheyne, Scottish physician. W. Stokes, Irish physician.

Chvostek's sign: tapping skin over facial nerve induces muscle twitching; seen in tetany and anxiety. F. Chvostek, Austrian surgeon.

Claude syndrome: ipsilateral oculomotor palsy with contralateral ataxia and chorea due to lesion in red nucleus. H. Claude, French neurologist and colleague of Lhermitte.

Cockayne syndrome: dwarfism, microcephaly, dermatitis, deafness, pyramidal and cerebellar signs. E. Cockayne, English paediatrician and entomologist.

Collet–Sicard syndrome: jugular foramen syndrome involving 9th to 12th cranial nerves). F. Collet, French otolaryngologist.

Creutzfeldt–Jakob disease: rapid-onset dementia due to abnormal prion protein. A. Jakob, German neuropathologist. H. Creutzfeldt, German pathologist.

Dandy–Walker syndrome: maldevelopment of foramina of Luschka and Magendie leading to hydrocephalus. W. Dandy, US neurosurgeon and temporary assistant to Cushing. A. Walker, US neurosurgeon.

Dejerine-Klumpke syndrome: lower brachial plexus palsy (waiter's tip sign). A. Dejerine-Klumpke, French neurologist.

Dejerine anterior bulbar palsy: anterior spinal artery occlusion; Dejerine–Landouzy dystrophy (FSH); Dejerine–Sottas neuropathy (HMSN III); and Dejerine–Thomas atrophy (OPCA). J. Dejerine, French neurologist and amateur boxer.

Dercum's disease: lipomas and neuropathy. F. Dercum, US neurologist.

Devic's disease: optic neuritis and myelopathy. E. Devic, French physician.

Duane's syndrome: developmental anomaly leading to contraction of the globe and narrowing of the palpebral fissure on attempted abduction of the affected eye. A. Duane, US ophthalmologist.

Duchenne muscular dystrophy: X-linked muscular dystrophy. G. Duchenne, eccentric peripatetic French neurologist who invented the punch muscle biopsy.

Eaton–Lambert myasthenic syndrome: weakness, post-tetanic facilitation, associated with voltage-gated calcium-channel antibodies. L. Eaton, US neurologist. E. Lambert, US neurophysiologist.

Edinger–Westphal nucleus: autonomic nucleus of oculomotor nerve. L. Edinger, German neurologist and hypnotist. C. Westphal, German neurologist who described Wilson's disease, the deep tendon reflex, and periodic paralysis. Mentored Pick and Wernicke.

Ekbom's syndrome: restless legs or delusional parasitosis. K. Ekbom, Swedish neurologist.

Erb–Duchenne paralysis: upper brachial plexus palsy. W. Erb, German neurologist and keen advocate of the tendon hammer.

Fabry's disease: angiokeratoma, painful neuropathy, stroke, acroparaesthesiae, and renal failure. J. Fabry, German dermatologist.

Fazio–Londe syndrome: pontobulbar atrophy. E. Fazio, Italian physician. P. Londe, French neurologist.

Foix–Alajouanine syndrome: subacute necrotizing myelopathy. C. Foix, French neurologist and lyricist. Pupil of Marie. T. Alajouanine, French neurologist.

Foster Kennedy syndrome: optic atrophy and contralateral papilloedema associated with frontal tumours. R. Foster Kennedy, Irish neurologist.

Fothergill disease: trigeminal neuralgia. J. Fothergill, English physician and abolitionist who coined the phrase 'I climbed on the backs of the poor to the pockets of the rich'.

Foville syndrome: gaze palsy, facial palsy, and contralateral hemiplegia due to lesion in the pons. A. Foville, French neurologist and Director of Asylums.

Friedreich's ataxia: autosomal recessive spinocerebellar degeneration. N. Friedreich, German neurologist, pupil of Virchow.

Froin's syndrome: high CSF protein secondary to spinal 'block'. G. Froin, French physician.

Froment's sign: flexion of thumb on attempting to hold a sheet of paper between index finger and thumb due to weakness of adductor pollicis. J. Froment, French physician.

Gelineau disease: narcolepsy. J. Gelineau, French physician.

Gerstmann's syndrome: right–left confusion, acalculia, finger agnosia due to dominant parietal lesion. J. Gerstmann, US neuropsychiatrist.

Gilles de la Tourette syndrome: tics. G. Gilles de la Tourette, French neurologist and pupil of Charcot.

Gordon reflex: compression of calf resulting in extension of the big toe in pyramidal lesions. A. Gordon, French neurologist.

Gowers' manoeuvre: inability to stand from sitting without using arms. W. Gowers, English neurologist and stenographer.

Gradenigo's syndrome: pain, deafness, and lateral rectus palsy. C. Gradenigo, Italian otolaryngologist.

Greenfield disease: metachromatic leucodystrophy caused by deficiency of aryl sulphatase A. J. Greenfield, English neuropathologist.

Guillain–Barré syndrome: acute demyelinating neuropathy. C. Guillain, French neurologist. J. Barré, French neurologist and colleague of Babinski.

Hallervorden–Spatz disease: autosomal recessive disorder with rigidity, dementia, and optic atrophy. J. Hallervorden, German neurologist and Nazi. H. Spatz, German neurologist.

Heidenhain variant: CJD with blindness. A. Heidenhain, German neurologist.

Hoffman syndrome: muscle hypertrophy and weakness seen in hypothyroidism. J. Hoffman, German neurologist.

Holmes' tremor: midbrain tremor. G. Holmes, Irish neurologist, keen gardener and golfer.

Hoover's sign: manoeuvre that may distinguish organic from hysterical hemiplegias. C. Hoover, US physician.

Horner's syndrome: ptosis and meiosis due to sympathetic lesion. J. Horner, Swiss opthalmologist who also established that red–green colour blindness was X-linked.

Huntington's disease: autosomal dominant neurodegenerative disease characterized by dementia and chorea. G. Huntington, US general practitioner.

Ishihara plates: test for colour blindness. S. Ishihara, Japanese ophthalmologist.

Jacksonian seizure: simple partial motor seizure. J. Hughlings Jackson, English neurologist and popularizer of the ophthalmoscope.

Jacod syndrome: optic atrophy, ophthalmoplegia, and trigeminal neuralgia due to lesion in petrosphenoid space. M. Jacod, French neurologist.

Jendrassik manoeuvre: reinforcement of deep tendon reflexes. E. Jendrassik, Hungarian physician.

Kayser–Fleischer ring: brown pigment in iris indicative of copper deposition in Wilson's disease. B. Kayser, German ophthalmologist. R. Fleischer, German physician.

Kernig's sign: flexion of the thigh and extension of the lower limb causing pain in the hamstrings in meningeal irritation. V. Kernig, Russian physician.

Kernohan syndrome: herniation of the temporal lobe causing traction on the contralateral cerebral peduncle and false localization as the weakness is in the ipsilateral limbs. J. Kernohan, Irish pathologist.

Korsakoff 's psychosis: loss of short-term memory usually due to alcoholism. S. Korsakoff, Russian neuropsychiatrist and humanist.

Kozhevnikov epilepsy: epilepsia partialis continua. A. Kozhevnikov, Russian neurologist and teacher of Korsakoff.

Krabbe's disease: globoid leucodystrophy. K. Krabbe, Danish neurologist.

Kufs' disease: ceroid neuronal lipofuscinosis. H. Kufs, German neurologist.

Kugelberg–Welander syndrome: spinal muscular atrophy (SMA), autosomal recessive, proximal anterior horn cell disorder. E. Kugelberg, M. Welander, Swedish neurologists.

Lafora body disease: progressive myoclonic epilepsy. G. Lafora, Spanish physician.

Lasègue's sign: pain and spasm induced by straight-leg raising in patients with lumbar pathology. E. Lasègue, French physician and flatmate of Claude Bernard.

Laurence–Moon–Biedl syndrome: retinitis pigmentosa, hypogonadism, and polydactyly. J. Laurence, English ophthalmologist. R. Moon, US ophthalmologist. A. Biedl, Czech physician.

Leber's optic atrophy: mitochondrial disease causing optic atrophy. T. von Leber, German ophthalmologist.

Leigh's syndrome: subacute necrotizing white matter disease of childhood. D. Leigh, English neuropathologist.

Lennox–Gastaut syndrome: myoclonic and atonic seizures of childhood. W. Lennox, US neurologist. H. Gastaut, French neurobiologist.

Lhermitte's sign: flexion of the neck causing electric shock-like sensation in cervical myelopathy. J. Lhermitte, French neurologist and theologian.

Luschka foramen: foramen of fourth ventricle. H. von Luschka, German anatomist.

Luysian bodies: subthalamic and thalamic nuclei. J. Luys, French neurologist and hypnotist.

Magendie foramen: fourth ventricular foramen F. Magendie, French physiologist and vivisectionist.

Marchiafava–Bignami syndrome: degeneration of corpus callosum usually due to alcoholism. E. Marchiafava, Italian neurologist. A. Bignami, Italian physician.

Marcus Gunn pupil: afferent pupillary defect. R. Marcus Gunn, Scottish ophthalmologist and fossil collector.

Melkersson–Rosenthal syndrome: facial palsy and fissured tongue. E. Melkersson, Swedish physician. C. Rosenthal, German neurologist.

Millard–Gubler syndrome: pontine lesion leading to facial and abducens palsies with contralateral hemiplegia. A. Millard, French physician. A. Gubler, French physician and botanist.

Miller Fisher syndrome: variant of Guillain–Barré syndrome characterized by ophthalmoplegia, ataxia, and areflexia. C. Miller Fisher, Canadian neurologist.

Mollaret meningitis: recurrent aseptic meningitis. P. Mollaret, French physician.

Monakow syndrome: hemiplegia, hemianaesthesia, and hemianopia due to thrombosis of the anterior choroidal artery. C. von Monakow, Russian neurologist.

Moniz sign: forced plantar flexion of the ankle leading to extension of the toes in pyramidal tract disease. A. Moniz, Portuguese neurologist and co-signatory to the Treaty of Versailles.

Foramen of Monro: foramen between lateral and third ventricles. A. Monro, Scottish anatomist.

Mott's law of anticipation: hereditary diseases appearing earlier in successive generations. F. Mott, English neuropathologist.

McArdle's syndrome: glycogen storage disease type V. B. McArdle, English neurologist.

MacCormac reflex: crossed adduction of contralateral thigh induced by eliciting the knee jerk in pyramidal tract disease. W. MacCormac, Irish surgeon.

Naffziger test: pressure on the jugular vein causes increased CSF pressure. H. Naffziger, US neurosurgeon.

Niemann–Pick disease: organomegaly and progressive dementia. A. Niemann, German paediatrician. L. Pick, German pathologist.

Nothnagel syndrome: ipsilateral oculomotor palsy and ataxia. H. Nothnagel, Austrian physician.

Ondine's curse: centrally mediated apnoea. Ondine, a legendary water nymph.

Oppenheim reflex: stroking medial side of tibia leading to extension of the great toe in pyramidal tract lesions. H. Oppenheim, German neurologist.

Pancoast syndrome: T1 root lesion usually caused by tumour at lung apex. H. Pancoast, US radiologist.

Parinaud's syndrome: dorsal midbrain lesion leading to failure of upgaze and light-near dissociation. H. Parinaud, French ophthalmologist.

Parkinson's disease: paralysis agitans J. Parkinson, English physician and pamphleteer. His house in Hoxton Square is now a nightclub.

Pick's disease: frontotemporal dementia. A. Pick, Czech physician and music lover.

Pringle disease: tuberous sclerosis. J. Pringle, English dermatologist.

Purkinje cells: cells of the cerebellar cortex. J. Purkinje, Bohemian physiologist and nationalist.

Queckenstedt test: compression of the internal jugular vein during a lumbar puncture to test patency of the subarachnoid space. H. Queckenstedt, German neurologist.

Radovici's sign: palmomental reflex. J. Radovici, Romanian neurologist.

Ramsay Hunt syndrome: myoclonic ataxia or facial nerve palsy induced by herpes zoster. J. Ramsay Hunt, US neurologist.

Raymond syndrome: abducens palsy and contralateral hemiplegia. F. Raymond, French neurologist and successor to Charcot.

Recklinghausen's disease: neurofibromatosis type I. F. von Recklinghausen, German pathologist.

Refsum's disease: retinitis pigmentosa, anosmia, neuropathy, and syndactyly caused by accumulation of phytanic acid. S. Refsum, Norwegian physician.

Riley–Day syndrome: familial dysautonomia. C. Riley, R. Day, US paediatricians.

Rolando fissure: central cerebral sulcus. L. Rolando, Italian anatomist and physician to Maria Theresa, Empress of Austria.

Romberg's sign: seen in vestibular disease and sensory ataxia where a patient cannot remain standing on eye closure. M. Romberg, German neurologist.

Sauvineau ophthalmoplegia: internuclear ophthalmoplegia. C. Sauvineau, French ophthalmologist and assistant to Parinaud.

Schwannoma: neurilemmoma. F. Schwann, German anatomist and Jesuit.

Sherrington's law: each posterior spinal nerve supplies its own dermatome. C. Sherrington, English neurophysiologist and Nobel prize winner.

Shy–Drager syndrome: multiple system atrophy. G. Shy, G. Drager, US neurologists.

Sjögren–Larsson syndrome: ichthyosis, ataxia, and mental retardation. T. Sjögren, T. Larsson, Swedish neurologists.

Snellen chart: visual acuity chart. H. Snellen, Dutch ophthalmologist.

Steele–Richardson–Olszewski syndrome: progressive supranuclear palsy. J. Steele, J. Richardson, J. Olszewski, US neurologists.

Steinert disease: myotonic dystrophy. H. Steinert, German physician.

Stellwag sign: infrequent blinking in Parkinson's disease. C. Stellwag, Austrian ophthalmologist.

Strachan's syndrome: painful neuropathy and deafness. W. Strachan, Scottish physician.

Sturge–Weber syndrome: neurocutaneous syndrome. W. Sturge, English physician and liberal. F. Weber, English physician and collector.

Sydenham's chorea: post-infectious chorea. T. Sydenham, English physician and Roundhead.

Sylvian aqueduct: cerebral aqueduct. F. Sylvius, Dutch physician.

Tapia syndrome: paralysis of vagus and hypoglossal nerves A. Tapia, Spanish physician.

Tay–Sachs disease: progressive dementia and retinal cherry-red spot caused by hexosaminidase A deficiency. W. Tay, English ophthalmologist and keen cyclist. B. Sachs, German physician.

Thomsen's disease: autosomal dominant myotonia congenita. A. Thomsen, Danish physician and sufferer from the disease.

Tinel's sign: tapping over carpal tunnel resulting in tingling in median nerve distribution. J. Tinel, French neurologist and member of the Resistance.

Todd's paresis: transient weakness following a focal epileptic seizure. R. Todd, Irish physician.

Tolosa–Hunt syndrome: orbital pseudotumour. E. Tolosa, Spanish neurosurgeon. W. Hunt, US neurosurgeon.

Turcot syndrome: familial intestinal polyps and gliomas. J. Turcot, Canadian surgeon.

Unverricht–Lundborg disease: Baltic myoclonus. H. Unverricht, German physician. H. Lundborg, Swedish physician.

Vernet's syndrome: paresis of glossopharyngeal, vagal, and accessory nerves. M. Vernet, French neurologist.

Villaret's syndrome: paresis of glossopharyngeal, vagal, accessory, and hypoglossal nerves with additional sympathetic involvement. M. Villaret, French neurologist.

Vogt–Koyanagi–Harada syndrome: poliosis, deafness, uveitis and meningitis. A. Vogt, Swiss ophthalmologist. Y. Koyanagi, E. Harada, Japanese ophthalmologists.

von Hippel–Lindau disease: cerebellar haemangioblastomas with retinal and renal angiomas. E. von Hippel, German ophthalmologist. A. Lindau, Swedish pathologist.

Wallenberg's syndrome: posterior inferior cerebellar artery thrombosis. A. Wallenberg, German neurologist.

Wallerian degeneration: degeneration of nerve fibre following axonotmesis. A. Waller, English physiologist.

Weber's syndrome: ipsilateral oculomotor palsy with contralateral hemiplegia due to midbrain lesion. H. Weber, German physician and founder of climatotherapy.

Werdnig–Hoffman disease: spinal muscular atrophy. G. Werdnig, Austrian neurologist. J. Hoffman, German neurologist.

Wernicke's encephalopathy: ophthalmoplegia, delirium, and ataxia due to thiamine deficiency. K. Wernicke, German physician.

West syndrome: infantile spasms. W. West, English physician.

Wilks syndrome: myasthenia gravis. S. Wilks, English physician.

Circle of Willis: arterial anastomosis at base of brain. T. Willis, English physician and Royalist.

Wilson's disease: hepatolenticular degeneration. S. Kinnier Wilson, US neurologist who advised 'Never believe what the patient says the doctor said'.

Appendix 4

Useful websites

Association of British Neurologists	<http://www.theabn.org>
Alzheimer's Society	<http://www.alzheimers.org.uk>
Ataxia	<http://www.ataxia.org.uk>
Brain and Spine Foundation	<http://www.brainandspine.org.uk>
British Association for the Study of Headache	<http://www.bash.org.uk>
British Epilepsy Association	<http://www.epilepsy.org.uk>
CMT International	<http://www.cmt.org.uk>
Driving and Licensing Authority	<http://www.dvla.gov.uk>
Directory of Genetic Disorders	<http://www.geneclinics.org/>
Dystonia Society	<http://www.dystonia.org.uk>
Encephalitis Support Group	<http://www.esg.org.uk>
Functional disorders	<http://www.neurosymptoms.org>
Gene testing laboratories in UK (Clinical Molecular Genetics Society)	<http://www.cmgs.org>
Genetic diseases	<http://www.equip.nhs.uk>
Guillain–Barré Syndrome Support	<http://www.gbs.org.uk>
ME Association	<http://www.meassociation.org.uk>
Migraine Trust	<http://www.migrainetrust.org>
Motor Neurone Disease Association	<http://www.mndassociation.org>
Multiple Sclerosis Society	<http://www.mssociety.org.uk>
Multiple System Atrophy	<http://www.msaweb.co.uk>
Muscular Dystrophy Campaign	<http://www.muscular-dystrophy.org>
Myasthenia Gravis Association	<http://www.crabby.demon.co.uk/mga>

Myotonic Dystrophy	℘ <http://www.mdsguk.org>
Narcolepsy Association	℘ <http://www.narcolepsy.org.uk>
National Society for Epilepsy	℘ <http://www.epilepsynse.org.uk>
National Stroke Association	℘ <http://www.stroke.org>
National Tremor Foundation	℘ <http://www.tremor.org.uk>
Neurofibromatosis Association	℘ <http://www.nfa-uk.org.uk>
Neuropathy Trust	℘ <http://www.neuropathy-trust.org>
OUCH (cluster headache)	℘ <info@ouch-uk.org>
Parkinson's Disease Society UK	℘ <http://www.parkinsons.org.uk>
PSP association	℘ <http://www.pspeur.org.uk>
Scope (cerebral palsy)	℘ <http://www.scope.org.uk>
Tourette Association	℘ <http://www.tsa.org.uk>
Trigeminal Neuralgia	℘ <http://www.tna-support.org> and ℘ <http://www.tna-uk.org.uk>
Wilson's support group	℘ <secretary@wilsons-disease.org.uk>
Tuberous Sclerosis	℘ <http://www.tuberous-sclerosis.org.uk>

Index

A

abacavir 257
abducens nerve (6) 10–12
abetalipoproteinaemia 147, 368
accessory nerve (11) 15
acetazolamide 248, 303
achalasia 412
aciclovir 372
acoustic nerve (8) 14
acoustic neuroma 474–83
acromegaly 440
action tremor 162
acute cord injury 112
acute disseminated encephalomyelitis (ADEM) 316
acute focal neurological deficit 78–9
acute neuromuscular weakness 56
differential diagnosis 57
acute subdural haematoma 99, 106
Addison's disease 438
adrenal gland dysfunction 438
adrenoleucodystrophy 368
AIDS see HIV/AIDS
alemtuzumab 318
alertness, testing 24
allodynia 270
almotriptan 232, 233
Alpers syndrome 364
alternating hand movements test 27
Alzheimer's disease 202–4
inherited 367
management 203
see also dementia
amantadine 261
amaurosis fugax 148
amitriptyline 235
amphotericin 377
ampicillin 123, 124
amyloid angiopathy 88
amyotrophic lateral sclerosis see motor neuron disease
Anderson's syndrome 302, 398
aneurysms
cerebral 460–2
fungal 461

pregnancy 456
saccular 581
traumatic intracranial 462
ankle jerks, absent 599
anosmia 4, 253
anterior cord syndrome 126
anterior horn-cell syndrome 126
anterior ischaemic optic neuropathy (AION) 148
anterograde memory testing 24
anti-NMDA receptor encephalitis 132–3
antibiotics, paralysis 406
anticholinergics 260
anticholinesterase overdose 406
antiemetics 232
antiepileptic drugs 218–22
migraine 232
teratogenicity 220
antiplatelet drugs 184–5
Anton's syndrome 149
aphasia 25, 26
progressive non-fluent 202, 206
apneustic breathing 408, 410
apomorphine 260
apraxia 26
aqueduct stenosis 514, 517
arachnoid cysts 512
arginase deficiency 368
Argyll Robertson pupil 9
arrested hydrocephalus 470
ARSACS (autosomal recessive spastic ataxia of Charlevoix-Saguenay) 147
arterial dissection, imaging 577
arteriovenous malformations 87
cerebral 464–5
pregnancy 456–7
aspirin 184, 232
astrocytoma 487, 488
ataxia 144–6
cerebellar 22, 144–6
episodic 302
Friedreich's see Friedreich's ataxia
hereditary 350, 351
multiple sclerosis 319

with oculomotor apraxia type 1 147
sensory 22, 146
with vitamin E deficiency 147
ataxia telangiectasia 147, 453
ataxic breathing 408, 410
atazanavir 374
atenolol 235
atheroembolism 184
atheroma, imaging 577
athetosis 166
atlanto-occipital dislocation 112
attention, testing 24
autoantibodies 428
autonomic function 559
autonomic neuropathy 336
autosomal dominant axonal neuropathy 353, 354
autosomal dominant cerebellar ataxias (ADCAs) 145
axillary nerve 40
axonal degeneration 270
axonal neuropathies 544
axonopathy 270
azathioprine 326–7

B

baclofen 244, 319
bacterial meningitis 235
Barthel Index 596
basal ganglia disorders 343
Becker's muscular dystrophy 356
cardiac pathology 400
Beevor's sign 599
belle indifference 385
benign paroxysmal positional vertigo (BPPV) 141, 344–5
benzylpenicillin 123, 124
Berardinelli–Seip congenital lipodystrophy 353
beri-beri 416
berry aneurysms 460–1
beta-blockers, migraine 235
bilateral scotoma 8
binasal hemianopia 8
bitemporal hemianopia 8
Biot's breathing 408, 410
bladder dysfunction 180
botulinum toxin A 234
botulism 406

brachial plexus 36
brain 32, 48, 49
brain death 564
brain injury 110
brainstem 48, 50
  infarction 141
  injury 408
  rule of 4 51
brainstem auditory evoked
  responses (BAERs) 565
brainstem death 394
brainstem myoclonus 169
breastfeeding, and
  epilepsy 225
Broca's aphasia 26
Brown–Séquard
  syndrome 126
Brown–Vialetto–von Laere
  syndrome 307
Bruns–Garland
  syndrome 277
burr holes 471, 476

C

C1 fracture
  (Jefferson) 112, 113
C2 fracture 112, 113, 116
C3–C7 fractures 114
cabergoline 259
CADASIL 209
cannabinoids 319
carbamazepine 219, 220
  trigeminal neuralgia 244
cardiac arrest, EEG 540
cardiac arrhythmias 396,
  401
cardiac disease 396–7, 398
cardiac pathology 400–1
cardiac surgery 397
cardiac syncope 136
cardiomyopathy 401
carotid artery
  dissection 192
  internal, stenosis 191
carpal tunnel
  syndrome 286–7
catheter angiography
  573–4
cauda equina 126
cavernoma 466, 467
cavernous angioma 89
cefotaxime 123, 124
ceftriaxone 123, 124
central cord syndrome 126
central disorders
  of ventilatory
  control 404, 408
cerebellar ataxia 22, 144–6

autosomal dominant 145
autosomal recessive 147
clinical signs 144
differential
  diagnosis 144, 145–6
inborn errors of
  metabolism 145
mitochondrial
  disorders 146
cerebellar
  degeneration 333, 334
cerebellar disorder 343
cerebellar ectopia 512–13
cerebellar infarction 141
cerebral aneurysms 460–2
  infectious 179
cerebral arteriovenous
  malformations 464–5
cerebral
  haemorrhage 178–9
cerebral herniation
  syndromes 128
cerebral metastases 479–80
cerebral vasculitis 193, 578
cerebral venous
  thrombosis 186–7
cerebrospinal fluid
  meningitis 123
  peripheral
    neuropathies 275,
    279
cerebrovascular
  disease see stroke
cervical disc prolapse 509
cervical facet
  dislocation 114–15,
  117, 118
cervical spine
  degenerative
    disorders 500–3
  trauma 584, 585
cervical spondylosis 500–3,
  508, 509
cervical spondylotic
  myelopathy 502
channelopathies 302–4
  cardiac pathology 398
Charcot–Marie–Tooth
  disease 352, 353
Cheyne–Stokes
  respiration 408, 410
Chiari malformation
  512–13, 516
chloramphenicol 123, 124
cholinesterase
  inhibitors 326
chorea 166
chronic inflammatory
  demyelinating
  polyneuropathy
  (CIDP) 278–81, 392
  management 279, 280

with monoclonal
  gammopathy 280–1
chronic progressive external
  ophthalmoplegia
  (CPEO) 365
chronic subdural
  haematoma 99
Churg–Strauss
  angiitis 428
ciclosporin 327
claw hand (main en
  griffe) 288
clindamycin 377
clinical neurophysiology
  523–68
  EEG see EEG
  EMG see EMG
  evoked potentials 312, 559
  nerve conduction
    studies see nerve
    conduction studies
  normal values 526,
    566, 567
clobazam 219
clonazepam 219, 319
clopidogrel 184
closed-angle glaucoma 148
cluster breathing 408, 410
cluster headache 241,
  242–3
coeliac disease 417
cognitive testing 24–8
  Mini-Mental State
    Examination
    (MMSE) 29
colloid cyst 494
coma 152–4
  aetiology 152
  classification 154
  EEG 540, 541
  general assessment 152
  Glasgow Coma Scale 95
  investigations 154
  neuroanatomy/
    neuropathology 152
  neurological
    assessment 152–3
  prognosis 156–7
  SSEPs 564
  see also loss of
    consciousness
combined anterior
  horn-cell pyramidal tract
  syndrome 126
communicating
  hydrocephalus 470
compound muscle action
  potential (CMAP) 523
computed tomography 570
  see also imaging
COMT inhibitors 261
concentration, testing 24

concentric needle electrode (CNE) 549, 550, 551
conduction block 401
conduction velocity 567
connective tissue disorders 428–30
constipation 414
contraception
    and epilepsy 224
    and migraine 236–7
conus medullaris 126
coordination, testing 18
cortical myoclonus 169, 564
corticobasal degeneration 254, 269
corticosteroids 279, 298
cranial cavity 32, 33
cranial nerves
    1 (olfactory) 4
    2 (optic) 6
    3 (oculomotor) 10–12
    4 (trochlear) 10–12
    5 (trigeminal) 10–12
    6 (abducens) 10–12
    7 (facial) 14
    8 (acoustic) 14
    9 (glossopharyneal) 15
    10 (vagus) 15
    11 (accessory) 15
    12 (hypoglossal) 15
cranial neuropathies 277
craniectomy 476
craniopharyngioma 474
craniotomy 476
Creutzfeldt–Jakob disease 210–13
    familial 367
    sporadic 210–12
    variant 212–13
cryptococcal meningitis 376, 377, 183
Cushing's response 400
Cushing's syndrome 400
cyproheptadine 235
cysticercosis 589–90
cytomegalovirus (CMV) 378, 589

D

Dandy–Walker malformation 513
Danon disease 398
dantrolene 319
darunavir 374
daytime sleepiness, excessive 158–61
debulking of intracranial tumours 476
deep tendon reflexes see tendon reflexes

degenerative spinal disorders see spinal disorders, degenerative
Dejerine–Sottas disease 352
delavirdine 374
delirium 90–2
dementia 198–200
    aetiology 198
    CADASIL 209
    clinical features 199–200
    epidemiology 198
    frontotemporal 206–7, 367
    HIV-associated 374
    inherited 367
    investigations 200
    Lewy body 208, 254
    Parkinson's disease 264
    semantic 207
    vascular 208
    see also Alzheimer's disease
demyelinating neuropathies 544
depression, Parkinson's disease 264
dermatology 444–50
    definitions 444
dermatomes
    anterior 19, 34
    posterior 20, 35
    upper and lower limbs 34, 35
dermatomyositis 298–300, 392
    management 298–300
developmental abnormalities 512–14
    imaging 516, 517, 518
developmental venous anomaly (DVA) 466
Devic's disease see neuromyelitis optica
dexamphetamine 161
diabetes mellitus 436
    diagnosis 276
diabetic cachectic neuropathy 277
diabetic lumbosacral radiculo-plexus-neuropathy 277
diabetic neuropathies 276–7
    classification 276–7
diabetic polyneuropathy 276
diabetic truncal radiculoneuropathy 277
diarrhoea 414
didanosine 374
diffuse axonal injury 101, 109

diffuse cerebral dysfunction 538–9
diffusion-weighted MRI 572
digital subtraction angiography 71, 74
dihydroergotamine 233
dipyridamole 184
dissociative non-epileptic attack disorder (NEAD) 226, 227
distal sensory peripheral neuropathy 375
Dix–Hallpike manoeuvre 342
dizziness
    neurological causes 342–3
    non-neurological causes 348
dominant hemisphere function 25, 27
donezepil 203
dopamin-responsive dystonia 363
dopamine agonists 259
dorsal root ganglionopathy 333, 336
downbeat nystagmus 599
dressing apraxia 28
driving, epilepsy 218
drug-induced conditions
    parkinsonism 257
    tremor 164
Duchenne's muscular dystrophy 356
    cardiac pathology 400
Duodopa® 261
dural arteriovenous fistula 468–9
dysaesthesiae 270
dysarthria 144
dysdiadokinesia 18, 144
dysmetria 144
dysphagia 412, 413
dysphasia 412
dystonia 170–1, 253
    inherited 363
dystonic tremor 163

E

ECG 398
EEG 526–7
    abnormal rhythms 530, 531, 532, 533
    activity 526
    continuous monitoring 540
    diffuse cerebral dysfunction 538–9
    display 526
    electrode placement 526
    epilepsy 534–5, 536, 537

EEG (Cont'd)
  intensive care
    unit 540, 541
  long-term monitoring 527
  recording 526–7, 528
  use/abuse 529
efavirenz 374
electrocardiogram see ECG
electroencephalography
  see EEG
electromyography see
  EMG
eletriptan 232, 233
emergencies 53–133
Emery–Dreifuss muscular
  dystrophy 358
  cardiac pathology 400
EMG 546
  abnormal patterns 548–51
  Guillain–Barré
    syndrome 554
  Lambert–Eaton myasthenic
    syndrome 558
  motor neuron disease 552
  muscle disorders 294–5,
    552, 553
  myasthenia gravis 325,
    556, 557
  radiculopathies 552
emtricitabine 374
encephalitis 333
  acute 130–1
  anti-NMDA
    receptor 132–3
  herpes simplex 381, 588
  limbic 131, 333, 334, 335
  viral 370–2, 371
encephalomyelitis
  acute disseminated 316
  with/without rigidity 334
endocarditis 396–7
endocrine disorders
  436–9
endocrine
  neuroanatomy 432,
    434
enfuvirtide 374
entacapone 261
ependymoma 498
epidermal naevus
  syndrome 449
epilepsy 136, 214–15, 304
  aetiology 214
  cardiac pathology 401
  classification 214–15
  clinical features 215
  driving 218
  EEG 534–5, 536,
    537
  imaging 221
  incidence 214
  investigations 215

juvenile myoclonic 215
  management 218–22
  pregnancy 224, 457–8
  status epilepticus 54–5
  in women 224–5
Epley's manoeuvre 346
eponyms 603
Epworth sleepiness
  scale 159
ergotamine 233, 243
essential tremor 162
etravirine 374
evoked potentials
  (EPs) 312, 559
  latencies 567
  somatosensory 562–4
excessive daytime
  sleepiness 158–61
extradural haematoma
  (EDH) 98, 106
eye movements 144
  extra-ocular 10
  pursuit/saccadic 10, 11
  reflex 155

F

F wave 523
Fabry's disease 368, 422
  cardiac pathology 398
facial nerve (7) 14
facioscapulohumeral
  muscular
    dystrophy 357–8
faecal incontinence 414
falls, Parkinson's
  disease 265
familial hemiplegic
  migraine 228
family history 2
fasciculation potentials,
  needle EMG 548
fatal familial insomnia 367
fatigue 320
Fazio–Londe syndrome 307
femoral nerve 44
fertility, and epilepsy 224
finger drop 599
fingolimod 318
flick sign 286
fluconazole 377
flucytosine 377
focal neurological
  syndromes, acute 78–9
focal neuropathies 544,
  545
folate deficiency 424
foot drop 22, 172–3
forearm exercise test 294
fosamprenavir 257
'freezing' 265
Friedreich's ataxia 147, 350

cardiac
    pathology 398, 401
frontal executive function 25
frontotemporal
  dementia 206–7, 367
frovatriptan 232, 233
Fukuda test 140
functional MRI 572
fundoscopy 8, 9
fungal aneurysms 461

G

gabapentin 219
  migraine 235
  spasticity 319
  trigeminal neuralgia 244
gait 22
  disturbances 22
  'freezing' 262
gait ataxia 144
galantamine 203
gangliosidoses 368
gastrointestinal motility
  disorders 412–13
gastroneurological
  disorders 412–14, 416–18
gastroparesis 412
gaze-evoked nystagmus 12
genetic neuropathies 352–5
gentamicin 124
germinoma 474
Gerstmann–Sträussler–
  Scheinker
    syndrome 145, 367
Glasgow Coma Scale 95
glatiramer acetate 318
glaucoma 148
glioblastoma 489
glioma 474, 478
gliomatosis cerebri 490
glossopharyngeal
  nerve (9) 15
glucagonoma 450
glycogen storage
  disease 401
Gottron's sign 292
Guillain–Barré
  syndrome 60–2, 392
  cardiac pathology 401
  EMG 554
  nerve conduction
    studies 554

H

haemangioblastoma 474,
  480–1, 493
haematological
  disorders 424–6
haemodialysis,
  complications 420–1

Haemophilus influenzae 122, 124
Hallpike's test 14, 342
Halmagyi test 599
hand movements, alternating 27
hand weakness/ paraesthesiae, unilateral 174–5
hangman's fracture 113–14, 116
head impulse test 139
head injury 94–6
  assessment 94
  classification 95
  complications 102
  Glasgow Coma Scale 95
  imaging 104, 105, 106, 107, 108, 109, 110, 583
  management 95–6, 98–102
  pathophysiology 94
  penetrating 100
  see also specific head injuries
head thrust test 599
headache
  acute (thunderclap) 64–5
  cluster 241, 242–3
  hypnic 241
  idiopathic stabbing 241
  migraine 228–9
  paroxysmal hemicrania 240, 241
  primary short-lasting 240, 241
  SUNCT 240, 241
  trigeminal neuralgia 241, 244–5
hemianopia 8
hemispatial neglect 28
hemispheric lesions 343
hereditary ataxias 350, 351
hereditary neuropathy with liability to pressure palsies 354–5
hereditary sensory and autonomic neuropathies 354
herpes simplex encephalitis 381, 588
hippocampal sclerosis 221
Hirschsprung's disease 412
history taking 1
  principles of 2
HIV encephalopathy 383, 588
HIV/AIDS 373
  neurological disorders 374–5
  opportunistic infections 376–9
hockey-stick sign 210–12

Hoehn and Yahr scale, modified 598
Holmes' tremor 163
Holmes–Adie pupil 9
homonymous hemianopia 8
Hoover's sign 599
hormone replacement therapy, and migraine 237
Horner's syndrome 9
Huntington's disease 362–3
hydrocephalus 343, 470–2
  arrested 470
  communicating 470
  non-communicating 470
  normal pressure 472
hyperaesthesia 270
hyperalgesia 270
hypercapnoea 402
hyperekplexia 302
hyperglycaemia 436
hyperkalaemic periodic paralysis 303
hypermagnesaemia 406
hyperparathyroidism 437
hyperpathia 270
hyperpituitarism 440
hyperprolactinaemia 440
hypertension, idiopathic intracranial 246–9
hypertensive haemorrhage 86
hyperthyroidism 437
hyperventilation 348
  central neurogenic 408, 410
hypnic headache 241
hypoaesthesia 270
hypocapnoea 402
hypoglossal nerve (12) 15
hypoglycaemia 436
hypokalaemia 56, 406
hypokalaemic periodic paralysis 303
hypomelanosis of Ito 449
hyponatraemia 441
hypoparathyroidism 437
hypophosphataemia 406
hypopituitarism 440
hyporeflexia 144
hypothalamus 432, 433
hypothyroidism 437
hypotonia 144
hypoxia 402

I
idiopathic intracranial hypertension 246–9
idiopathic stabbing headache 241
imaging
  cavernoma 467

Creutzfeldt–Jakob disease 211
degenerative spinal disorders 508, 509, 510, 511
developmental abnormalities 516, 517, 518
epilepsy 221
head injury 104, 105, 106, 107, 108, 109, 110, 583
infections 380, 381, 382, 383, 588
intracranial haemorrhage 86, 87, 88, 89, 582
intracranial tumours 475, 484, 485, 486, 487, 488, 489, 490, 491, 492, 493, 494, 586
limbic encephalitis 335
MELAS 366
multiple sclerosis 312, 314, 315
multiple system atrophy 256
neurosarcoidosis 317
parkinsonian syndromes 255
spinal injuries 116, 117, 118, 119, 120, 584
spinal tumours 496, 497, 498, 499
stroke 181, 188, 189, 190, 191, 192, 193, 194, 195, 196, 197, 576
subarachnoid haemorrhage 70, 71, 72, 73, 74, 75, 76, 580–1
immune reconstitution syndromes (IRIS) 378, 589
immunoglobulin, IV 279, 327, 392–3
inborn errors of metabolism 145
inclusion body myositis 298, 299
  management 300
incontinentia pigmenti 453–4
indinavir 257
infections
  bacterial meningitis 235
  imaging 380, 381, 382, 383, 588
  post-head injury 101
  shunts 198
  viral encephalitis 370–2
inferior quadrantanopia 8

inflammatory bowel
disease 417
insulin neuritis 277
interferon beta 318
intracerebral
haematoma 100
intracranial haemorrhage
84–5, 178–9
imaging 86, 87, 88,
89, 582
management 183
intracranial pressure,
raised 128, 129
intracranial tumours 474–7
imaging 475, 484, 485,
486, 487, 488, 489,
490, 491, 492, 493,
494
management
475–7, 478–83
intramedullary
metastasis 499
iron deficiency anaemia 424
isoniazid 124

J

jaw supporting sign 599
junctional scotoma 8
juvenile myoclonic
epilepsy 215

K

Kallman's syndrome 4
Kearns–Sayre syndrome 365
cardiac
pathology 398, 401
Kennedy's syndrome 307
kidney
hereditary disorders 422
neurological
complications 420–1
transplantation 421
Kleine–Levin syndrome 158
Korsakoff syndrome 416
Kurtzke expanded disability
status scale 595
Kussmaul breathing 408

L

labyrinthine infarction 141
lacosamide 219
lacunar stroke 180
Lafora disease 398, 401
Lambert–Eaton myasthenic
syndrome 333, 337, 406
EMG 558
nerve conduction
studies 558

lamivudine 374
lamotrigine 219, 220
trigeminal neuralgia 244
Leber's hereditary optic
neuropathy 149,
365, 398
leukaemia 425
levetiracetam 219, 220
levodopa 254, 258
Lewy body
dementia 208, 254
Lhermitte's sign 599
limb–girdle muscular
dystrophy 356, 357
cardiac pathology 400
limbic encephalitis 131,
333, 334, 335
voltage-gated potassium
channel associated 131
*Listeria
monocytogenes* 122, 124
lithium 243
long QT syndrome 396,
397, 401
lopinavir 374
loss of consciousness
136–7
aetiology 136
diagnosis 137
investigations 137
see also coma
lower limbs
dermatomes 34, 35
examination 16–22
innervation 42, 43, 44,
45, 46, 47
SSEPs 562
Lown–Ganong–Levine
syndrome 398
lumbar canal stenosis
505–6, 599
lumbar disc
prolapse 504–5, 510
lumbar puncture 123, 248,
388–90, 599
lumbosacral plexus 42, 43
Luria three-step test 27
lymphoma, primary
CNS 478–9, 491

M

macro-orchidism 440
magnetic resonance
angiography 572
magnetic resonance
imaging 571–2
diffusion-weighted 572
functional 572
see also imaging
magnetic resonance
spectroscopy 572

malignant hyperthermia
syndrome 302
malignant middle
cerebral territory
syndrome 183
maraviroc 374
median nerve 38, 567
melanoma, metastasis 492
MELAS 146, 365, 366
cardiac pathology 398,
401
memantine 203
memory testing 24
Ménière's disease 340
meningioma 474, 478,
484, 497
meningitis 122–5, 380
bacterial 235
causative organisms 122
cerebrospinal fluid in
123
cryptococcal 376, 377
cutaneous signs 446
imaging 588
treatment 123–4, 125
tubercular 124, 588,
590, 591
menopause, and
migraine 237
menstrual migraine 236
MERRF 146, 352, 365
cardiac
pathology 398, 401
metabolic diseases,
inherited 368
cardiac pathology 398
metachromatic
leucodystrophy 368
methotrexate 327
methylphenidate 161
methysergide 235, 243
metoprolol 235
microscopic polyangiitis
428
migraine 228–9, 302
clinical features 228–9
differential diagnosis 230
epidemiology 228
familial hemiplegic 228
IHS criteria 231
investigations 230
management 232–3, 234
menstrual 236
pathophysiology 228
pregnancy 238
prophylaxis 234, 235
triggers 229
variants 229
in women 236–8
Mini-Mental State
Examination (MMSE)
29

mitochondrial disorders
  cardiac pathology
    398, 401
  cerebellar ataxia 22,
    144–6
  inherited 364, 365
mitochondrial myopathy,
  neuropathy, GI
  involvement
  encephalopathy
  (MNGIE) 352, 365
mitoxantrone 318
Miyoshi's myopathy 357
modafinil 161
monoamine oxidase
  inhibitors 261
monoclonal
  gammopathy 278–81
mononeuropathies 277
motor conduction
  velocity 523
motor neuron disease
  306–7
  aetiology 306, 307
  clinical features 306
  EMG 552
  investigations 308
  management 308–9
  mimics of 307
  nerve conduction
    studies 552
motor neuron
  syndromes 336
movement disorders,
  inherited 362–3
multifocal motor neuropathy
  with conduction
  block 282, 392
multiple myeloma 425
multiple sclerosis 310–11,
  392
  clinical features 310–11
  course 311
  diagnosis 312, 313
  differential diagnosis 316
  epidemiology 310
  imaging 312, 314, 315
  investigations 312
  management 318–20
  pathogenesis 310
  pregnancy 457
  SSEPs 564
multiple system
  atrophy 254, 256, 266–7
muscle biopsy 295
muscle disorders 292
  channelopathies 302–4
  classification 292
  clinical features 292
  EMG 294–5, 552, 553
  HIV-associated 375
  inherited 292, 356–8

investigations 294–5
nerve conduction
  studies 294–5
muscle strength 16, 18
muscular dystrophies
  cardiac pathology 398,
    400, 401
  molecular diagnosis 295
musculocutaneous nerve 37
myasthenia gravis 324–5,
  392, 406
  clinical features 324
  differential diagnosis 325
  EMG 325, 556, 557
  epidemiology 324
  investigations 325
  management 326–8, 329
  with MuSK antibodies 330
  nerve conduction
    studies 556, 557
  ocular 325, 328
  pathophysiology 324
  in women 328
myasthenic syndromes see
  Lambert–Eaton
  myasthenic syndrome;
  myasthenia gravis
mycophenolate mofetil 327
myelography 574
myoclonus 168–9, 333,
  335, 338
myokymia 549
myopathic gait 22
myopathies see muscle
  disorders
myotomes 17
myotonia congenita 303
  EMG 550, 551
myotonic dystrophy 360–1
  cardiac pathology 398

N

nadolol 235
naratriptan 232, 233
narcolepsy 160–1
NARP (neuropathy–ataxia–
  retinitis pigmentosa) 146
natalizumab 318
National Institutes of Health
  Stroke Scale 81
neck flexion extension
  weakness 599
needle EMG 546
Neisseria meningitidis 124
nelfinavir 374
nerve action potential 523
nerve biopsy 275
nerve conduction
  studies 274, 542–3
  Guillain–Barré
    syndrome 554

Lambert–Eaton myasthenic
  syndrome 558
motor nerves 567
motor neuron disease 552
muscle disorders 552, 553
myasthenia
  gravis 556, 557
peripheral
  neuropathies 274, 278,
    544, 545
radiculopathies 552
sensory nerves 567
neurilemmoma 474
neuroanatomy 31–52
  brain 32, 48, 49
  brainstem 48, 50
  cranial cavity 32, 33
  dermatomes see
    dermatomes
  innervation
    lower limbs 42, 43, 44,
      45, 46, 47
    upper limbs 36, 37,
      38, 39, 40
  spinal cord 52
neurocutaneous
  melanosis 449
neurocutaneous syndromes,
  inherited 452–4
neuroendocrine
  syndromes 442
neurofibroma 474, 496
neurofibromatosis 452
neurogenetic disorders 349
  genetic
    neuropathies 352–5
  hereditary
    ataxias 350, 351
  hereditary metabolic
    diseases 368
  inherited dementias 367
  inherited mitochondrial
    disorders 364, 365
  inherited movement
    disorders 362–3
  inherited
    myopathies 356–8
  myotonic dystrophy see
    myotonic dystrophy
neurological disability scales
  Barthel Index 596
  Kurtzke expanded disability
    status scale 595
  modified Hoehn and Yahr
    scale 598
  Rankin stroke disability
    scale 598
neurological examination
  bedside cognitive
    testing 24–8
  cranial nerves see
    cranial nerves

neurological examination (Cont'd)
general 3
Mini-Mental State Examination (MMSE) 29
upper and lower limbs 16–22
neuromyelitis optica 316, 322–3
neuromyotonia, EMG 548
neuronavigation 476
neuronopathy 270
neuropathic pain 270
neuropathic tremor 163
neuropathy, cutaneous signs 447
neuropathy, ataxia, retinitis pigmentosa (NARP) 365
neuropsychiatric-cutaneous syndromes 449–50
neuroradiology 569–90
cerebrovascular disease 576–8
cervical spine trauma 584, 585
CNS infections 588–90
diagnostic 570–5
head injury 583
interventional 575
intracranial haemorrhage 582
intracranial tumours 586
subarachnoid haemorrhage 580–1
see also imaging
neurosarcoidosis 316, 317
neurosurgery 459–521
nevirapine 377
Niemann–Pick disease 368
non-communicating hydrocephalus 470
non-dominant hemisphere function 28
non-epileptic attack disorder 226, 227
Nonaka myopathy 357
normal pressure hydrocephalus 472
nuclear isotope studies 574–5
nutritional deficiency syndromes 416–17
nystagmus 11–12, 144
downbeat 599
positional 345
spontaneous 138–9

O

obstructive sleep apnoea/hypopnoea syndrome 160

obturator nerve 45
ocular myopathy 398
oculomotor nerve (3) 10–12
palsy 9
odontoid peg fractures 113, 119
olfactory nerve (1) 4
oligoclonal bands 312
Ondine's curse 408
ophthalmoplegia, internuclear 600
ophthalmoplegic migraine 229
Oppenheim's dystonia 363
opsoclonus, myoclonus and ataxia 333, 335
optic nerve (2) 6
optic neuritis 150
oral contraception and epilepsy 224
and migraine 236
organophosphate poisoning 406
orientation, testing 24
orphenadrine 260
orthostatic hypotension 266
orthostatic tremor 163
oxcarbazepine 219
trigeminal neuralgia 244
oxybutynin 264, 267, 319–320

P

pain perception 559
palatal tremor 164
papilloedema 247
paradoxical embolic stroke 180
paraesthesiae 174–5, 270
paramyotonia congenita 303
paraneoplastic disorders 332, 333
central nervous system 334–5
investigations and management 338
peripheral nervous system 336–7
see also individual disorders
paraproteinaemias 426
parathyroid dysfunction 437
parkinsonian gait 22
parkinsonism/Parkinson's disease 250–1, 599
aetiology 250
associated problems 264–5
causes 250
clinical features 252–3
diagnosis 252
differential diagnosis 254

drug treatment 258–61
drug-induced 257
epidemiology 250
exclusion criteria 252
inherited 362
investigations 255
pathophysiology 251
surgical options 262–3
vascular 254
paroxysmal hemicrania 240, 241
Parsonage–Turner syndrome 174
past medical history 2
pellagra 416, 450
penetrating head injuries 100
pergolide 259
perilymph fistula 141
periodic limb movement disorder 161
periodic paralysis 401
peripheral labyrinthine disorder 342
peripheral neuropathy 270–1
chronic 272–3
clinical examination 271
diabetic 276–7
diagnosis 272–3
history 270
HIV/AIDS-associated 375
investigations 274–5
nerve conduction studies 274, 544, 545
see also specific conditions
peroneal nerves 47
phaeochromocytoma 438
Phalen's sign 292
phenobarbital 219, 224
phenytoin 219, 220
trigeminal neuralgia 244
piracetam 219
pituitary disorders 436–41
pituitary gland 433, 434
pituitary microadenoma 485
pizotifen 235
plasma cell dyscrasias 425–6
plasma exchange 279, 327
plasmacytoma 426
POEMS syndrome 442
POLG1 330
polycystic kidney disease 422
polymyositis 298–300, 392, 406
management 298–300
polyradiculopathy 375
porphyria 449
positron emission tomography (PET) 574

posterior column syndrome 126
posterolateral column syndrome 126
postural hypotension 136
postural instability 265
pramipexole 259
prednisolone 243, 326
pregabalin 219
pregnancy
  aneurysm 456
  arteriovenous malformation 456–7
  epilepsy 224, 457–8
  migraine 238
  multiple sclerosis 457
  subarachnoid haemorrhage 456
primary lateral sclerosis see motor neuron disease
prion diseases 367
progressive bulbar palsy see motor neuron disease
progressive multifocal leucoencephal-opathy 378, 589
progressive muscular atrophy see motor neuron disease
progressive supranuclear palsy 254, 268
propranolol 235
Proteus syndrome 449
proximal myotonic myopathy 356
pseudo-obstruction 413
psychogenic tremor 164
psychosis, Parkinson's disease 264
pupils
  abnormalities 9
  reactions 8
pyrazinamide 124
pyridostigmine 326
pyridoxine 124
pyrimethamine 377

Q

quadrantanopia 8

R

radial nerve 40
radiculopathies
  EMG 552
  nerve conduction studies 552
radiography 570
  see also imaging
raltegravir 374
Rankin stroke disability scale 598
rasagiline 261
Refsum's disease 4
renal see kidney
respiratory failure 402, 404, 405, 406
  central disorders of ventilatory control 408
retinal migraine 229
retinopathy 333, 335
retrograde memory testing 24
rhabdomyolysis 54, 294, 406
rheumatoid arthritis 428, 429
rheumatoid factor 428
rhombencephalitis 335
rifampicin 124
Riley–Day syndrome (familial dysautonomia) 355
riluzole 308
Rinne's test 14
ritonavir 374
rituximab 327
rivastigmine 203
rizatriptan 232, 233
Romberg's sign 22, 146, 271, 342, 385
ropinirole 259
rotigotine 259
rule of 4 51

S

saccular aneurysms 581
salivation, Parkinson's disease 265
SANDO 352
saquinavir 257
Schwannoma 474
sciatic nerve 46
scleroderma 428
scorpion bite 406
scotoma 8
Segawa's disease 363
segmental demyelination 270
seizures 101
  cutaneous signs 449
  non-epileptic attack disorder 226, 227
  see also epilepsy
selegiline 161, 261, 264
semantic dementia 207
Semont's manoeuvre 347
sensory ataxia 22, 146
sensory ataxia neuropathy, dysarthria, ophthalmoplegia (SANDO) 365
sensory conduction velocity 523
sensory nerve action potential (SNAP) 543
sensory neuropathy/neuronopathy, subacute 333, 336
sensory testing 18
serotonin antagonists 235
sex hormone dysfunction 439
shawl sign 298
shellfish poisoning 406
short-cycle periodic breathing 408
shoulder shrug 599
shunts, complications of 473
sickle cell disease 425
single-photon emission computed tomography (SPECT) 575
Sjögren's syndrome 4, 429
  autoantibodies 428
skull fracture, basal 101
sleep disorders
  Epworth sleepiness scale 159
  excessive daytime sleepiness 158–61
  narcolepsy 160–1
  obstructive sleep apnoea/hypopnoea syndrome 160
  Parkinson's disease 264
  periodic limb movement disorder 161
small fibre studies 559
snake bite 406
social history 2
sodium valproate see valproic acid
solifenacin 180
somatization disorders 177–386
somatosensory evoked potentials 562–4
space-occupying lesions 98
spastic
  paraparesis 22, 142–3
    aetiology 142
    clinical features 142
spider bite 406
spinal cord 52
  acute injury 112
  compression 127
  disorders 126
  infarct 197
spinal disorders, degenerative
  cervical spine 500–3
  imaging 508, 509, 510, 511
  thoracic/lumbar spine 504–6
spinal dysraphism (spina bifida) 514, 518

spinal injuries 112–15
  acute cord injury 112
  C1 fracture
    (Jefferson) 113
  C1/C2 fracture 112, 116
  C2 fracture 113
  cervical facet
    dislocation 114–15,
    117, 118
  hangman's
    fracture 113–14, 116
  imaging 116, 117, 118,
    119, 120, 584
  instability 112
  odontoid peg
    fractures 113, 119
  rehabilitation 115
  subaxial (C3–C7)
    fractures 114
  thoracolumbar
    fractures 115
spinal interneuritis 334
spinal metastases 499
spinal myoclonus 169
spinal tumours 496, 497,
  498, 499
SSEPs see somatosensory
  evoked potentials
status epilepticus 54–5
  complications 54
  management 55
stavudine 257
Steele–Richardson–Olszewski
  syndrome 254, 268
stereotaxy 476
stiff person syndrome 333
straight sinus thrombosis 194,
  195, 196
Streptococcus pneumoniae
  122, 124
stroke 178–81
  aetiology 178–9
  clinical features 179–80
  cutaneous signs 448
  imaging 181, 188, 189,
    190, 191, 192, 193,
    194, 195, 196, 197, 576
  investigations 180
  management 80–3, 182–3
    thrombolysis 83
  and migraine 236–7
  National Institutes of
    Health Stroke Scale 81
  prevention 184–5
  risk factors 179
Sturge–Weber syndrome
  453
subarachnoid haemorrhage
  53–69, 179
  cardiac pathology 398, 400
  Fisher classification 68

imaging 70, 71, 72, 73, 74,
  75, 76, 580–1
management 67
pregnancy 456
traumatic 100
WFNS grading system 68
subdural haematoma 106,
  107, 108, 473
  acute 99
  chronic 99
sulphadiazine 377
sumatriptan 198, 232
SUNCT 240, 241
superior quadrantanopia 8
sural nerve 567
surgery
  cardiac 397
  epilepsy 222
  parkinsonism/Parkinson's
    disease 262–3
  thymectomy 327–8
  trigeminal neuralgia 245
syncope
  cardiac 136
  vasovagal 136
syringomyelia 520, 521
systemic lupus
  erythematosus
  428–9, 449
  autoantibodies 428

T

Tangier's disease 368
task-specific tremor 163
temperature perception 559
tendon reflexes 21
tenofovir 374
Tensilon® (edrophonium)
  test 325
teratoma 474
thoracic disc prolapse 504
thoracolumbar
  fractures 115
thrombolysis 83
thunderclap headache 64–5
thymectomy 327–8
thyroid dysfunction 437
thyrotoxic storm 437
tiagabine 219
tibial nerve 46, 567
tick paralysis 406
tics 165
timolol 235
Tinel's sign 172, 173, 174
tipranavir 374
tizanidine 319
tolterodine 319
tone 16
topiramate 219, 220
  migraine 235

toxoplasmosis 376, 377,
  382, 589
transient visual
  obscurations 148
transtentorial
  herniation 408
trauma
  cervical spine 584, 585
  head injury see
    head injury
traumatic intracranial
  aneurysms 462
tremor 144, 162–4
  classification 162
  drug-induced 164
  dystonic 163
  essential 162
  Holmes' 163
  multiple sclerosis 319
  neuropathic 163
  palatal 164
  primary orthostatic 163
  psychogenic 164
  task-specific 163
  trigeminal nerve (5) 14
trigeminal
  neuralgia 241, 244–5
    drug treatment 244
    surgical options 245
trihexyphenidyl 260
triptans 232, 233
trochlear nerve 10–12
tubercular meningitis 124,
  588, 590, 591
tuberculoma 590
tuberous sclerosis 452
tumours see intracranial
  tumours

U

ulnar nerve 39
ulnar neuropathy 288–90
ultrasonography 570–1
  see also imaging
unsteadiness
  neurological causes
    342–3
  non-neurological
    causes 348
Unterberger's test 14, 140,
  342
upper limbs
  dermatomes 34, 35
  examination 16–22
  innervation 36, 37,
    38, 39, 40
  SSEPs 562, 563
uraemic
  encephalopathy 420
uraemic neuropathy 420

V

vacuolar myelopathy 374
vagus nerve (10) 15
  stimulation 222
valproic acid 219, 220
  migraine 235
vancomycin 124
vascular dementia 208
vasculitic neuropathy
  284–5
vasculitides 428–30
vasovagal syncope 136
venous thrombosis 577–8
ventricular hypertrophy 401
ventricular tumours 481–2
verapamil 243
vertebral canal stenosis
  511
vertebrobasilar
  migraine 229
vertigo 138–41, 340
  aetiology 138
  benign paroxysmal
    positional 141, 344–5
  benign recurrent 229
  clinical features 138–40
  differential diagnosis 141
  management 140
vestibular neuritis 141

vestibular Schwannoma
  474–83, 486
viral encephalitis 370–2
vision loss
  acute 148–9
  bilateral transient 148
  monocular transient 148
  non-progressive
    bilateral 149
  non-progressive
    unilateral 148–9
  sudden onset with
    progression 149
visual acuity 6
visual evoked
  responses 560, 561
visual field 6
  defects 6–8
vitamin B1 deficiency 416
vitamin B3 deficiency 416
vitamin B6 deficiency 416
vitamin B12 deficiency
  416–17, 424
vitamin D deficiency 417
vitamin E
  deficiency 147, 417
voltage-gated potassium
  channel associated
  limbic encephalitis
  131

von Hippel–Lindau
  disease 422, 453

W

Waldenström's
  macroglobulinaemia 426
Wallerian degeneration 270
Weber's lateralization
  test 14
websites 611–12
Wegener's
  granulomatosis 428
Welander's myopathy 357
Wernicke's aphasia 26
Wernicke's encephalopathy
  416
Whipple's disease 418
women
  epilepsy 224–5
  migraine 236–8
  myasthenia gravis 328

Z

zalcitabine 257
zidovudine 257
zolmitriptan 232, 233
zonisamide 219